DIMENSIONAL DIAGNOSIS

The Guilford Series in Personality and Psychopathology

Christopher J. Hopwood, *Series Editor*

Psychology and psychiatry are transitioning from categorical models of mental disorders to evidence-based dimensional models that integrate personality and psychopathology. This series presents reader-friendly resources on all aspects of dimensional models. Practitioners will find trustworthy guides on assessment, diagnosis, and intervention. Students and researchers will find summaries of cutting-edge findings in this vibrant area. Books in this series are carefully crafted to guide contemporary research and clinical practice.

Practitioner's Guide to the Alternative Model for Personality Disorders
Bo Bach, Christopher J. Hopwood, Erik Simonsen, and Robert F. Krueger

Dimensional Diagnosis: Practical and Conceptual Issues in the Integration of Personality and Psychopathology
Christopher J. Hopwood and Carla Sharp, Editors

ALSO AVAILABLE

Mentalizing in Psychotherapy: A Guide for Practitioners
Carla Sharp and Dickon Bevington

Multimethod Clinical Assessment
Christopher J. Hopwood and Robert F. Bornstein, Editors

DIMENSIONAL DIAGNOSIS

Practical and Conceptual Issues in the Integration of Personality and Psychopathology

EDITED BY

Christopher J. Hopwood
Carla Sharp

THE GUILFORD PRESS
New York London

A Division of Guilford Publications, Inc.
www.guilford.com

Printed in the United States of America

This book is printed on acid-free paper.

For product and safety concerns within the EU, please contact *GPSR@taylorandfrancis.com,* Taylor & Francis Verlag GmbH, Kaufingerstraße 24, 80331 München, Germany.

Last digit is print number: 9 8 7 6 5 4 3 2 1

Library of Congress Cataloging-in-Publication Data is available from the publisher.

ISBN 978-1-4625-6238-1 (cloth)

To my dad, from whom I came,
through some fortuitous combination
of nature and nurture, never to associate
working hard with hard work;
my mom, who passed along her sensitivity;
and JB, who showed me the value
of kindness and perspective

—C. J. H.

To Milla and Phoebe,
who are the best of teachers

—C. S.

About the Editors

Christopher J. Hopwood, PhD, is Professor of Personality Psychology at the University of Zurich, Switzerland. Dr. Hopwood is Associate Editor of the *Journal of Personality Assessment* and the *Journal of Psychopathology and Clinical Science*, and Editor-in-Chief of the journal *Psychology of Human–Animal Intergroup Relations*. He is the 2018 recipient of the Theodore Millon Grant in Personality Psychology from the American Psychological Foundation, among other honors. Dr. Hopwood's research interests include personality assessment and development, interpersonal processes, psychopathology, and human–animal relations.

Carla Sharp, PhD, is John and Rebecca Moores Professor of Clinical Psychology and Associate Dean for Faculty and Research at the University of Houston, where she is also Director of the Adolescent Diagnosis Assessment Prevention and Treatment (ADAPT) Center and the Developmental Psychopathology Lab. Dr. Sharp holds adjunct positions at University College London in the United Kingdom and the University of the Free State in South Africa. Her work has significantly advanced scientific understanding of personality pathology in youth. She is a recipient of the Mid-Career Investigator Award from the North American Society for the Study of Personality Disorders and the Award for Achievement in the Field of Severe Personality Disorders from the Borderline Personality Disorder Resource Center.

Contributors

Shayan Asadi, MS, Department of Psychology, University of Michigan, Ann Arbor, Michigan

Arielle Baskin-Sommers, PhD, Departments of Psychology and Psychiatry, Yale University, New Haven, Connecticut

Cassandra L. Boness, PhD, Center on Alcohol, Substance Use, and Addictions, University of New Mexico, Albuquerque, New Mexico

Jennifer L. Callahan, PhD, ABPP, Department of Psychology, School of Behavioral and Brain Sciences, The University of Texas at Dallas, Richardson Texas

Nicole Casali, PhD, Department of Criminology, Max Planck Institute for the Study of Crime, Security and Law, Freiburg, Germany

Sarah E. Cecil, BA, Clinic for Emotional Health, Department of Psychology, University of Kentucky, Lexington, Kentucky

Christopher C. Conway, PhD, Department of Psychology, Fordham University, New York, New York

Patrick W Corrigan, PsyD, Department of Psychology, Illinois Institute of Technology, Chicago, Illinois

Colin G. DeYoung, PhD, Department of Psychology, University of Minnesota, Minneapolis, Minnesota

Johannes C. Ehrenthal, PhD, Department of Psychology, University of Cologne, Cologne, Germany

Christoph Flückiger, PhD, Swiss/GermanBPP, Institute of Psychology, Clinical Psychology II, University of Kassel, Kassel, Germany

Miriam K. Forbes, PhD, School of Psychological Sciences, Macquarie University, Sydney, New South Wales, Australia

Anna Hartford, PhD, Department of Philosophy, Unit for Social and Political Ethics, Stellenbosch University, Stellenbosch, South Africa

Adele M. Hayes, PhD, Department of Psychological and Brain Sciences, University of Delaware, Newark, Delaware

Sabine C. Herpertz, Dr. med, Department of General Psychiatry, University Hospital Heidelberg, Heidelberg, Germany

Alexandra Hines, MS, Clinic for Emotional Health, Department of Psychology, University of Kentucky, Lexington, Kentucky

Christopher J. Hopwood, PhD, Department of Psychology, University of Zurich, Zurich, Switzerland

Susanne Hörz-Sagstetter, PhD, Department of Clinical Psychology and Psychotherapy, Psychologische Hochschule Berlin, Berlin, Germany

Sierra A. Iwanicki, PhD, Research and Development, Psychological Assessment Resources, Lutz, Florida

Eranda Jayawickreme, PhD, Department of Psychology and Program for Leadership and Character, Wake Forest University, Winston-Salem, North Carolina

Tyra Jones, BA, Department of Psychology, University at Buffalo, Buffalo, New York

Leonie Kampe, PhD, MSc, Department of Psychological Diagnostics, International Psychoanalytic University Berlin, Berlin, Germany

Rowan Kemmerly, MA, Department of Psychology, Rutgers University, Newark, New Jersey

André Kerber, BSc, DiplPsych, PhD, Department of Clinical Psychological Intervention, Freie Universität Berlin, Berlin, Germany

Vardha Kharbanda, MA, Department of Psychology, Illinois Institute of Technology, Chicago, Illinois

Robert F. Krueger, PhD, Department of Psychology, University of Minnesota, Minneapolis, Minnesota

Madeline L. Kushner, MS, Clinic for Emotional Health, Department of Psychology, University of Kentucky, Lexington, Kentucky

Benjamin B. Lahey, PhD, Department of Public Health Sciences, University of Chicago, Chicago, Illinois

Brendan Lam, BA, Department of Psychology, Yale University, New Haven, Connecticut

Anna Lichtwarck-Aschoff, PhD, Faculty of Social Sciences, Department of Pedagogical and Educational Sciences, University of Groningen, Groningen, The Netherlands

Donald R. Lynam, PhD, Department of Psychological Sciences, Purdue University, West Lafayette, Indiana

Kristian E. Markon, PhD, Department of Psychology, University of Minnesota, Minneapolis, Minnesota

Giorgia Michelini, PhD, Department of Biological and Experimental Psychology, Queen Mary University of London, London, England, United Kingdom

Joshua D. Miller, PhD, Department of Psychology, University of Georgia, Athens, Georgia

Leslie C. Morey, PhD, Department of Psychological and Brain Sciences, Texas A&M University, College Station, Texas

Janan Mostajabi, MS, Department of Psychology, University of Michigan, Ann Arbor, Michigan

Thomas Munder, PhD, Department of Psychology, University of Kassel, Kassel, Germany

Sharon M. Nelson, PhD, Psychology Department, The Pennsylvania State University, University Park, Pennsylvania

Sienna Nielsen, MS, Department of Psychology, University of Michigan, Ann Arbor, Michigan

Merlijn Olthof, PhD, Faculty of Social Sciences, Department of Pedagogical and Educational Sciences, University of Groningen, Groningen, The Netherlands

Samuel Paskewitz, PhD, Department of Psychology, Yale University, New Haven, Connecticut

Sarah L. Pedersen, PhD, Department of Psychiatry, University of Pittsburgh, Pittsburgh, Pennsylvania

Nathaniel L. Phillips, MS, Department of Psychology, University of Georgia, Athens, Georgia

Holly E. Poore, PhD, Department of Psychiatry, Robert Wood Johnson Medical School, West Piscataway, New Jersey

Paula Marie Powe, MD, Department of Psychiatry, University of Pittsburgh, Pittsburgh, Pennsylvania

Juliette L. Ratchford, PhD, Department of Psychology and Program of Leadership and Character, Wake Forest University, Winston-Salem, North Carolina

Craig Rodriguez-Seijas, PhD, Department of Psychology, University of Michigan, Ann Arbor, Michigan

Camilo J. Ruggero, PhD, Department of Psychology, School of Behavioral and Brain Sciences, The University of Texas at Dallas, Richardson, Texas

Shannon Sauer-Zavala, PhD, Clinic for Emotional Health, Department of Psychology, University of Kentucky, Lexington, Kentucky

Stephen M. Schueller, PhD, Department of Psychological Science, University of California–Irvine, Irvine, California

Carla Sharp, PhD, Department of Psychology, University of Houston, Houston, Texas

Leonard J. Simms. PhD, Department of Psychology, University at Buffalo, Buffalo, New York

Dan J. Stein, MD, PhD, DPhil (deceased), SAMRC Unit on Risk and Resilience in Mental Disorders, Department of Psychiatry and Neuroscience Institute, University of Cape Town, Cape Town, Western Province, South Africa

Trevor Sanchez Stevens, BA, Department of Psychological and Brain Sciences, University of Delaware, Newark, Delaware

Isabel Thielmann, PhD, Department of Criminology, Max Planck Institute for the Study of Crime, Security and Law, Freiburg, Germany

Rachel A. Vaughn-Coaxum, PhD, Department of Psychiatry, School of Medicine, University of Pittsburgh, Pittsburgh, Pennsylvania

Irwin D. Waldman, PhD, Department of Psychology, Emory University, Atlanta, Georgia

Frances Wang, PhD, Department of Psychiatry, University of Pittsburgh, Pittsburgh, Pennsylvania

Monika A. Waszczuk, PhD, Department of Psychology, Rosalind Franklin University of Medicine and Science, North Chicago, Illinois

Theresa L. Welles, PhD, Psychology Department, The Pennsylvania State University, University Park, Pennsylvania

Thomas A. Widiger, PhD, Psychology Department, University of Kentucky, Lexington, Kentucky

Sylia Wilson, PhD, Institute of Child Development, University of Minnesota, Minneapolis, Minnesota

Aidan G. C. Wright, PhD, Department of Psychology and Eisenberg Family Depression Center, University of Michigan, Ann Arbor, Michigan

Charlotte S. Zell, BA, Department of Psychology, University of Houston, Houston, Texas

Contents

CHAPTER 1

Introduction

Christopher J. Hopwood, Carla Sharp,
and Robert F. Krueger

It is very easy to find articles in the mental health literature that begin with a paragraph lamenting the downsides of categorical diagnosis (e.g., comorbidity, heterogeneity, and arbitrary cutoffs) and championing the virtues of dimensional alternatives. Many of the chapters in this book start that way. This is now a general consensus in the field: Dimensional models better reflect the current state of knowledge about the structure of psychopathology than categorical models. The premise of this book is that despite this, it is not exactly clear how the transition from categorical to dimensional models should occur, in both research and the clinic. There are things to think about, issues to work out, challenges that may yet be unforeseen, and sources of inertia to overcome. This book is an attempt to create space for dialogue about these issues that is both progressive and reflective.

In this introductory chapter, we define categorical and dimensional concepts, situate this book in the historical context of the transition to personality-based dimensional diagnosis of psychopathology, highlight how new conceptions of diagnosis raise a host of issues that need to be resolved in the transition to a more evidence-based model of mental health problems, and frame our approach to this book.

Categorical and Dimensional Models

Before going further, it is important to define our terms because categorical and dimensional are not always used in the same way. By categorical, we mean the diagnostic model that was established in the DSM-III

American Psychiatric Association, 1980). In this model, most mental health constructs are conceptualized as polythetic categories in which disorders are understood as syndromes with some number of symptoms and diagnosis is based on a patient meeting some predetermined number of symptom criteria. For example, the DSM assumes that major depressive disorder is a syndrome with nine possible symptoms and a patient with five of those nine "has" it. Disorders in this model are grouped into chapters by designated experts based on similarity of phenomenology or inferred etiology. There are other possible categorical systems for psychiatric taxonomy (e.g., prototype approaches), but given the pervasiveness of the DSM (and the *International Classification of Diseases,* which uses a very similar model, albeit with a dimensional approach to personality disorder diagnosis), this is generally what people mean when they write about the "categorical model."

Dimensional can mean at least three things (Hopwood et al., 2023). First it can mean that the diagnostician could simply sum the symptoms of a diagnosis to get a continuous score. For example, rather than using a cutoff of five to determine whether a person "has" depression, the severity of that person's depression could be described on a scale from one to nine. Second, it can mean that the indicators of a diagnostic construct would fit a one-dimensional factor model. Many criteria sets in the DSM would not meet this definition of dimensional. Third, it can mean that, as a collection, all the diagnostic constructs can be conceptualized within a hierarchy of dimensions whose relations are established empirically. This third meaning is strongly rooted in factor-analytic methods and is the basis for the increasingly popular Hierarchical Taxonomy of Psychopathology (HiTOP; Kotov et al., 2017) model. Because the third meaning of dimensional most directly solves or at least explains the problems of comorbidity and heterogeneity that are common complaints about the categorical model (Krueger et al., 2018), it is a stronger basis for comparison, and it is what we mean when we use "dimensional model." Here again, we note there are other approaches to thinking about taxonomy that are congenial to the dimensional perspective or at least have the potential to improve on polythetic categories (Eaton et al., 2023; Zachar & Kendler, 2007), but in this book we focus on the comparison between categorical and dimensional models.

Back to the Future: Personality as a Basis for Taxonomy

In the mid-20th-century taxonomy, personality and psychopathology were closely aligned in Western mental health care. For instance, the psychoanalytic and neo-psychoanalytic theories that dominated psychiatry understood symptoms as embedded within personality structure (Fenichel, 1945; Menninger, 1963). Likewise, the psychological assessment tradition that dominated clinical psychology used "personality assessment" instruments such as the MMPI or Rorschach to conduct diagnostic evaluations (Rappaport et al., 1945). However, in the late 20th century personality and psychopathology came to be seen as largely distinct. This was due to the influences of the neo-Kraepelinian descriptive psychiatry on diagnosis in the form of the DSM (e.g., Feighner et al., 1972; see Kendler et al., 2010) and brief cognitive, behavioral, and pharmacological interventions that focused on symptom change (Wilson, 1993). The main area of overlap between personality and psychopathology during this era was understood to involve personality disorder concepts, which were thought of as involving personality features that were so problematic that they caused clinically significant dysfunction and distress (Millon, 1983). In other words, personality was seen as distinct from psychiatric symptoms.

In the beginning of the 21st century the pendulum began swinging back to more integrative models, albeit in a less psychoanalytic and more psychometric form. Personality played an important role in the transition from categorical to dimensional models for three interrelated reasons. The first is methodological: Contemporary dimensional models like HiTOP are based on factor-analytic methods that are common in personality psychology (Ringwald et al., 2023). The second is empirical: The number and nature of higher-order dimensions in factor analyses of mental health constructs, personality disorders, and personality traits are very similar (Markon et al., 2005; Soodla et al., 2025; Wright & Simms, 2015), supporting the use of personality models to organize psychopathology. The third is historical: Personality disorders have been at the cutting edge of this debate and were the first to formally transition to dimensional models in the DSM-5 and ICD-11 (Krueger, 2013), arguably setting the stage for a reenvisioning of psychiatric taxonomy writ large (Krueger et al., 2018).

Issues in the Transition from Categorical to Dimensional Diagnosis

Although significant differences in perspective remain, there is now a general sentiment favoring the value of this rapprochement in the empirical literature, which can be summarized under the rubric of "dimensional diagnosis." Nevertheless, the fieldwide shift toward dimensional diagnosis is complex. The fact that most scholars agree that dimensional models are superior to categorical models does not mean that they agree among themselves or the applied clinical community on what dimensional models should look like, how they should be implemented, or how briskly the transition should occur.

A total reformulation of psychiatric taxonomy raises both practical issues in implementing dimensional models in the clinic and conceptual issues in the way in which psychopathology is thought about and studied. On the practical side, how can dimensional models of diagnosis be applied in different clinical settings? How does dimensional diagnosis change how we think about psychotherapy technique and training? Could dimensional diagnosis help with problems such as stigma and inclusion? Conceptual issues include questions such as what are the differences between personality and psychopathology and what are personality disorders if personality and all mental disorders share a common structure? What does developmental and genetic research have to say about the integration of personality and psychopathology? What are the implications of dimensional diagnosis for research on psychopathology, epidemiology, and psychotherapy? How can we understand neurodevelopmental and cognitive disorders that have not been extensively studied in conjunction with other forms of psychopathology?

Format and Content of This Book

There is significant debate regarding how to understand the general issue of how personality is related to psychopathology and what this means for dimensional diagnosis as well as how to answer questions like these. The goal of this book is to provide a forum for productive discussion of these practical/clinical and conceptual/research issues. To encourage rigorous and thoughtful exchange, different topics are addressed by pairs of author teams. Thus, each chapter has two parts; references for both parts will be found at the end of each chapter. Authors were selected who would be likely to have different perspectives on their topic and asked to lean into those differences so that different perspectives would be represented. Each contribution was organized around three specific questions within each topic to ensure a shared focus. As a group, the authors are generally sanguine about the advantages of dimensional diagnosis, but they focus on different strengths, offer different kinds of suggestions about how to move forward, and identify a variety of challenges along the path of progress. Here, in reflecting on these differing perspectives within and across chapters, we highlight overarching themes and questions that emerged, perhaps pointing to an agenda for the next generation of research on dimensional diagnosis.

A first theme that emerged is one grappled with by Morey and Simms and Jones in Chapter 2—that is, the dilemma of determining "caseness" in dimensional diagnosis. Dimensional diagnosis, by its very nature, does not group individuals, with downstream implications for study designs, epidemiology, and intervention. The issue of "caseness" is revisited in Chapter 8, with Conway arguing for a clean departure from study designs in which individuals are grouped (e.g., case–control designs). Baskin-Sommers et al. recommend a more flexible approach by which constructs derived from formal statistical modeling can be used to arrange psychopathology indicators into dimensions, categories, or combinations of the two. "Caseness" is also of concern in Chapter 11, which addresses the challenges of dimensional diagnosis for epidemiology. Stein and Hartford explain the philosophical roots of the problem, and like Baskin-Sommers et al., they argue for an integrative solution. Markon provides out-of-the-box solutions and considers the effect of characterizing distributions rather than frequencies—the former of course not being contingent on "caseness." Either way, for dimensional diagnosis to be routinely used in clinical practice, it is likely that some balance between the variable-centered approaches typical of dimensional diagnosis and the person-centered approaches characteristic of categorical diagnosis will be needed. As Morey states, "it is important to remember that it is ultimately at the level of the person where important decisions are to be made" (p. 18).

A second overarching theme relates to how dimensional diagnosis can innovate intervention. In Chapter 3, Callahan offers an intriguing model for how HiTOP superspectra, spectra, and dimensions could be mapped onto different therapeutic techniques across therapeutic modalities and Flückiger highlights the potential of dimensional diagnosis to shift a focus from deficit- to strength-based intervention by focusing on emphasizing the positive pole of typical–atypical continua. Chapter 4 builds on these proposals by highlighting the advantages of dimensional diagnosis for more effective intervention (Sauer-Zavala et al.) and by making the point that psychodynamic psychotherapies have always relied on dimensional diagnosis (Hörz-Sagstetter and Kampe). Both author groups in Chapter 12 discuss ways in which dimensional models fundamentally change the way we think about psychotherapy research, and in Chapter 15, Thielmann and Casali and Jayawickreme et al. show the value of interventions that leverage basic (as opposed to extreme, maladaptive) traits also in nonclinical populations. We are encouraged by these proposals but acknowledge that research in this area is still nascent, necessitating calls for research that uses dimensional diagnosis in treatment trials and/or a translation of existing therapeutic approaches using the language of dimensional diagnosis.

A third overarching theme concerns how the relative dearth of treatment outcome literature for dimensional diagnosis may affect the training of clinicians, which is constrained by strict standards for what may be taught as evidence-based practice. In Chapter 5, both Ruggero and Callahan and Nelson et al. argue for the need for faster incorporation of research into curricula as well as frontline clinical practice, where most clinical training practica occur. We concur and hope to see more intentional and explicit integration of dimensional diagnosis in the training of mental health professionals.

A fourth theme and an area where a robust empirical basis is slowly emerging is in evaluating the advantages of dimensional diagnosis for reducing stigma. In Chapter 6, Lahey cogently explains the potential of dimensional diagnosis and Corrigan and Kharbanda review literature demonstrating its advantages. Similar to the research–practice and research–training gaps described above, Chapter 6 highlights a research–public knowledge gap, which if addressed, can play a significant role in further reducing stigma associated with mental illness. The potential for destigmatization for minority populations is further elaborated in Chapter 7 with convincing arguments by Pederson et al. However, Asadi et al. cautions that for dimensional diagnosis to reach its full potential, it will have to be properly contextualized in its sociocultural context. As yet, not enough research has evaluated the applicability of dimensional diagnosis across diverse groups.

The last theme that emerges across chapters is a conceptual one. It is fair to say that a leading dimensional approach to diagnosis and one promoted by several authors in this volume is a dispositional trait-based approach—sometimes referred to as the personality—psychopathology-spectrum approach, of which HiTOP is a good example. In Chapter 9, Lahey and Zell and Sharp tackle the implications of the personality–psychopathology-spectrum approach from a developmental point of view. Lahey promotes the idea that a pure trait dispositional approach is adequate and desirable to explain all psychopathology but contends that traits and psychopathology may have different causal influences. Zell and Sharp argue that when considering developmental continuities and discontinuities, dispositional trait-based approaches are inadequate to fully explain the onset and/or course of psychopathology. They call for a broader view and understanding of personality that goes beyond traits—most notably to explicitly include self and identity function in its definition. Poore and Waldman in Chapter 10 expand on Lahey's thesis, concluding that although genetic influences on personality and psychopathology appear to overlap substantially, this overlap is incomplete, with evidence that environmental influences also differ in these domains. Although generally supportive of the personality–psychopathology-spectrum approach promoted by Lahey, Poore, and Waldman, Waszczuk, in her review of the genetic research in Chapter 10, agrees with Zell and Sharp when she cautions that it remains unclear whether this formulation holds across developmental stages and specific traits. The tension on how best to understand "personality" in personality–psychopathology-spectrum approaches continues in Chapters 13 and 14. In Chapter 13, DeYoung and Krueger distinguish "symptoms" of psychopathology from traits by determining that symptoms become traits when they are persistent and severe—a position supported by the pure dispositional trait approach espoused by Miller et al. in Chapter 14 who view traits as pathological when they are persistent, precocious, and pervasive. However, De Young and Krueger then expand the classic personality–psychopathology approach beyond traits to add characteristic adaptations as a second layer of personality derived from traits in transaction with the environment. They further expand the definition of psychopathology as frustrated goal pursuit, adaptation, and attainment—which they term "dysfunction." The expansion of the personality construct beyond traits is also promoted by Herpertz in Chapter 13, albeit through the lens of the level-of-personality-functioning construct of the alternative model of personality disorder—arguably the only explicit dimensional diagnostic system currently in DSM-5 (with its associated version in ICD-11). Like Zell and Sharp in Chapter 9, Herpertz homes in on the process—and capacity-oriented aspects of personality presumed to be distinct from traits—that is, "the capability to reflect on one's characteristic ways of thinking, feeling, and behaving, to be aware of one's agency, to have knowledge of the goals and motives that drive one's behavior and social interaction with others, and to be able to see oneself from the perspective of others." This expanded approach aligns with Wright and Mostjabi's argument in Chapter 14 for the predominance of self and interpersonal functioning in understanding personality (and personality disorder) and further shows up in Chapter 16 where Wilson and Michelini and Forbes attempt to integrate developmental and neurocognitive disorders into trait-based dimensional systems, encouraging us to consider capacities beyond the level of descriptive (self-reported) traits. Together, there seems to be some preoccupation with the limitations of traits, potentially calling for an expanded definition of the traditional personality–psychopathology-spectrum approach.

Conclusion

The era of polythetic categories that began with DSM-III served a useful purpose in mental health practice and research, but there is now sufficient evidence that it is invalid in some basic ways, has not significantly advanced mental health, and is problematic for most scholars and practitioners such that transitioning to a different paradigm seems inevitable.

Some view dimensional models like HiTOP as the best contender, but arguably still in its translational infancy. This book highlights remaining empirical, conceptual, and practical questions to be addressed to move this agenda forward. The transition from categorical to dimensional models has the potential to improve mental health care and research (Conway et al., 2019), but it will be challenging. With some notable exceptions, a lot of the literature on this topic has had a cheerleading quality that presumably stems from the well-intentioned motive to push the field forward but risks glossing over the various practical and conceptual challenges associated with reformulating psychiatric diagnosis. We believe that it is a good time to create spaces, like this volume, where some of these challenges are discussed by some of the people who are at the forefront of diagnostic research and practice and that thoughtful reflection and discussion will ultimately stimulate progress toward better ways to classify mental health problems.

REFERENCES

American Psychiatric Association. (1980). *Diagnostic and statistical manual of mental disorders* (3rd ed.). Author.

Conway, C. C., Forbes, M. K., Forbush, K. T., Fried, E. I., Hallquist, M. N., Kotov, R., . . . Eaton, N. R. (2019). A hierarchical taxonomy of psychopathology can transform mental health research. *Perspectives on Psychological Science, 14*(3), 419–436.

Eaton, N. R., Bringmann, L. F., Elmer, T., Fried, E. I., Forbes, M. K., Greene, A. L., . . . Waszczuk, M. A. (2023). A review of approaches and models in psychopathology conceptualization research. *Nature Reviews Psychology, 2*(10), 622–636.

Feighner, J. P., Robins, E., Guze, S. B., Woodruff, R. A., Winokur, G., & Munoz, R. (1972). Diagnostic criteria for use in psychiatric research. *Archives of General Psychiatry, 26*(1), 57–63.

Fenichel, O. (1945). *The psychoanalytic theory of neurosis*. Norton.

Hopwood, C. J., Morey, L. C., & Markon, K. E. (2023). What is a psychopathology dimension? *Clinical Psychology Review, 106*, 102356.

Kendler, K. S., Muñoz, R. A., & Murphy, G. (2010). The development of the Feighner criteria: A historical perspective. *American Journal of Psychiatry, 167*(2), 134–142.

Kotov, R., Krueger, R. F., Watson, D., Achenbach, T. M., Althoff, R. R., Bagby, R. M., . . . Zimmerman, M. (2017). The hierarchical taxonomy of psychopathology (HiTOP): A dimensional alternative to traditional nosologies. *Journal of Abnormal Psychology, 126*(4), 454–477.

Krueger, R. F. (2013). Personality disorders are the vanguard of the post-DSM-5.0 era. *Personality Disorders: Theory, Research, and Treatment, 4*(4), 355–362.

Krueger, R. F., Kotov, R., Watson, D., Forbes, M. K., Eaton, N. R., Ruggero, C. J., . . . Zimmermann, J. (2018). Progress in achieving quantitative classification of psychopathology. *World Psychiatry, 17*(3), 282–293.

Markon, K. E., Krueger, R. F., & Watson, D. (2005). Delineating the structure of normal and abnormal personality: An integrative hierarchical approach. *Journal of Personality and Social Psychology, 88*(1), 139–157.

Menninger, K. (1963). *The vital balance: The life process in mental health and illness*. Viking Penguin.

Millon, T. (1983). The DSM-III: An insider's perspective. *American Psychologist, 38*(7), 804–814.

Rappaport, D., Gill, M. M., & Schaefer, R. (1945). *Diagnostic psychological testing*. Year Book.

Ringwald, W. R., Forbes, M. K., & Wright, A. G. (2023). Meta-analysis of structural evidence for the hierarchical taxonomy of psychopathology (HiTOP) model. *Psychological Medicine, 53*(2), 533–546.

Soodla, H. L., Lehto, K., Kõiv, K., Vainik, U., Akkermann, K., & Mõttus, R. (2025). Assessing the overlap of personality traits and internalizing psychopathology using multi-informant data: Two sides of the same coin? *Journal of Psychopathology and Clinical Science, 134*(4), 400–413.

Wilson, M. (1993). DSM-III and the transformation of American psychiatry: A history. *American Journal of Psychiatry, 150*(3), 399–410.

Wright, A. G., & Simms, L. J. (2015). A metastructural model of mental disorders and pathological personality traits. *Psychological Medicine, 45*(11), 2309–2319.

Zachar, P., & Kendler, K. S. (2007). Psychiatric disorders: A conceptual taxonomy. *American Journal of Psychiatry, 164*(4), 557–565.

CHAPTER 2

What does dimensional diagnosis mean for clinical assessment?

One of the biggest challenges in mental health is bridging bench and bedside. Although there is significant momentum in favor of dimensional models in the research literature, uptake of these models in clinical practice has been slow. How should dimensional models inform clinical assessment? We asked experts three questions related to this theme.

How should mental disorders be assessed?

How should diagnostic cutoffs be established?

What is the role of factor-based models for applied clinical assessment?

Morey emphasizes subtle distinctions between meanings of the word "dimension" and, in particular, the difference between acknowledging that most evidence supports mental health concepts as continua and arguing that psychopathology is dimensional according to stricter (e.g., factor-analytic) conceptualizations of that word. Simms and Jones highlighted issues in clinical assessment that go beyond the link between factor-analytic models and applied assessment, such as the importance of multimethod data and the distinction between mental health problems and associated impairments. Both sets of authors agreed that identifying cases along continua is both necessary and arbitrary and offered different solutions for establishing clinical cutoffs. Their views differed mostly regarding the role of factor analysis. Morey had fundamental questions about its role in past discovery and future taxonomy, whereas Simms and Jones framed it as a primary approach that may need to be supplemented around the edges.

PART I

Dimensional diagnosis and clinical assessment

LESLIE C. MOREY

In this section, we are asked to comment on what dimensional diagnosis means for clinical assessment, with a particular focus on three specific issues. During my career, I've provided comments on each of these three issues, and in the interest of brevity as well as transparency I will begin my comments on each topic with a brief summary and citation of previous writings where I've offered some discussion on these topics. I reference "transparency," as it is entirely possible that my view on these topics might differ now from what I wrote 20 or 30 years ago. Over the course of academic writings that has spanned 6 decades, my beliefs have sometimes changed, with a prime example involving noteworthy instability in my optimism (or lack thereof) around the utility of multivariate methods for solving crucial problems in clinical assessment and diagnosis. Thus, the following comments often link to previous statements that I have made on these topics that may provide a more in-depth examination of them, along with some brief commentary on the extent to which these views have demonstrated temporal stability, a characteristic presumed but certainly not assured.

How Should Mental Disorders Be Assessed?

Certainly by the time that my *Personality Assessment Inventory* (Morey, 1991) was developed, I had arrived at the conclusion that mental disorders should be assessed along a continuum, where I argued that a "strictly qualitative approach to diagnosis does not accurately reflect the inherently 'fuzzy' nature of most concepts in mental health" (Morey, 1991, p. 64) and went on to point out that this "may hold true regardless of whether most clinical disorders are categorical or dimensional in nature" (p. 64). For example, if mental health concepts are categorical "prototypes" (e.g., Rosch, 1978), the degree to which a given observation resembles the conceptual prototype reflects a continuum that itself is likely to provide critical information in case formulation, even while the underlying concept is categorical. Thus, my presumption continues to be that there is meaningful valid dimensional variance in all mental health concepts such that they must be assessed dimensionally to avoid significant loss of information.

As a demonstration, we were able to use the Collaborative Longitudinal Personality Study (Gunderson et al., 2000) to provide one of the more comprehensive estimates of just how much information is lost by categorizing personality disorder concepts. This study afforded the opportunity to compare the use of the DSM categorical formulation of personality disorder as opposed to converting the formulation of those same constructs to dimensions by simply adding up the number of diagnostic indicators met by each participant at their initial assessment—for example, contrasting the diagnosis of borderline personality disorder using a "at least 5 of 9 indicators required" with a score that ranged from zero to nine of these indicators met. Across 10 different indicators of predictive validity for the 10-year outcome of study participants, the average amount of variance predicted by the categorical version of the DSM personality disorder concepts was less than a third of that predicted by the dimensionalized version (Morey et al., 2012). To me, such findings provide a rather convincing argument that such concepts must be assessed as continua.

How Should Diagnostic Cutoffs Be Established?

Even when faced with compelling evidence that there is significant dimensional variance in a mental health, it often becomes necessary to provide a threshold for determining "caseness" because many of the implications of these concepts lead to dichotomous decisions: Should this individual receive treatment? Should they be hospitalized? Are they competent to stand trial? Within the personality disorders field in particular, there has been considerable skepticism about such thresholds being "arbitrary" (e.g., Cooper et al., 2010), as they tend to rely on simplistic algorithms (e.g., more than half of all possible symptoms) that have no inherent scientific basis. However, I have previously argued (Morey, 2021; Hopwood et al., 2023) that designating a diagnostic threshold on a clinical continuum is not necessarily arbitrary because there can be scientific justifications for doing so. This perception of arbitrariness may be driven by the field's heavy reliance on statistical methods that assume linear relationships and normal distributions for our variables of interest, but a scientific rationale for a diagnostic threshold can sometimes be found in the nonlinearity and non-normality of our phenomena of interest. In various fields of medicine, potential thresholds on continuous assessments can be identified where there is a nonlinear change in expected outcomes or relationships with other variables of critical importance. Two examples of this involve establishing caseness in diabetes and hypertension, where the continuous indicators of HbA1c and diastolic blood pressure, respectively, demonstrate ranges where mortality risk increases exponentially rather than linearly. Such points of inflection provide a meaningful scientific basis for establishing a threshold.

With respect to potential non-normality of distributions, evidence of multimodality such as a significant second mode found at an extreme could reflect a natural threshold between "cases" and the general population. For example, in conducting research over the years with the PAI Infrequency (INF) scale, a validity scale used to detect problematic responding, it has been typical to find a distribution with a pronounced positive skew but also presenting with a distinct secondary mode, particularly in samples that may have limited motivation to respond carefully, such as undergraduate samples or anonymous online participants. When such modes are observed, the point of rarity between this secondary mode and the rest of the population provides a natural breakpoint for establishing "case" membership, in this instance whether test responses should be considered valid. Given the important implications of establishing caseness for mental health concepts, there has been limited research dedicated to pursuing questions such as nonlinearity or non-normality in these concepts. To date there is little evidence to support the existence of such meaningful thresholds for dimensions in psychopathology.

The absence of such evidence precludes the use of the natural properties of the dimension to guide caseness determination, but that does not necessarily mean that the field must then rely on "arbitrary" rules. More typically, the guiding principles involve the selection ratio—namely, what percentages of "cases" for a particular concept make sense in terms of societal resources and community norms. For example, although the pharmaceutical industry might support a threshold that suggests that 90% of the general population requires treatment for depression, such a rule would stretch both the available resources for mental health treatment and our definition of "within normal limits." A similar example can be found in the early application of intelligence measures, such as Yerkes's work with the Army during World War I where their testing procedures identified roughly half of recruits as intellectually disabled—a result that was greeted with appropriate skepticism by the Army. As a result, conventions for some constructs have evolved that invoke distributional properties, such as being 1.5 (e.g., learning disorder) or 2.0 (e.g., intellectual disability) standard deviations from the population mean. Despite the appearance of being objective and scientifically based, those arguably arbitrary thresholds have achieved acceptance primarily because the resulting selection ratio has been judged to be appropriate. It must be noted that adopting such conventions for all mental health concepts would result in very similar prevalence of "cases" despite that constructs such as schizophrenia, somatization, or adjustment problems may have distinctly different implications for functioning and need for intervention. As noted in Hopwood et al. (2023), "Absent natural thresholds, this determination becomes an ethical or sociopolitical question, having to do with factors such as how much concern a society has with mental health problems, considerations regarding the balance between providing care and stigmatizing human variability, the resources a society has to help people with mental health difficulties, and the value placed on treating every person the same way" (p. 8).

What Is the Role of Factor-Based Models for Applied Clinical Assessment?

Nearly 20 years ago, I offered the following brief conclusion on this topic: "It is my belief that the factor analysis of scale scores is virtually useless in the construct validation of multidimensional clinical measures in the absence of a well-articulated theory of the classificatory relations (Skinner, 1981) among the different constructs" (Morey, 1995, p. 399). This view persists to this day. The presumption that constructs in mental health all consist of groups of indicators that demonstrate high degrees of linear interrelationships that then are additively aggregated and which are presumably independent of other such groups of indicators, continues to strike me as an instance of trying to make nature conform to our methods rather than the other way around. Factor analysis and internal consistency reflect a presumption that substantial intercorrelations among indicators of a given concept are critical for the measurement of that construct, but such intercorrelations are neither necessary nor sufficient as an indicator of either reliability, in a test–retest sense, or validity. Moreover, as pointed out by Loevinger (1954) more than half a century ago, high indicator intercorrelations can actually work against validity, particularly content validity.

Just because an investigator *can* perform a factor analysis of clinical indicators doesn't necessarily mean that they *should*. These techniques can play an important role in data reduction and have their place as a tool in exploring the properties of applied clinical assessment measures, but this place is more descriptive than evaluative—a measure having a simple factorial structure or having high internal consistency isn't necessarily "good" or "bad." Rather, it describes properties of the measure than may or may not align with theoretical expectations for the measure. As an example, I have encountered more than one "critique" of the PAI Inconsistency scale (ICN), which is designed to measure inconsistent responding across the instrument, with the criticism being that the scale has a "bad" coefficient alpha: Are we thus to conclude that a measure of inconsistency is problematic because the indicators are not consistent?

Aside from my misgivings about the significance ascribed to factor analysis in the development and validation of clinical measures, I would also note that as a tool of discovery, I believe that the yield of factor analyses has been overestimated. This is not to say that models that have emerged from the factor analysis tradition have no validity or utility; rather, I would suggest that factor analysis was not really necessary for the articulation of these dimensions. Consider the dimensions of the five-factor model (FFM), perhaps the most studied factor-analytic model in the discipline. It is difficult to argue that factor analysis was critical in the process of discovery for these constructs. Eysenck, arguably the first to describe factor analyses that yielded the initial two dimensions of the FFM, noted that those results corresponded to two dimensions of psychopathology, the degree of neuroticism and the hysteria versus dysthymia distinction, that were already well established in the psychiatric literature by the time he conducted those analyses in the 1940s. The Extraversion/Conscientiousness and Agreeableness dimensions strongly resemble the interpersonal continua of agency and communion that were described in detail by Sullivan (1953) and Leary (1957), without any assistance from factor analysis. There is less harmony than might be expected from the fifth dimension in the FFM (Schwaba & Thalmayer 2024), but whether one concludes that it reflects intelligence, poor reality testing, conformity, or something else, it is hard to argue that those constructs would not have been discovered without the contribution of factor analysis.

Conclusion

The evidence is mounting steadily against a conclusion that most mental health concepts are categories where a given individual is either a member of a category or not. It seems clear that people differ by degree on most of these concepts and that considering it as an either/or distinction loses much of what we can infer about such a person as a result. The field has simply gathered too much data that contradicts a dichotomous categorical approach to excuse the general exclusion of dimensional models from the diagnostic nomenclature. Nonetheless, I would encourage the field to turn similar falsification efforts toward many of the assumptions and methods that have evolved in psychology around dimensional approaches such as the belief that summing putative indicators by definition produces a "dimension" with specific implications of that term (Hopwood et al., 2023), that high intercorrelations among these indicators are required for the resulting continuum to have significant implications or validity, that a factor analysis of these indicators will invariably lead to insights about the nature of the phenomena, or that our emphases should be on developing a taxonomy of variables rather than of people (Revelle, 2024). With respect to the latter, it is important to remember that it is ultimately at the level of the person where important decisions are to be made—and each person is a combination of myriad critical variable dimensions. It is not adequate to devote full attention to identifying and understanding dimensions in isolation—the field must go beyond such rudiments to arrive at a better understanding of the implications of various configurations of these dimensions. It is unwise to presume that all relevant phenomena in mental health are additive, linearly related, and normally distributed, even though the field's preferred statistical tools make such assumptions. These dimensions likely interact in highly complex ways, and the distribution of people in this multivariable space is unlikely to be multivariate normal. Complex interactions between these variables will probably prove to be the rule rather than the exception; inconsistency of observed relationships over time may be a fact of nature and not measurement error; and the distributions of clinical problems in this space are likely to involve local densities, the centroids of which may be meaningfully described as categories. Although I generally believe that multivariate methods have an important place in the study of taxonomy in mental health, the derivation of factorial models of cross-sectional mental health symptoms does not seem to have led to significant changes in our understanding of etiology or treatment of such problems in the 80-plus years that such models have been produced. Even a noted empiricist such as Meehl (1957) felt strongly that as researchers, we must use our heads as well as formulas, and part of doing so involves an openness to other approaches and to insights provided by theory and not just by methods. Ideally, the application of approaches from different complementary angles can converge to yield a deeper understanding of how to best conceptualize clinical problems.

PART II

Implementation of dimensional factor-based models of psychopathology in clinical practice

LEONARD J. SIMMS and TYRA JONES

Dimensional models of psychopathology have gained considerable traction in psychopathology and assessment research in recent years, but their uptake into clinical practice has been slow. The move toward dimensional psychopathology models reflects a long-known recognition of the complexities of mental health disorders as they traditionally have been classified, such as psychiatric comorbidity and within-diagnosis heterogeneity, and that models based on categorical understandings of psychopathology don't fit psychiatric symptom data particularly well (Clark et al., 1995; Kotov et al., 2017). Central to this evolution are recent models like the hierarchical taxonomy of psychopathology (HiTOP; Kotov et al., 2017) and the research domain criteria (RDoC; Insel et al., 2010) initiatives, which emphasize the importance of understanding mental disorders along multiple dimensional spectra rather than as distinct psychiatric entities. The models differ in important ways—HiTOP advocates for a dimensional understanding of symptoms at different levels of specificity or generality (i.e., broad psychiatric spectra down to narrow-band symptoms and traits), whereas RDoC seeks to bridge the gap between biology and behavior, focusing on core psychopathology-relevant dimensions that cut across traditional psychiatric disorders.

Regardless of model, the shift to dimensional models raises critical questions about how mental disorders should be assessed, the criteria for establishing diagnostic cutoffs, and the role of factor-based models in applied clinical assessment. In this discussion, we briefly provide our perspectives on these interrelated questions. Addressing these questions should help guide dissemination and implementation work and provide a clearer roadmap for clinical translation efforts. It is important to note that despite these questions and their associated challenges, research suggests that clinicians find dimensional models of psychopathology acceptable or even preferable for communicating (e.g., Glover et al., 2012; Morey et al., 2014).

How Should Mental Disorders Be Assessed?

Recent literature reveals important insights about how best to assess mental disorders. In short, assessment of psychopathology should (1) involve the use of multiple methods when possible (e.g., self-report, interview, collateral reports, behavioral data), (2) be based on dimensional models rather than those rooted in binary diagnostic categories, (3) be rooted in modern transdiagnostic models rather than antiquated psychiatric diagnoses, and (4) disentangle the descriptive features of psychopathology from the impairments that those features may cause (i.e., separating severity from style).

Multiple Methods

Using dimensional models of psychopathology in clinical practice ideally occurs with a multifaceted approach that integrates various assessment methods to capture the complexity of an individual's mental health. Using multiple methods—such as self-report questionnaires, structured clinical interviews, collateral reports from family or friends, and direct behavioral observations—provides a more comprehensive understanding of the patient's experiences and challenges. Self-report measures offer valuable insights into the individual's subjective experiences but often are prone to response biases (e.g., Huprich & Bornstein, 2007) and potential insight issues (e.g., Carlson & Oltmanns, 2015). Structured interviews permit a value-added and more nuanced assessment of the severity and contextual relevance of psychiatric symptoms (Banerjee et al., 2009; Brauer & Sendatzki, 2024; Stepp et al., 2005). Collateral reports from others who know patients well also can reveal important incremental information about how symptoms manifest across settings, including the extent to which symptomatology is accompanied by significant distress or impairment (e.g., Oltmanns & Turkheimer, 2009). Behavioral data (e.g., direct behavioral observations, ecological momentary assessment responses) also provide evidence of functioning, allowing clinicians to observe real-world interactions and behaviors. A multimethod approach involves clinicians using several of these methods to enhance diagnostic accuracy, develop a more complete contextual understanding of the patient's problems, and inform treatment planning by creating a richer more layered view of an individual's psychopathology and psychosocial functioning.

Dimensions versus Categories

The emphasis on dimensional models rather than binary categories represents a significant advancement in the assessment of mental health disorders. Traditional categorical systems (e.g., DSM-5, ICD) can lead to oversimplification and may not fully capture the variability of an individual's symptoms (e.g., Kotov et al., 2017). Dimensional models, including HiTOP and RDoC most recently, advocate for evaluating symptoms along a continuum, thus acknowledging the gradations of psychopathology (e.g., Krueger et al., 2018). Such dimensional approaches allow clinicians to more precisely understand the *degree* of a given patient's psychopathology, and these approaches have shown considerable evidence of incremental validity over traditional categorical approaches (e.g., Markon et al., 2011) and thus have the potential to lead to more precise estimates of psychopathology and more nuanced treatment plans.

Transdiagnostic Models

Transdiagnostic models are those that include underlying psychiatric dimensions that cut across traditional diagnostic boundaries (e.g., anxiety vs. depression) that often fail to reflect shared underlying mechanisms across disorders. Modern psychiatric classifications are transdiagnostic and thus should be the basis of clinical assessment efforts. Transdiagnostic models focus on common dimensions such as emotion regulation, cognitive styles, and interpersonal functioning, which enable clinicians to address core psychiatric issues that transcend specific diagnoses (Insel et al., 2010). Such an approach encourages a more holistic understanding of mental health, as it promotes interventions that target shared pathways rather than simply treating surface-level symptoms.

Severity versus Style

Last, differentiating between severity and style in clinical assessments is crucial for effective practice. Severity pertains to the intensity and effects of symptoms, whereas style refers to the individual's characteristic patterns of thoughts, feelings, and behavior used to cope with distress (Hopwood et al., 2011). Distinguishing these features aids case conceptualization and treatment planning. For example, a patient experiencing high levels of anxiety may have learned to employ adaptive coping strategies (e.g., cognitive restructuring, relaxation), whereas another patient with more moderate anxiety might employ maladaptive coping strategies (e.g., avoidance, harmful substance use), resulting in greater impairment. Thus, the severity–style distinction allows clinicians to develop more accurate diagnostic conclusions and case conceptualizations that disentangle the nature of psychiatric features from the associated impairments, which should lead to more nuanced and personalized treatment plans.

How Should Diagnostic Cutoffs Be Established?

Establishing diagnostic cutoffs in dimensional models of psychopathology presents significant challenges, primarily because traditional criterion thresholds generally lack empirical support and fail to accurately "carve nature at its joints" with respect to psychopathology, resulting in categories that obscure the underlying dimensionality of mental health conditions (Kotov et al., 2017). Arbitrary diagnostic thresholds can lead to misclassification of patients, as they may not correspond to meaningful distinctions in symptom severity or functional impairment.

To address these challenges, a viable solution involves measuring psychopathology features along evidence-based dimensions and implementing a system of graded intensity thresholds. Each dimension of psychopathology can be broken down into levels of severity such as "within normal limits"(WNL), "a little," "moderate," and "extreme." Ideally, these thresholds would be informed by community and clinical reference groups (i.e., norms), providing a reference point for assessing individual symptom severity. Of equal importance is ensuring that reference groups for these graded intensity thresholds should be inclusive and reflect the diversity (e.g., ethnic, racial, gender, and sexual minority) of the full populations within which the measure is to be used clinically. Research has begun to delineate graded interpretive ranges for some measures (Stasik-O'Brien et al., 2019), but much more is needed to cover the full range of psychiatric dimensions. Moreover, although it will take time to transition to an evidence-based set of graded thresholds, the resulting ranges and cut points may be helpful specifically with precision medicine "stepped-care" models (e.g., van Straten et al., 2015) in which different grades of disorder are associated with unique prescriptions for treatment.

Along with graded intensity thresholds, given the argument above about separating diagnostic severity versus style, it also is important to assign impairment labels for each dimension. These labels, such as "none," "mild," "moderate," and "severe," can provide valuable context regarding the functional effects of symptoms. Requiring that a dimension be coded as moderate or higher on both the intensity and impairment scales would provide clinicians with a threshold for diagnostic purposes. This dual coding system allows for a more complete and disentangled assessment of an individual's psychopathology. An example of this actually appears in DSM-5 with respect to intellectual disability classification, which requires evidence of both statistically low intellectual performance and associated psychosocial impairment.

Of note, impairment thresholds could also be applied at not only the level of individual dimensions but also a global transdimensional level. Doing this would enable clinicians to evaluate how multiple dimensions interact and contribute to an individual's overall level of functioning.

What Is the Role of Factor-Based Models for Applied Clinical Assessment?

Factor-based models play a crucial role in applied clinical assessment by providing cleaner diagnostic targets that are relatively homogenous and distinctive, especially when compared to traditional psychiatric classifications. Whereas conventional diagnostic systems, such as the DSM-5, often present overlapping diagnostic categories with considerable comorbidity, factor-based models are well suited to clarifying these distinctions by identifying underlying transdiagnostic dimensions of psychopathology (Kotov et al., 2017). For instance, HiTOP is based on decades of factor-analytic evidence showing how psychiatric symptoms and features aggregate at different levels of abstraction (i.e., broad spectra down to narrow-band traits and symptom dimensions). Such a multilevel factor-based model permits clinicians to assess and intervene at the level that makes the most sense for the clients they are serving. For example, HiTOP's spectrum level might be a particularly useful assessment target if the goal is to evaluate patients for some of the newer transdiagnostic treatment approaches, such as Barlow's (2011) unified protocol, which is targeted at a wide range of psychiatric presentations that are relevant to HiTOP's internalizing spectrum. Similarly, additional adjustments to such treatments might be facilitated by assessing narrower factor-based dimensions within the HiTOP model (e.g., subfactors or narrow-band traits/symptoms).

However, factor-based models are not without limitations. They can encounter difficulties, particularly in classifying extreme base rate clinical phenomena, such as psychotic features, severe externalizing behaviors, and suicidality. These conditions might not fit neatly into the dimensional structures proposed by factor models, as their rarity or severity can lead to inconsistent findings across different studies (Krueger et al.,

2018). Consequently, the reliability of factor-based models is contingent on the robustness of the data from which they are derived. Models based on multiple samples with adequate size and diverse diagnostic representation are more likely to yield valid psychiatric dimensions, ensuring that the resulting classifications are reflective of real-world clinical phenomena rather than the result of severity-based factor-analytic results. Thus, it is important for researchers to prioritize replicability and comprehensive sampling when developing factor-based classification models.

In cases where factor-analytic studies yield contradictory structural classification evidence, human expertise and the input of expert committees become critical. Although statistical methods provide valuable insights, they cannot fully replace clinical judgment, particularly when faced with ambiguous or conflicting data. Expert committees guided by clear and open standards and procedures can synthesize findings across studies, consider the clinical relevance of different dimensions, and ultimately provide guidance on how to navigate discrepancies. For example, the HiTOP Consortium has a Revisions Workgroup, whose job it is to adjudicate the evidence needed to make changes to the official model. To that end, The Revisions Workgroup has published a clear set of procedures, rooted in open-science principles, that will be used to guide their work (Forbes et al., 2024). Such rigor is especially important when factor-analytic results are inconsistent or ambiguous.

Summary and Conclusions

Despite the challenges inherent in dimensional factor-based models of psychopathology, the process of clinical assessment should be firmly rooted in evidence-based classifications of psychopathology, which largely are dimensional in nature. By prioritizing evidence-based dimensional models, there is great potential for clinicians to enhance the accuracy and effectiveness of their assessments, leading to improved patient outcomes. Of course, the evidence for this final statement is mainly in the form of a promissory note, as much work is needed to facilitate the translation of dimensional psychopathology models into clinical practice (e.g., Ruggero et al., 2019).

PART I REFERENCES

Cooper, L. D., Balsis, S., & Zimmerman, M. (2010). Challenges associated with a polythetic diagnostic system: Criteria combinations in the personality disorders. *Journal of Abnormal Psychology, 119,* 886–895.

Gunderson, J. G., Shea, M. T., Skodol, A. E., McGlashan, T. H., Morey, L. C., Stout, R. L., . . . Keller, M. (2000). The Collaborative Longitudinal Personality Disorders Study. I: Development, aims, design, and sample characteristics. *Journal of Personality Disorders, 14,* 300–315.

Hopwood, C. J., Morey, L. C., & Markon, K. E. (2023). What is a psychopathology dimension? *Clinical Psychology Review, 106,* 102356.

Leary, T. (1957). *Interpersonal diagnosis of personality.* Ronald Press.

Loevinger, J. (1954). The attenuation paradox in test theory. *Psychological Bulletin, 51,* 493–504.

Meehl, P. E. (1957). When shall we use our heads instead of the formula? *Journal of Counseling Psychology, 4*(4), 268–273.

Morey, L. C. (1991). *The Personality Assessment Inventory: Professional manual.* Psychological Assessment Resources.

Morey, L. C. (1995). Critical issues in construct validation: Comment on Boyle and Lennon (1994). *Journal of Psychopathology & Behavioral Assessment, 17*(4), 393–401.

Morey, L. C. (2021, April). *Determining caseness in a dimensional system of psychopathology.* Paper presented at the meetings of the Hierarchical Taxonomy of Psychopathology Consortium (online).

Morey, L. C., Hopwood, C. J., Markowitz, J. C., Gunderson, J. G., Grilo, C. M., McGlashan, T. H., . . . Skodol, A. E. (2012). Comparison of alternative models for personality disorders, II: 6-, 8-, and 10-year follow-up. *Psychological Medicine,42*(8), 1705–1713.

Revelle, W. (2024). The seductive beauty of latent variable models: Or why I don't believe in the Easter Bunny. *Personality and Individual Differences, 221,* 112552.

Rosch, E. (1978). Principles of categorization. In E. Rosch & B. B. Lloyd (Eds.), *Cognition and categorization.* Erlbaum.

Schwaba, T., & Thalmayer, A. G. (2024, July 3). Openness/intellect: The weirdest trait in the Big Five world? *https://doi.org/10.31234/osf.io/wnzy4*

Skinner, H. A. (1981). Toward the integration of classification theory and methods. *Journal of Abnormal Psychology, 90,* 68–87.

Sullivan, H. S. (1953). *The interpersonal theory of psychiatry.* Norton.

PART II REFERENCES

Banerjee, P., Gibbon, S., & Huband, N. (2009). Assessment of personality disorder. *Advances in Psychiatric Treatment, 15*(5), 389–397.

Barlow, D. H., Farchione, T. J., Fairholme, C. P., Ellard, K. K., Boisseau, C. L., Allen, L. B., & Ehrenreich-May, J. (2011). *Unified protocol for transdiagnostic treatment of emotional disorders: Therapist guide.* Oxford.

Brauer, K., & Sendatzki, R. (2024). The interview as an assessment method in psychology. In C. Junker (Ed.), *Inspecting the interview: A companion* (pp. 137–160). De Gruyter.

Carlson, E. N., & Oltmanns, T. F. (2015). The role of metaperception in personality disorders: Do people with personality problems know how others experience their personality? *Journal of Personality Disorders, 29*(4), 449–467.

Clark, L. A., Watson, D., & Reynolds, S. (1995). Diagnosis and classification of psychopathology: Challenges to the current system and future directions. *Annual Review of Psychology, 46,* 121–153.

Forbes, M. K., Ringwald, W. R., Allen, T., Cicero, D. C., Clark, L., DeYoung, C. G., . . . Wright, A. G. (2024). Principles and procedures for revising the hierarchical taxonomy of psychopathology. *Journal of Psychopathology and Clinical Science, 133*(1), 4–19.

Glover, N. G., Crego, C., & Widiger, T. A. (2012). The clinical utility of the Five Factor Model of personality disorder. *Personality Disorders: Theory, Research, and Treatment, 3,* 176–184.

Hopwood, C. J., Malone, J. C., Ansell, E. B., Sanislow, C. A., Grilo, C. M., McGlashan, T. H., . . . Morey, L. C. (2011). Personality assessment in DSM-5: empirical support for rating severity, style, and traits. *Journal of Personality Disorders, 25*(3), 305–320.

Huprich, S. K., & Bornstein, R. F. (2007). An overview of issues related to categorical and dimensional models of personality disorders assessment. *Journal of Personality Assessment, 89*(1), 3–15.

Insel, T., Cuthbert, B., Garvey, M., Heinssen, R., Pine, D. S., Quinn, K., . . . Wang, P. (2010). Research domain criteria (RDoC): Toward a new classification framework for research on mental disorders. *The American Journal of Psychiatry, 167*(7), 748–751.

Kotov, R., Krueger, R. F., Watson, D., Achenbach, T. M., Althoff, R. R., Bagby, R. M., . . . Zimmerman, M. (2017). The hierarchical taxonomy of psychopathology (HiTOP): A dimensional alternative to traditional nosologies. *Journal of Abnormal Psychology, 4,* 454–477.

Krueger, R. F., Kotov, R., Watson, D., Forbes, M. K., Eaton, N. R., Ruggero, C. J., . . . Zimmermann, J. (2018). Progress in achieving quantitative classification of psychopathology. *World Psychiatry, 17*(3), 282–293.

Markon, K. E., Chmielewski, M., & Miller, C. J. (2011). The reliability and validity of discrete and continuous measures of psychopathology: A quantitative review. *Psychological Bulletin, 137*(5), 856–879.

Morey, L. C., Skodol, A. E., & Oldham, J. M. (2014). Clinician judgments of clinical utility: A comparison of DSM-IV-TR personality disorders and the alternative model for DSM-5 personality disorders. *Journal of Abnormal Psychology, 123*(2), 398–405.

Oltmanns, T. F., &Turkheimer, E. (2009). Person perception and personality pathology. *Current Directions in Psychological Science, 18,* 32–36.

Rhodes, M., & Baron, A. (2019). The development of social categorization. *Annual Review of Developmental Psychology, 1,* 359–386.

Ruggero, C. J., Kotov, R., Hopwood, C. J., First, M., Clark, L. A., Skodol, A. E., . . . Zimmerman, J. (2019). Integrating the hierarchical taxonomy of psychopathology (HiTOP) into clinical practice. *Journal of Consulting and Clinical Psychology, 87,* 1069–1084.

Stasik-O'Brien, S. M., Brock, R. L., Chmielewski, M., Naragon-Gainey, K., Koffel, E., McDade-Montez, E., . . . Watson, D. (2019). Clinical utility of the Inventory of Depression and Anxiety Symptoms (IDAS). *Assessment, 26*(5), 944–960.

Stepp, S. D., Trull, T. J., Burr, R. M., Wolfenstein, M., & Vieth, A. Z. (2005). Incremental validity of the Structured Interview for the Five-Factor Model of Personality (SIFFM). *European Journal of Personality, 19*(4), 343–357.

van Straten, A., Hill, J., Richards, D. A., &Cuijpers, P. (2015). Stepped care treatment delivery for depression: A systematic review and meta-analysis. *Psychological Medicine, 45*(2), 231–246.

CHAPTER 3

What does dimensional diagnosis mean for conceptualizing psychotherapy processes?

The disconnection between diagnosis and treatment, and in particular psychotherapy process, has long been lamented by clinicians and researchers. There is a common view that diagnosis communicates little about how to engage with clients in psychotherapy. Could dimensional models help? In this chapter, we asked experts three questions about the meaning of dimensional diagnosis for conceptualizing psychotherapy processes.

Are there associations between psychotherapy processes and dimensions of psychopathology?

How can dimensional models be used to help us understand variation in psychotherapists?

Could the transition to dimensional diagnosis open new avenues for understanding, applying, and training psychotherapy processes?

Callahan argues that dimensional models can be used to align treatment strategies with different levels and dimensions, that therapists can use the same dimensional frameworks to both diagnose their clients and think about how to match or adjust their style to their client presentations, and that a dimensional perspective fundamentally shifts training away from diagnostically targeted approaches to a focus on the whole person, including variation within diagnostic categories. Flückiger draws on recent research from his team showing that considering transdiagnostic factors such as worry can make formulation and intervention more effective and efficient, that some therapists are more able to develop an alliance with their clients than others regardless of the client's diagnosis, and that the strength-based approaches that may be encouraged by dimensional models are effective therapeutic techniques. He also provides a case example to illustrate that most assessment measures already integrate dimensional and categorical thinking, although progress in connecting these measures to diagnosis and treatment is needed. Both authors present sanguine views about the potential for dimensional models to improve conceptualizations of therapy process while also pointing to important areas of research that are needed to fulfill this potential.

PART I

Rethinking psychotherapy processes in a dimensional framework

Jennifer L. Callahan

For over a century, psychotherapy has evolved through shifting paradigms, each promising greater precision in understanding and treating mental illness. Yet, despite these advances, fundamental questions remain about whether the field has been moving toward greater clarity or merely reorganizing its assumptions. In its early days, psychotherapy was highly unstructured, with clinicians relying on trial and error to determine what worked for individual patients. Over time, recurring insights coalesced into theoretical orientations, leading to broad traditions—psychodynamic, humanistic, behavioral, and cognitive. However, instead of fostering cohesion, this systemization led to competing schools of thought, each claiming superiority, with theoretical divides running increasingly deep both within and between orientations.

By the 1950s, psychotherapy's fragmentation faced a serious challenge when Eysenck (1952) argued that treatment based on theoretical orientation was no more effective than spontaneous recovery. This critique prompted empirical research into the effectiveness of psychotherapy, culminating in meta-analyses (e.g., Smith & Glass, 1977) that reinforced what became known as the Dodo Verdict[1]—the finding that

[1]The verdict is a nod to *Alice's Adventures in Wonderland* (Carroll, 1865), where the Dodo organizes a nonsensical event called the Caucus Race. The race has no clear rules, and participants run in random directions until the Dodo arbitrarily declares it over. As there is no real winner, the Dodo announces, "Everybody has won, and all must have prizes." In psychotherapy research, this analogy captures not only the idea that no single approach consistently outperforms others but also the broader critique that psychotherapy practice, much like the Caucus Race, lacked clear rules and was arbitrarily driven by theoretical allegiance instead of empirical evidence.

most therapies produced equivalent outcomes, calling into question whether orientation-driven treatment selection was justified (Luborsky et al., 1975). At the same time, the 1950s also saw the introduction of the *Diagnostic and Statistical Manual of Mental Disorders* (DSM; American Psychiatric Association, 1952), which provided a standardized classification system for diagnosing mental disorders. As a categorical framework, DSM facilitated research comparing disorder-driven treatments and resulted in a proliferation of psychotherapy research aligned with the DSM structure. By the 1980s, DSM-III (American Psychiatric Association, 1980) introduced operationalized symptom-based criteria, further strengthening the link between categorical diagnosis and treatment selection. Coupled with the influence of Smith and Glass's (1977) meta-analysis, which heightened the focus on empirical validation, these shifts cemented a drive in psychotherapy research toward identifying treatments that could be empirically matched to specific diagnoses. By the late 1990s, this movement culminated in the empirically supported treatments (ESTs) initiative, which formally codified the idea that specific disorders required distinct interventions (Chambless et al., 1998). Across those developments, psychotherapy was guided by either allegiance to theoretical orientation or diagnostic models that categorized mental illness into discrete disorders. But what if this entire framework—this brief history of therapy—has been built on faulty assumptions about how mental health treatment works? What if we have been working within a system that obscures meaningful patterns rather than refining our understanding?

In this chapter, I argue that it is time to reconsider not just how we diagnose mental illness but also how we conceptualize psychotherapy itself. A dimensional framework offers a way forward—one that moves beyond static categories and intervention protocols. To explore this, three questions will be addressed: How do psychotherapy processes align with dimensions of psychopathology? How can dimensional models improve our understanding of therapist variability? And could shifting to dimensional diagnosis open new avenues for applying and training psychotherapy processes?

Psychotherapy Processes and Dimensions of Psychopathology

A primary advantage of dimensional case conceptualization is its emphasis on shared mechanisms across conditions. The hierarchical taxonomy of psychopathology's (HiTOP) hierarchical structure (Kotov et al., 2017) introduces a novel flexibility into therapeutic intervention, aligning closely with the established phase model of psychotherapy, which has been broadly supported by research and refined in various ways since its seminal publication (Howard et al., 1993). Essentially, successful courses of psychotherapy appear to be marked by three interconnected change processes: remoralization (improvement in hope and motivation), symptom remediation (alleviation of acute symptoms), and rehabilitation (restoration of functioning impaired by symptoms). The HiTOP's hierarchical conceptualization complements this understanding, allowing therapists to map interventions dynamically onto the patient's evolving needs across the course of psychotherapy.

When need for remoralization is evident, therapists can be directed to focus on *superspectra* involvement, with interventions directed toward instilling hope, enhancing motivation, and managing immediate distress to quickly reduce acute suffering and foster clients' belief in the possibility of improvement. For example, motivational interviewing (MI) can be used to strengthen clients' intrinsic motivation for change, whereas solution-focused brief therapy (SFBT) may highlight strengths and past successes to build hope. Hope therapy can offer structured strategies to enhance future-oriented thinking, and behavioral activation (BA) can encourage engagement in meaningful activities to improve mood and increase agency. Cognitive restructuring techniques from cognitive-behavioral therapy (CBT) can help challenge hopeless thoughts, and crisis intervention strategies such as grounding exercises and distress tolerance skills can be used to provide immediate relief. Mindfulness-based interventions, including self-compassion and breath-focused techniques, can assist in emotional regulation, and narrative therapy techniques help clients reframe their experiences in ways that emphasize resilience. Prioritizing the therapeutic alliance can foster motivation and engagement, and psychoeducation on recovery trajectories can normalize distress while reinforcing optimism about treatment outcomes.

When change processes need to focus on symptom remediation, HiTOP *spectra* can guide tailored symptom-management strategies for more flexible and effective interventions. For instance, across the internalizing spectrum are shared underlying mechanisms related to negative affect and avoidance (Forbes et al., 2016). Treatments such as cognitive restructuring, behavioral activation, and exposure therapy are widely recognized for targeting these shared dimensions. Similarly, the externalizing spectrum includes impulsivity, substance use, and aggression, which are best addressed by interventions targeting behavioral control, emotion regulation, and reinforcement strategies (Krueger et al., 2016). Dialectical behavior therapy (DBT) and contingency management, for example, can provide transdiagnostic benefits across externalizing expressions. As yet another example, the thought disorder spectrum encompasses cognitive-perceptual dysregulation, suggesting a need for psychotherapy to focus on the change processes of reality testing, social skills training, or cognitive remediation (Morrison et al., 2014).

For some patients, long-term gains are likely unsustainable without attending to maladaptive *trait-level* dimensions such as emotional dysregulation, cognitive rigidity, or maladaptive interpersonal patterns. Dialectical behavior therapy can be used to target emotional dysregulation through skills training in distress tolerance, emotion regulation, and interpersonal effectiveness. Cognitive remediation therapy (CRT) can help address cognitive rigidity by improving cognitive flexibility and problem-solving skills. Schema therapy may be useful in modifying deeply ingrained maladaptive interpersonal patterns by identifying and restructuring core beliefs developed in early life. Additionally, mentalization-based therapy (MBT) can be effective for patients with difficulties in understanding and responding to social and emotional cues, whereas acceptance and commitment therapy (ACT) can promote psychological flexibility, reducing avoidance behaviors and fostering long-term adaptation. Although not an exhaustive consideration of how changes processes can be mapped dimensionally, these examples are intended to highlight the flexibility created by a dimensional nosology in guiding intervention strategies based on shared mechanisms across conditions.

Using Dimensional Models to Understand Variation in Psychotherapists

Just as patients exhibit meaningful variability in symptom dimensions, therapists differ in their competencies, interpersonal styles, and adaptability, factors that shape treatment effectiveness in nuanced ways (Flückiger et al., 2018; Wampold, 2015). Although psychotherapy research has often treated therapist effects as relatively uniform, growing evidence suggests these differences may account for significant variance in patient outcomes, sometimes exceeding the contribution of specific treatment modalities (Wampold, 2015). Therapist variability can be explicitly mapped onto a dimensional framework, offering meaningful ways to align therapist traits with specific patient profiles. For example, therapists' interpersonal traits can reflect dimensions such as antagonism versus agreeableness or detachment versus warmth, significantly influencing their effectiveness in alliance building, intervention flexibility, and countertransference management. A dimensional conceptualization of therapist characteristics such as these holds promise for nuanced therapist–patient matching that improves patient treatment outcomes. For illustration, consider three therapist characteristics[2]—alliance-building, intervention flexibility, and countertransference management—each of which has been identified as particularly influential in shaping psychotherapy outcomes (Flückiger et al., 2018; Wampold, 2015).

First, a therapist's ability to build rapport is one of the strongest predictors of psychotherapy success, but alliance building is not a uniform skill. Some therapists naturally connect with a broad range of clients, whereas others are more effective with clients who have specific symptom profiles. Those high in warmth and agreeableness may form strong alliances with internalizing clients, whereas more assertive or structured therapists may connect better with externalizing individuals. Effective alliance building depends on the match between therapist traits and patient symptom dimensions. Second, intervention flexibility—the ability to adjust techniques based on patient needs—is another critical factor in treatment success. Therapists who are high in conscientiousness may excel with structured, protocol-driven approaches, benefiting patients with impulsivity or cognitive disorganization, whereas those high in cognitive flexibility may be better suited for complex, multidimensional cases. However, both rigid adherence to protocols and excessive flexibility can undermine effectiveness, highlighting the need for a tailored approach. Third, managing countertransference is also crucial, particularly with emotionally dysregulated patients. Therapists with greater emotional stability are better equipped to handle intense emotional reactions, whereas those prone to high negative affect may require specific training to manage therapeutic interactions effectively. Rather than suppressing emotional responses, therapists should refine their ability to regulate and use them constructively, recognizing that countertransference, like patient symptoms, exists along a continuum.

Project MATCH (1993), often cited as evidence against patient matching, highlights the limitations of categorical approaches. Its failure to identify significant patient–treatment matches stemmed from focusing solely on patient attributes while overlooking therapist characteristics such as emotional stability, conscientiousness, and interpersonal warmth. As a result, likely meaningful therapist–patient interactions were obscured. A dimensional perspective could encourage therapists to better align their trait expressions with patient needs to reduce variability in treatment outcomes across their patients. For instance, a highly

[2]Although these dimensions do not represent the full range of therapist variability, they provide a foundation for understanding how therapist factors intersect with patient needs.

conscientious and emotionally stable therapist may be particularly effective for impulsive dysregulated patients, whereas a warm and interpersonally sensitive therapist may best support socially withdrawn individuals. A dimensional matching approach leverages therapist strengths to optimize patient outcomes through more precise data-driven pairings.

New Avenues for Understanding, Applying, and Training Psychotherapy Processes

Traditional psychotherapy, typically shaped by diagnostic categories and/or a provider's theoretical orientation, limits flexibility in addressing individual patient needs. Given the significant variability in symptom presentation, it is unrealistic to assume that a therapist's orientation-driven approach will suit every patient or that those with the same diagnosis require identical treatments. For example, two patients diagnosed with posttraumatic stress disorder may exhibit vastly different dimensional profiles—one presenting with hyperarousal and externalizing behaviors such as anger and impulsivity but the other displaying emotional avoidance and internalizing traits like withdrawal and depressive symptoms. A dimensional approach goes beyond selecting the right intervention and instead requires modifying the entire therapeutic process including timing, pacing, sequencing, and therapist–patient interaction strategies. Dimensional models could refine common psychotherapy processes by improving case conceptualization, increasing intervention flexibility, and enhancing therapist decision making. To illustrate, the first patient may benefit from structured skills-based interventions that target impulse control, emotion regulation, and trauma exposure, whereas the second may require gradual relationally focused processes that emphasize emotional engagement, relief from depressive symptoms, and carefully paced trauma processing. In approaching psychotherapy in such a manner, dimensional models inherently reshape treatment priorities and session structure. A therapist using a dimensional approach must continuously assess which symptoms or traits are most pressing or most responsive to intervention at a given moment and respond accordingly. By conceptualizing psychotherapy as a fluid, evolving process, therapists can strategically sequence interventions to align with a patient's dimensional profile and treatment trajectory. This adaptive approach essentially personalizes treatment to better address the underlying barriers to treatment engagement and lasting change.

Ultimately, a process-driven approach extends beyond patient treatment and holds implications for therapist development and training, fundamentally reshaping how clinicians learn to conceptualize and implement psychotherapy processes. A dimensional framework shifts the focus toward therapist flexibility, real-time clinical decision making, and adaptive intervention delivery. It becomes more necessary to train in psychotherapy processes that develop the therapist's ability to pivot intervention strategies, even midsession, based on evolving dimensional needs. Instead of following a predetermined order of techniques, therapists must be able to determine when and how to introduce interventions (e.g., exposure techniques, cognitive restructuring, relational repair, or behavioral activation) in response to real-time assessment. Equally important is developing a therapists' skill in the pacing and titration of emotional work, ensuring that they recognize when to intensify or slow down interventions based on the patient's distress tolerance and symptom interplay. Managing countertransference also becomes central in a dimensional model, as therapists must identify and regulate their own biases and reactions toward different symptom dimensions—whether frustration with cognitive rigidity or overengagement with high emotionality.

Conclusion

Dimensional models of psychopathology fundamentally reshape psychotherapy processes at every level, from case conceptualization to intervention selection, session structure, and therapist training. They require a shift away from static category-driven treatments toward a dynamic continuously evolving approach tailored to symptom dimensions, patient engagement patterns, and therapist responsiveness. This is not merely an incremental improvement but a paradigm shift—one that fully realizes a question first posed by Gordon Paul (1967, p. 111): "What treatment, by whom, is most effective for this individual with that specific problem, and under which set of circumstances?"

Paul's question emerged in response to a crisis in psychotherapy research, as the field had become fragmented by competing theoretical orientations. His challenge was not simply to compare therapies but to move beyond orientation-driven treatment and rigorously investigate what worked for whom and under what conditions. This call for research ultimately led to the evidence-based treatment movement and the push for ESTs in the 1990s. However, in aligning itself with categorical nosology, psychotherapy research narrowed its scope, shifting from an open exploration of therapy effectiveness to a model that linked specific interventions to specific diagnoses. Although the field moved past theoretical disputes, it ultimately replaced them with a framework that treated diagnostic categories as the primary determinant of treatment selection.

More than 50 years later, it is time to revisit Paul's question. This is not to dismiss the progress that has been made but to recognize that its original intent was constrained by a diagnostic system that prioritized disorder categories over symptom dimensions. Studies that were meant to investigate the effectiveness of psychotherapy emphasized classification over individualized symptom profiles, refining treatments for disorders rather than individuals. The transition to a dimensional framework does not negate the past half-century of research. Instead, it provides an opportunity to reinterpret its findings in a way that aligns more closely with clinical reality.

In many ways, the possibilities opened by a dimensional approach are not entirely new. They reflect a return to core principles of psychotherapy. Before theoretical schools and diagnostic frameworks formalized treatment structures, psychotherapy was inherently personalized. It was built on the understanding that each patient is unique and so too must be the therapeutic process. Although fields such as precision medicine now emphasize individualized treatment as an innovation, psychotherapy has long recognized that no two patients are exactly alike. No two therapists are exactly alike either. The challenge today is not to reinvent psychotherapy. It is to modernize and formalize what has always been at the heart of its effectiveness: its ability to adapt to the individual in front of us.

PART II

Dimensional diagnoses

Bringing research and practice together

CHRISTOPH FLÜCKIGER

Since the early days of mental illness classification (Meyer, 1912), various models have focused on the psychological, biological, and social levels of analysis and have developed different types of assessment approaches that have emphasized either internal, patient-centered or external, clinician-centered variations. The HiTOP model (e.g., Kotov et al., 2017) highlights the hierarchically structured multidimensionality of mental health conditions as a possible way to account for commonalities and specificities of the psychological, biological, and social situation of each single patient. This chapter provides answers to the three questions that structure this section by briefly presenting an exemplary research example for each question and by providing a further pragmatic clinical illustration for the third question.

Are There Associations between Psychotherapy Processes and Dimensions of Psychopathology?

This question will be answered using the example of pathological worrying. In the DSM and International Classification of Diseases (ICD), pathological worrying can be seen as one of the main symptoms of generalized anxiety disorder (GAD) that distinguishes it from other anxiety disorders. In contrast, the HiTOP model highlights the potential relevance of pathological worrying as a transdiagnostic feature of a broader distress factor.

We carried out a systematic review and meta-analysis that looked at the link between worry and mental health by summarizing data from all available studies found in the literature (Vîslă et al., 2022). In the case of the DSM/ICD model, it could be hypothesized that worry and poor mental health is particularly highly correlated in GAD populations. In contrast, if the association persists across anxiety and depression samples, this would suggest a higher hierarchical level (related to the distress factor) in the HiTOP model. By analyzing data from 138 correlational samples, we found a strong link between worry and poor mental health (with a correlation coefficient of .53), although there was a lot of variation in the results. The link was not significantly different regardless of whether the studies involved people with a GAD or major depressive disorder, supporting a conception of worry as a common symptom in the distress factor. However, we also found that worry and mental health are less strongly linked in older populations, suggesting that the quality of worry changes over the life course and possibly also the threshold for perceiving "real" or pathological worry (e.g., Miloyan et al., 2014). Overall, our findings support the need to treat severe worry regardless of whether a person has been diagnosed with GAD or depression. Such a view has pragmatic clinical implications in the sense that interventions for worry could be considered as a therapeutic option not only in the treatment of GAD but also for distressed samples more generally (e.g., Baik & Newman, 2023; Flückiger et al., 2022).

To answer the above question directly, yes, in the case of worry it seems very helpful for clinicians to know that pathological worry is a distress state that can be observed and consequently treated not only in individuals suffering from GAD. One might argue that such challenges in the categorical allocation could be pragmatically managed by formulating comorbidities. However, not every distressed patient with worrying symptoms will get a full GAD diagnosis so there is a risk that the worries are not recognized as such. The main point from a clinical perspective is that the clinical nuances can be mapped more precisely in the HiTOP model, which is often not possible with the traditional dichotomous diagnoses (present/absent). Our meta-analytic data indicate that worrying related to negative mental health is present not only in GAD but also in samples with depression and other anxiety disorders.

How Can Dimensional Models Be Used to Help Us Understand Variation in Psychotherapists?

This question will be answered using the example of the alliance–outcome association. The alliance is the most studied outcome-related process characteristic worldwide (Wampold & Flückiger, 2023). As part of the American Psychological Association-Task Force "Psychotherapy

Relationships That Work" (Norcross & Lambert, 2018), we conducted a comprehensive systematic search and meta-analysis integrating 300 empirical manuscripts investigating about 30,000 psychotherapies, with the majority of studies (80%) being conducted in North America (Flückiger et al., 2018). Overall, there is a moderate predictive correlation of 8% explained variance (r = .28; confidence interval .26 ≤ r ≤ .23) between the alliance measured mostly once during therapy and the therapy outcome (at the end of therapy). Strong therapist effects were found; that is, in general there are therapists that have therapeutic skills to build better alliances with a variety of patients in comparison to others and this variation in therapists predicts psychotherapy outcomes (Del Re et al., 2021).

Further moderator analyses also indicated comparable alliance–outcome correlations across mental disorders, except for substance use samples that indicated slightly lower associations (r = .18; Flückiger et al., 2013, 2018). Interestingly, the very same samples of substance use disorders (SUDs) also indicated a much higher percentage of ethnic minorities. Particularly, there was a very high rate of Black participants in the SUD samples (r = .86). This confounder was unexpected, as in the general population there is not a general tendency for ethnic minorities and Black people in particular to show substantially higher prevalence for SUD. Overall, the present results exemplify the complexity and multidimensionality of psychotherapeutic diagnostics, processes, and outcomes. In the present case, without simultaneous consideration of both aspects (i.e., SUD or ethnic minority status and in combination with further potential moderators), the interpretation of each aspect would likely lead in very different directions.

To answer the question posed above directly, yes, in the case of alliance some psychotherapists are able to build better alliances across many (complex) mental health conditions than others. A balanced multidimensional understanding of mental illness may help therapists develop an individualized understanding of each patient and engage in collaborative therapeutic qualities. The example of the substance abuse and ethnic minorities subfactor impressively underlines the importance of a multifaceted effort to understand mental health conditions. An overly simplified and decontextualized understanding of disorder-specific interpretations would support stereotypical interpretations. Multidimensional models may help to get a differentiated understanding of each patient that covers a comprehensive analysis of the patient's psychosocial participation and integrates further aspects such as the existing abilities, skills, individual dispositions, preferences, social support, and therapy goals of the individual patient and their environment.

Could the Transition to Dimensional Diagnosis Open New Avenues for Understanding, Applying, and Training Psychotherapy Processes?

This question will be answered using the example of strength-based methods (SBMs), a superordinate term that covers approaches such as strength-based, resilience-oriented, and positive interventions in psychotherapy. In psychotherapy, SBMs focus not only on compensating negative mental states but also on capitalizing on an individual's strengths to promote positive mental health and using it for therapeutic progress. The World Health Organization (2022) defines mental health as "a state of mental well-being that enables people to cope with the stresses of life, realize their abilities, learn well and work well, and contribute to their community." Positive mental health includes, for example, (1) how satisfied someone is with their life, how much joy they feel, and the positive emotions they experience daily; (2) accepting oneself, growing personally, and finding meaning in life; and (3) being part of social networks and having fulfilling relationships (Iasiello et al., 2022; Schürmann et al., 2023). From this point of view, dimensional models are focused not only on understanding the negative aspects of mental health but also on obtaining a differentiated assessment of the positive poles of mental health, bearing in mind that traditionally, there is a natural interest in the negative poles of mental health in clinical contexts.

There is initial empirical evidence that working with SBM contributes to the effectiveness of psychotherapy. As part of the American Psychological Association Task Force "Skills and Methods" (Hill & Norcross, 2023), we executed a systematic review and narrative synthesis encompassing eight studies that evaluated SBMs during psychotherapy sessions and their immediate effects on treatment outcomes (Flückiger et al., 2023). Additionally, we performed a systematic review and a multilevel comparative meta-analysis to contrast strength-based bona fide psychotherapy with other forms of bona fide psychotherapy in posttreatment scenarios, analyzing 57 effect sizes derived from nine studies. The findings revealed that despite varied methodological approaches, the pattern observed in the process–outcome studies consistently indicated that SBM was correlated with therapy success at the session level. The comparative meta-analysis yielded a weighted mean overall effect size of $g = 0.17$ (confidence interval: $0.03 \leq g \leq 0.31$), suggesting a small yet statistically significant benefit of strength-based psychotherapies. The heterogeneity of the effect sizes was found to be nonsignificant, indicating reasonable consistency across studies. These results underscore that SBMs are not merely a coincidental aspect of treatment advancement but rather may play a distinct and beneficial role in enhancing psychotherapy outcomes (Flückiger et al., 2023). Dimensional models, which capture client weaknesses and strengths, therefore may allow for a diagnostic system that encourages clinicians to incorporate SBMs in treatment planning.

Clinical Illustration

Figure 3.1 illustrates the clinical potential of dimensional models using a common output of the Symptom Checklist 90 (Derogatis et al., 1999), one of the most commonly used clinical self-reports to assess mental health concerns. Even though clinical questionnaires usually refer to more traditional psychopathological categories (such as the Symptom Checklist 90), they assess these qualities in a differentiated dimensional way (also see Flückiger et al., 2016). It is not uncommon to use cutoff values in clinical self-reports to validate observer-based diagnoses. Whereas this is an applaudable step to integrate patient perspectives into clinical assessments, such an interpretation strategy would not use the full potential of a well-constructed dimensional self-report. In Figure 3.1, the patient reached the cutoff values for depression and paranoid ideation. The experienced clinician's diagnostic judgment that the patient was suffering from depressive symptoms was confirmed. In addition, the clinician could not recognize any paranoid symptoms. However, this potential discrepancy did not particularly worry the clinician, as the items capture inner strangeness. The patient confirmed that she attributed the strangeness to the fact that it was the first time in her life that she had experienced such strong feelings and that these feelings seemed quite strange and unfamiliar to her. The patient commented that it was rather relieving and reassuring to know that these feelings were not as familiar to her as they were to her friend, who had been experiencing periods of severe depressive stages for years.

One of the most astonishing statements, however, was that the patient reported that she no longer went outside so much and was withdrawing at home. Looking at the anxiety scale, she does not actually feel like an anxious person and enjoys meeting her best friends, especially Muriel. Even though the therapist did not respond much to this during the session, she was appropriately surprised that the patient reported three sessions later that she had now met Muriel again for the first time in 6 months and that the meeting had made her extremely happy. She spoke enthusiastically about the evening. Such sudden gains often experienced early in therapy are a common and well-documented phenomenon in distressed patients (Shalom & Aderka, 2020). This brief clinical

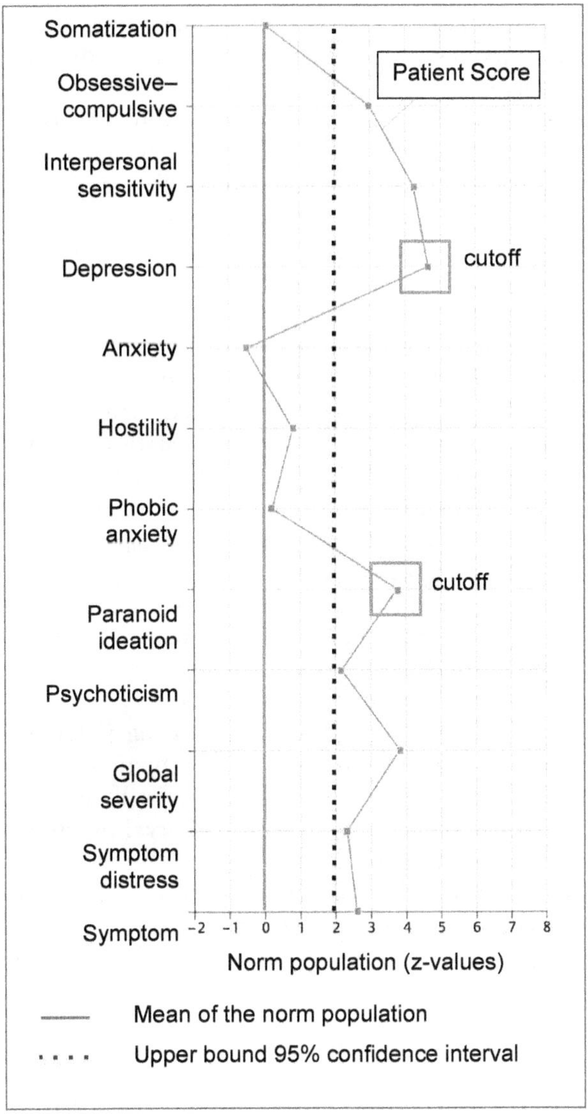

FIGURE 3.1. Interpretation of the Symptom Checklist 90 as dimensional versus categorical information.

example illustrates that a collaborative understanding of dimensional questionnaires provides excellent opportunities to gain a nuanced clinical understanding of a patient's case.

To answer the question posed above directly, yes, the transition to dimensional assessment of mental health opens new avenues and has the potential to bring together and systematize different diagnostic traditions. Whereas psychological questionnaires are usually constructed to assess a dimensional understanding of a particular psychological concepts, existing classification systems attempt to formulate clear criteria for distinguishing clinical from subclinical and nonclinical populations. These hard criteria are often relevant to the extent to which psychotherapy is or is not funded by health insurers in many European countries, for example. From this perspective, there is self-evident interest to create clear, simple, and easily communicable classification systems that define a mental disorder with "disease value." This external communication often runs counter to a differentiated clinical perspective during treatment. Overall, dimensional models meet the desire of many clinicians for differentiated clinical assessments.

It is a common standard in psychological assessments to elaborate multiple dimensional constructs simultaneously. Furthermore, there is a long tradition in psychotherapy research of capturing the individual psychology of a person in a very differentiated way. This can involve the use of various assessments, including integrating judgments of closely related persons of the patient that refer to both clinical and nonclinical concepts. Psychotherapy diagnostics are (and should be) not independent of the common standards of assessment in general psychology, ensuring that broad and careful psychodiagnostics are conducted. The transformation process to bring dimensional models into clinical classification systems is not yet complete and demands openness and innovation in the future.

PART I REFERENCES

American Psychiatric Association. (1952). *Diagnostic and statistical manual of mental disorders*. Author.

American Psychiatric Association. (1980). *Diagnostic and statistical manual of mental disorders* (3rd ed.). Author.

Carroll, L. (1865). *Alice's adventures in wonderland*. Macmillan.

Chambless, D. L., Baker, M. J., Baucom, D. H., Beutler, L., Calhoun, K. S., Crits-Christoph, P., . . . Woody, S. R. (1998). Update on empirically validated therapies, II. *The Clinical Psychologist, 51*(1), 3–16.

Eysenck, H. J. (1952). The effects of psychotherapy: An evaluation. *Journal of Consulting Psychology, 16*(5), 319–324.

Flückiger, C., Del Re, A. C., Wampold, B. E., & Horvath, A. O. (2018). The alliance in adult psychotherapy: A meta-analytic synthesis. *Psychotherapy, 55*(4), 316–340.

Forbes, M. K., Tackett, J. L., Markon, K. E., & Krueger, R. F. (2016). Beyond comorbidity: Toward a dimensional and hierarchical approach to understanding psychopathology across the life span. *Development and Psychopathology, 28*(4, pt. 1), 971–986.

Howard, K. I., Lueger, R. J., Maling, M. S., & Martinovich, Z. (1993). A phase model of psychotherapy outcome: Causal mediation of change. *Journal of Consulting and Clinical Psychology, 61*(4), 678–685.

Kotov, R., Krueger, R. F., Watson, D., Achenbach, T. M., Althoff, R. R., Bagby, R. M., . . . Zimmerman, M. (2017). The hierarchical taxonomy of psychopathology (HiTOP): A dimensional alternative to traditional nosologies. *Journal of Abnormal Psychology, 126*(4), 454–477.

Krueger, R. F., Markon, K. E., Patrick, C. J., & Iacono, W. G. (2016). Externalizing psychopathology in adulthood: A dimensional-spectrum conceptualization and its implications for DSM-V. *Journal of Abnormal Psychology, 114*(4), 537–550.

Luborsky, L., Singer, B., & Luborsky, L. (1975). Comparative studies of psychotherapies: Is it true that "everybody has won and all must have prizes"*Archives of General Psychiatry, 32*(8), 995–1008.

Morrison, A. P., Turkington, D., Pyle, M., Spencer, H., Brabban, A., Dunn, G., . . . Hutton, P. (2014). Cognitive therapy for people with schizophrenia spectrum disorders not taking antipsychotic drugs: A single-blind randomised controlled trial. *The Lancet, 383*(9926), 1395–1403.

Paul, G. L. (1967). Strategy of outcome research in psychotherapy. *Journal of Consulting Psychology, 31*(2), 109–118.

Project MATCH Research Group. (1993). Project MATCH: Rationale and methods for a multisite clinical trial matching patients to alcoholism treatment. *Alcoholism: Clinical and Experimental Research, 17*(6), 1130–1145.

Smith, M. L., & Glass, G. V. (1977). Meta-analysis of psychotherapy outcome studies. *American Psychologist, 32*(9), 752–760.

Wampold, B. E. (2015). How important are the common factors in psychotherapy? An update. *World Psychiatry, 14*(3), 270–277.

PART II REFERENCES

Baik, S. Y., & Newman, M. G. (2023). The transdiagnostic use of worry and rumination to avoid negative emotional contrasts following negative events: A momentary assessment study. *Journal of Anxiety Disorders, 95*, 102679.

Del Re, A. C., Flückiger, C., Horvath, A. O., & Wampold, B. E. (2021). Examining therapist effects in the alliance–outcome relationship: A multilevel meta-analysis. *Journal of Consulting and Clinical Psychology, 89*(5), 371–378.

Derogatis, L. R., & Savitz, K. L. (1999). The SCL-90-R, Brief Symptom

Inventory, and matching clinical rating scales. In M. E. Maruish (Ed.), *The use of psychological testing for treatment planning and outcomes assessment* (2nd ed., pp. 679–724). Erlbaum.

Flückiger, C., Carratta, K., Del Re, A. C., Probst, G., Vîslă, A., Gómez Penedo, J. M., & Wampold, B. E. (2022). The relative efficacy of bona fide cognitive behavioral therapy and applied relaxation for generalized anxiety disorder at follow-up: A longitudinal multilevel meta-analysis. *Journal of Consulting and Clinical Psychology, 90*(4), 339–352.

Flückiger, C., Del Re, A. C., Horvath, A. O., Symonds, D., Ackert, M., & Wampold, B. E. (2013). Substance use disorders and racial/ethnic minorities matter: A meta-analytic examination of the relation between alliance and outcome. *Journal of Counseling Psychology, 60*(4), 610–616.

Flückiger, C., Del Re, A. C., Wampold, B. E., & Horvath, A. O. (2018). The alliance in adult psychotherapy: A meta-analytic synthesis. *Psychotherapy, 55*(4), 316–340.

Flückiger, C., Munder, T., Del Re, A. C., & Solomonov, N. (2023). Strength-based methods: A narrative review and comparative multilevel meta-analysis of positive interventions in clinical settings. *Psychotherapy Research, 33*(7), 856–872.

Flückiger, C., Znoj, H., & Vîslă, A. (2016). Detecting information processing bias toward psychopathology: Interpreting Likert scales at intake assessment. *Psychotherapy, 53*(3), 284–290.

Hill, C. E., & Norcross, J. C. (2023). Research evidence on psychotherapist skills and methods: Foreword and afterword. *Psychotherapy Research, 33*(7), 821–840.

Iasiello, M., Van Agteren, J., Schotanus-Dijkstra, M., Lo, L., Fassnacht, D. B., & Westerhof, G. J. (2022). Assessing mental wellbeing using the Mental Health Continuum—Short Form: A systematic review and meta-analytic structural equation modelling. *Clinical Psychology: Science and Practice, 29*(4), 442–456.

Kotov, R., Krueger, R. F., Watson, D., Achenbach, T. M., Althoff, R. R., Bagby, R. M., . . . Zimmerman, M. (2017). The hierarchical taxonomy of psychopathology (HiTOP): A dimensional alternative to traditional nosologies. *Journal of Abnormal Psychology, 126*(4), 454–477.

Meyer, A. (1912). General reviews and summaries pathopsychology and psychopathology. *Psychological Bulletin, 9*(4), 129–145.

Miloyan, B., Byrne, G. J., & Pachana, N. A. (2014). Age-related changes in generalized anxiety disorder symptoms. *International Psychogeriatrics, 26*(4), 565–572.

Norcross, J. C., & Lambert, M. J. (2018). Psychotherapy relationships that work III. *Psychotherapy, 55*(4), 303–315.

Schürmann-Vengels, J., Troche, S., Victor, P. P., Teismann, T., & Willutzki, U. (2023). Multidimensional assessment of strengths and their association with mental health in psychotherapy patients at the beginning of treatment. *Clinical Psychology in Europe, 5*(2), e8041.

Shalom, J. G., & Aderka, I. M. (2020). A meta-analysis of sudden gains in psychotherapy: Outcome and moderators. *Clinical Psychology Review, 76*, Article 101827.

Vîslă, A., Stadelmann, C., Watkins, E., Zinbarg, R. E., & Flückiger, C. (2022). The relation between worry and mental health in nonclinical population and individuals with anxiety and depressive disorders: A meta-analysis. *Cognitive Therapy and Research, 46*(3), 480–501.

Wampold, B. E., & Flückiger, C. (2023). The alliance in mental health care: Conceptualization, evidence and clinical applications. *World Psychiatry, 22*(1), 25–41.

World Health Association. (2022). *Fact sheet: Mental health.* Retrieved from *https://url43.mailanyone.net/scanner?m=1vFBfT-000000006vw-2FJI&d=4%7Cmail%2F90%2F1762003200%2F1vFBfT-000000006vw-2FJI%7Cin43g%7C57e1b682%7C21691412%7C8436362%7C69060B2FE9828FB9F026CD9D26EDC38D&o=%2Fphtw%3A%2Fwtsnhw.%2F.itwotlheph-oatt%2Ficlenasm%23a-hathtel1_bat%3Db&s=IOeQ8Ma74gJJXJFq1gJyBge9BKM*

CHAPTER 4

What does dimensional diagnosis mean for conceptualizing psychotherapy technique?

A shift toward dimensional diagnosis portends a fundamental change in the way psychotherapy technique is conceived. Rather than interventions designed to target specific disorders, interventions would need to be organized around dimensions. This could confer certain opportunities: For instance, just as mental health problems can be organized hierarchically such that broad dimensions can be parsed into narrower ones, specific psychotherapy techniques also cluster into broader classes of intervention. However, psychotherapy researchers and practitioners have built an entire infrastructure around categorical diagnostic approaches, and thus this shift also foretells difficult practical and cultural challenges. In this section, we asked experts to answer three questions about the implications of dimensional diagnosis for psychotherapy technique:

Given that psychotherapy technique is currently organized largely around specific disorders, how does the transition to dimensional diagnosis affect the way we think about therapy technique?

How can the transition to dimensional diagnosis promote and support integrative models of psychotherapy technique?

How does dimensional diagnosis fit with the way clinicians already practice?

Sauer-Zavala et al. come from a perspective that integrates cognitive-behavioral and trait-based approaches. They are relatively hopeful about the opportunities for integration to make treatment more parsimonious, personalizable, and potent. Although they recognize some practical challenges, they also emphasize that many psychotherapists often think dimensionally despite the categorical diagnostic scheme and for this reason are optimistic that the transition might be easier than it may seem. Hörz-Sagstetter and Kampe highlight that the psychodynamic perspective from which they come has been dimensional all along. They concentrate on personality functioning, a fundamental psychodynamic construct that defines modern conceptions of personality disorder, and demonstrate via two cases its importance for tailoring treatments.

PART I

Targeting higher-order dimensions of personality

A potent, parsimonious, and personalizable approach to addressing psychopathology

SHANNON SAUER-ZAVALA, MADELINE L. KUSHNER, ALEXANDRA HINES, and SARAH E. CECIL

Many have articulated how a shift to a dimensional system of classification will result in a more valid understanding of psychopathology relative to categorical approaches (e.g., *Diagnostic and Statistical Manual of Mental Disorder, Fifth Edition, Text Revision* [DSM-5-TR; American Psychiatric Association, 2022]; Andrews, 1996; Blashfield et al., 2014). Such a shift also has the potential to significantly streamline treatment for mental health conditions. In the prevailing system, patients are assigned categorical diagnoses and treated with the associated protocol(s), creating a large training burden for clinicians who must learn numerous discrete interventions to provide empirically supported care (McHugh et al., 2009). Additionally, most patients do not fit neatly within these diagnostic categories (i.e., subthreshold symptoms, comorbidity; Bosman et al., 2019), suggesting that our disorder-specific approach to treatment does not align with real-world clinical presentations. Dimensional models of psychopathology with higher-order elements that can account for comorbidity among conditions and point to a limited number of treatment targets can address these barriers to widespread dissemination of research-supported mental health care.

Proposals for Incorporating Personality into Psychotherapy

For a dimensional diagnostic system to be widely adopted by the field, its translation to clinical practice must be clear. Several groups (e.g.,

Mullins-Sweatt et al., 2020; Ruggero et al., 2019) have made recommendations for how the information gleaned from dimensional models can be used by clinicians, although uptake may be limited for several reasons. First, most of the treatment recommendations that are based on higher-order dimensions (spectra, personality traits) match each trait (e.g., antagonism) to existing interventions (e.g., interpersonal effectiveness in dialectical behavior therapy); however, there is limited empirical support that the existing tools actually affect personality. Second, most of the proposals for how to integrate dimensional classification in the therapy have been limited to personality disorders (i.e., Hopwood, 2018; Mullin-Sweatt et al., 2020), with limited relevance for more prevalent conditions that are also clearly mediated by higher-order temperamental domains (e.g., emotional disorders). Finally, when more comprehensive recommendations that apply to a broader range of psychopathology have been forwarded (i.e., Bach & Presnall-Shvorin, 2020), treatment recommendations are made at the facet level (Hagerty, 2023; Ruggero et al., 2019). Given that each of the five broad domains of personality is composed of six facets (e.g., neuroticism is composed of anxiety, depression, anger, self-consciousness, impulsiveness, and vulnerability), this approach would yield 30 distinct treatment approaches. Although this number of interventions is far fewer than the number of protocols required to address each DSM diagnosis, it may still result in significant therapist burden (i.e., time and costs associated with learning a large number of treatments). Additionally, it is not clear that the facets organized beneath a broad personality domain are functionally distinct, warranting discrete treatment approaches.

A Dimensional Personality-Based *Treatment* ***System***

A dimensional system of *treatment* that focuses on the domain or spectra level (i.e., higher-order personality traits) has the potential to result in parsimonious, potent, and personalizable care. Although personality traits have historically been thought to remain stable across the lifespan (Roberts & DelVecchio, 2000; Soto et al., 2011), emerging evidence suggests that improvements in the five-factor model (FFM) domains occur naturalistically and more quickly in the context of psychological treatment (Roberts et al., 2017; Bleidorn et al., 2022). Moreover, when personality traits are directly targeted (e.g., Sauer-Zavala, Southward, Fruhbauerova, et al., 2023; Hudson et al., 2019; Magidson et al., 2014) improvements on these domains are more robust relative to when treatment is focused at the symptom level (Sauer-Zavala et al., 2021).

Personality-Based Treatment Is More Parsimonious

As noted previously, the disorder-specific approach to treatment, exemplified by the DSM system, results in approximately 50 separate treatments that correspond to each diagnostic category. Additionally, single-disorder protocols do not adequately address comorbid conditions and create a costly training burden for clinicians (McHugh & Barlow, 2010) In contrast, targeting higher-order FFM dimensions that account for symptoms of various disorders has the potential to parsimoniously lead to simultaneous symptom improvement across a range of conditions. For example, neuroticism-focused treatment (Barlow et al., 2018) is associated with significant improvements in anxiety, depressive, obsessive–compulsive, trauma and stressor-related, and eating disorders (Cassiello-Robbins et al., 2020; Sakiris & Berle, 2019) and is adept at addressing comorbidity among them (Steele et al., 2018). Extending these findings to the remaining FFM domains, a clinician may need to be proficient in only up to five personality-based approaches to competently address the broad range of commonly presenting psychological conditions.

Personality-Based Treatment Is Personalizable

An intervention system based on the higher-order domains of the FFM also has the potential to be easily tailored according to each patient's deficits. Dimensional personality profiles can be created for each patient and used to select the personality-based modules corresponding to the specific mechanisms that maintain symptoms for that patient (Samuel & Widiger, 2006; Sauer-Zavala et al., 2002; Sauer-Zavala et al., 2022). For example, borderline personality disorder (BPD) is located on multiple FFM domains (Neuroticism, Agreeableness, Conscientiousness; Ball et al., 1997; Costa & McCrae, 1990); however, due to heterogeneity in this condition, not all patients with BPD will display maladaptive levels of all three FFM domains (Sauer-Zavala, Southward, Fruhbauerova, et al., 2023). Thus, different combinations of personality-based treatment modules would be warranted. For example, BPD compass, a personality-focused intervention, was designed to be modular such that skills for neuroticism, antagonism, and disinhibition could be presented in isolation (Sauer-Zavala, Southward, Fruhbauerova, et al., 2023); thus, a patient with elevated neuroticism would receive only the module corresponding to that trait, whereas someone with difficulties in all three BPD-relevant traits would receive the full treatment package. Additionally, because comorbid disorders in the same FFM domain can be considered manifestations of shared underlying mechanisms rather than discrete categorical phenomena, (Brown & Barlow, 2018) an intervention system based on the FFM can also be used to develop personalized treatments for patients with co-occurring conditions.

Personality-Based Treatment Is More Potent

Treatment targeting the mechanisms that maintain symptoms should result in more precise, and therefore potent, care (Kazdin, 2006, 2009). For example, a patient who engages in substance use may do so because they want to dampen strong negative emotions (i.e., high neuroticism) or because they are seeking the rewarding sensations that substances produce regardless of consequences (i.e., low conscientiousness). A one-size-fits-all treatment for substance use disorder may not adequately address these different processes maintaining a particular patient's symptoms. Moreover, when a patient's range of difficulties are explained by more than one personality-based mechanism, an intervention system with modules for each FFM domain may represent a potent and parsimonious approach because modular treatments demonstrate improved efficiency relative to traditional care (Weisz, 2012).

Translation to Practice

If the field shifts from using categorical systems of classification to one of the proposed dimensional approaches, it is important to consider how the day-to-day practice of therapists will be affected. Currently, for many practitioners the provision of a yes/no diagnosis is necessary for insurance reimbursement (at least in the United States). For therapists to accept a new system, the process for how dimensional ratings translate to being reimbursed for services will need to be clearly articulated. Beyond this bureaucratic aspect of psychotherapy, understanding and treating clients based on core processes that underlie symptoms is probably more in line with how most therapists practice relative to "treating a DSM diagnosis." As noted previously, clinicians in routine practice are less likely to use empirically supported protocols that have been proven efficacious in clinical trials. However, many therapists do subscribe to evidence-based practice—that is, applying transdiagnostic therapeutic elements (e.g., cognitive restructuring, values identification, assertiveness training) to a range of patient difficulties rather than following a diagnosis-specific protocol. Thus, pulling from a limited number of treatment modules (tied to higher-order dimensions of personality) that can be applied broadly to a range of symptoms is largely consistent with the evidence-based practice approach. If anything, a personality-based model of classification may assist with conceptualization and strategy selection. For therapists who provide more supportive care due to well-documented barriers to uptake for empirically supported/evidence-based practice, reducing the training burden to five personality-based treatment modules may improve the likelihood that research-supported therapeutic strategies are adopted.

Conclusions

For a transition to dimensional classification to be accepted by clinicians, it must improve care for people experiencing mental health difficulties. By focusing on the higher-order elements included in proposed dimensional models, clinicians need learn only five or six personality-focused treatment modules, significantly streamlining care. Moreover, by personalizing the modules each patient receives based on the higher-order factors maintaining their symptoms, treatment may be more potent (targeting idiographic maintaining factors) and parsimonious (clients get the skills they need, without extra elements).

PART II

Addressing basic dimensions of personality functioning

A classic yet contemporary conceptualization of personality pathology

SUSANNE HÖRZ-SAGSTETTER and LEONIE KAMPE

Dimensional models of personality functioning have been a central concept for understanding and treating personality disorders in psychodynamic conceptualization for many years (e.g., Fonagy & Bateman, 2006; Kernberg, 1984). With the more recent introduction of the alternative model of personality disorders (AMPD) in DSM-5 (American Psychiatric Association, 2013) and its adaptation to ICD-11 (World Health Association, 2019; Tyrer et al., 2011), functional impairments in core dimensions of personality have become the focus of diagnosing personality disorders and a central target for goals and techniques in psychotherapy. Thereby, therapeutic approaches not only seek to improve personality functioning and personality traits but also rely on these dimensional approaches for tailoring specific strategies and techniques. In this chapter, a brief overview of classic and contemporary dimensional models of personality impairments is given before describing how therapeutic approaches can address functional deficits.

Dimensional Psychodynamic Models of Personality Functioning

With the recent changes in DSM-5 and ICD-11 diagnostic models for personality pathology, a dimensional approach to underlying impairments in functioning has been introduced in the international classification systems to replace current categorical symptom-based models. In criterion A of the AMPD, these dimensions are divided into aspects of the self (dimensions identity and self-direction) and interpersonal relatedness (dimensions empathy and intimacy; Bender et al., 2011). Empirically based moderate impairment across these dimensions of functioning is the main criterion for diagnosing personality disorders. In addition to this dimension of severity, Criterion B of the DSM-5 alternative model assesses a set of traits that describe the types of problems presented (American Psychiatric Association, 2013). Also, in ICD-11 (World Health Organization, 2019), intrapersonal and interpersonal functioning has been included as the main criterion to assess severity of personality disorder pathology. This diagnostic perspective provides the ability to diagnose each person's specific personality problems, and it also assesses a dimension of severity for subthreshold personality pathology (Blüml & Doering, 2021) that is useful for clinicians (Sharp & Wall, 2021). This new approach not only improves known shortcomings of the prevailing categorical approach but also provides useful therapeutic implications for clinical practice (Bach & Simonsen, 2021).

This perspective has a long tradition in psychodynamic thinking (Hörz-Sagstetter et al., 2021). Already in the early model of personality organization (Kernberg, 1967), the diagnosis of underlying pathology has been a central source for understanding, diagnosing, and treating personality disorders. Stemming from psychoanalytic theory, the model diagnoses impairment in the dimensions of identity, primitive defense mechanisms, and capacity for reality testing (Kernberg, 1981). Borderline personality organization is characterized by severe identity diffusion, the use of mainly primitive defenses (meaning splitting-based, interpersonal, and projective automatic processes for regulating emotional distress), and varying deficits in the ability for reality testing. This definition of functional impairment defines our understanding of personality disorders and has been trailblazing for specific psychotherapeutic strategies and techniques (Kernberg, 1984).

Later psychodynamic approaches, such as the operationalized psychodynamic diagnostic system (OPD Task Force, 2008), also offer a dimensional model for assessing impairments in personality functioning, developing treatment plans, and evaluating changes. In this model, which empirically has been shown to go beyond the assessment of symptoms (Vierl et al., 2024), the level of personality structure is conceptualized as the availability of basic psychological functions. Four structural dimensions are described (i.e., perception, regulation, communication, and attachment), each of which consists of a self-related and an object-related subdimension. The diagnostic approaches from the OPD-system and the Level of Personality Functioning Scale (LPFS) from the DSM-5 alternative model also converge empirically (Zimmermann et al., 2013).

Studies have shown that the dimensional approach to personality impairment has specific therapeutic implications (Bach & Simonsen, 2021; Hörz-Sagstetter et al., 2021). These concern not only the goals of psychotherapy but also tangible strategies and techniques, which will be introduced next.

Goals and Mechanisms of Change in Treating Impairments in Personality Functioning

Less impairment in personality functioning is a core predictor for psychoemotional stability, social-economic integration and success, and overall life satisfaction (Kocjan et al., 2021; Waszczuk et al., 2022). The construct of personality functioning is perceived as a clinically helpful perspective for the assessment of severity of pathology that goes beyond symptom-oriented diagnoses not only in patients with personality disorders but also in those who are members of other clinical groups (Bach & Tracy, 2022; Wendt et al., 2024). For patients with personality disorders, it is known that more functional impairments are associated with more comorbidities, overall symptoms, and subjective experience of distress (Clark et al., 2018; Rentrop et al., 2014) and are also associated with poorer treatment outcomes (Koelen et al., 2012). Impairment in personality functioning implies lower abilities to regulate internal processes, drives, and emotions as well as relationships, conflicts, attachment, and empathic relatedness (Biberdzic et al., 2024; Hörz et al., 2009; Ohse et al., 2024). It is therefore a central target in psychotherapy to address functional deficits and tailor specific treatments that seek to help personality improvement and to make this a central outcome criterion. To date, many studies have shown that after specific treatment, not only the symptoms but also the level of functioning significantly improve (Clarkin et al., 2007, 2018; Diamond et al., 2014, 2023; Huber et al., 2013; Levy et al., 2006).

Furthermore, specific dimensions of functioning like defense mechanisms have demonstrated incremental value related to specific difficulties of personality disorders (Kampe et al., 2018; Ohse et al., 2024). The dimensional diagnostic approach offers a distinct picture of areas of impairment as well as psychological resources, yielding an individual diagnostic profile: Whereas one patient with overall moderate impairment can be relatively functional in interpersonal relationships but struggling with controlling impulses, goals, and directions, another patient at the same level of impairment can show little impairment of self-direction but significant problems in leading empathic and intimate relationships. With a dimensional diagnostic approach, specific areas of impairment can quickly be identified and become the individualized goal of a patient's custom-made therapy. Techniques are based on these broader dimensions of functioning, in particular interpersonal functioning, instead of on working on symptoms or traits (Hutsebaut, 2023).

Dimensional Treatment Techniques Addressing Impairments of Personality Functioning

Focusing on specific impairments of personality dimensions means moving beyond categorical disorders. Several treatment approaches stemming from the psychodynamic tradition have developed manuals that focus not only on specific disorders but also impairments of personality functioning. Transference-focused psychotherapy (TFP) was originally developed for the treatment of borderline personality disorder (Clarkin et al., 1999), but in its further evolution it has been applied to a larger patient population, and in its current manual, it generally targets treating self and interpersonal functioning, represented in the entry criteria of both the DSM-5 and ICD-11 systems (Caligor et al., 2018; Clarkin et al., 2021). Specific treatment techniques are directed at impairments in self-functioning; for example, a focus on identity pathology is set by clarifying and integrating additional aspects of a patient's self-image to improve an impoverished sense of self. As an example of treating difficulties of interpersonal functioning, a TFP therapist will focus on the extreme and/or distorted mental representations of others that often lead to relationship conflicts and breakdowns. The techniques applied are repeated clarification of these internalized relationship patterns, asking for other aspects of the objects and, consequently, gradually obtaining more diverse and integrated representations of others. The personality dimensions on which the framework of TFP is based are empirically closely associated with the LPFS of the DSM-5 AMPD (Kampe et al., 2018) and can therefore also be used to study changes in personality functioning.

Other psychodynamic approaches like mentalization-based therapy (MBT; Bateman & Fonagy, 2004; Bateman et al., 2023) also use a transdiagnostic and dimensional approach to improve impairments in personality functioning. Here, a focus is set on impairments of mentalization that subserve self- and interpersonal functioning and therefore might moderate treatment outcome (Luyten et al., 2024). The ability to mentalize is a concept akin to the empathy dimension of the DSM-5 AMPD; thus, a focus on this aspect of personality functioning is expected to improve impairments of personality functioning.

Clinical Application: Case Examples[1]

To illustrate the development of treatment strategies based on the dimensional diagnostic assessment, two case examples from the validation study of the German Structured Clinical Interview of SCID-5-AMPD-I will be described (Ohse et al., 2022). The SCID-5-AMPD-I (Bender et al., 2018; German version: Hörz-Sagstetter et al., 2025) assesses personality functioning by examining the four AMPD domains (identity, self-direction, empathy, intimacy), each based on three subdomains, on a scale ranging from 0 (*no impairment*) to 4 (*extreme impairment*) (cf. Figure 4.1). In Case Example 1, a patient with moderate to severe impairment is presented. The overall level of functioning was rated at moderate to severe impairment (score of 2 or 3); the dimensional diagnostic approach reveals distinct areas of functional impairment (Figure 4.1).

The diagnostic interview, conducted with the SCID-5-AMPD-I (Bender et al., 2018), revealed areas of moderate and severe impairment. In the identity section, the patient presents an overall weak sense of autonomy and inner emptiness. Their definition of inner and interpersonal boundaries is overall weak; they tend to overidentify with others while fluctuating between overidentifying and pushing other people away for independence. Their self-worth is easily influenced and destabilized by events or other people, and their self-evaluation may oscillate between unrealistic forms of self-aggrandizement and severe self-contempt or extreme self-devaluation and hatred. In terms of interpersonal functioning, the patient shows severe impairment in their capacities for empathy, especially in understanding and recognizing the experience and motives of other people. Areas of self-direction and closeness to other people also show impairment: Emotion regulation depends on positive evaluation by others, and threats to self-esteem can trigger strong negative emotions such as anger and shame. Close relationships are sought to satisfy needs for appraisal and self-regulation, and they have an unrealistic expectation of being perfectly understood by others.

This diagnostic approach is highly informative for treatment planning: First, as described by Bach and Simonsen (2021), severe impairment hints toward a patient who will mostly benefit from individual therapy with a strong focus on the therapeutic relationship. Their regulatory impairments should be addressed with a clearly articulated therapeutic contract, and the therapist should be aware of impulsive self-harm tendencies or aggression toward other people, including the therapist. Furthermore, this diagnostic approach offers an individual profile for

[1] Case materials are composites of several profiles from our study for anonymity.

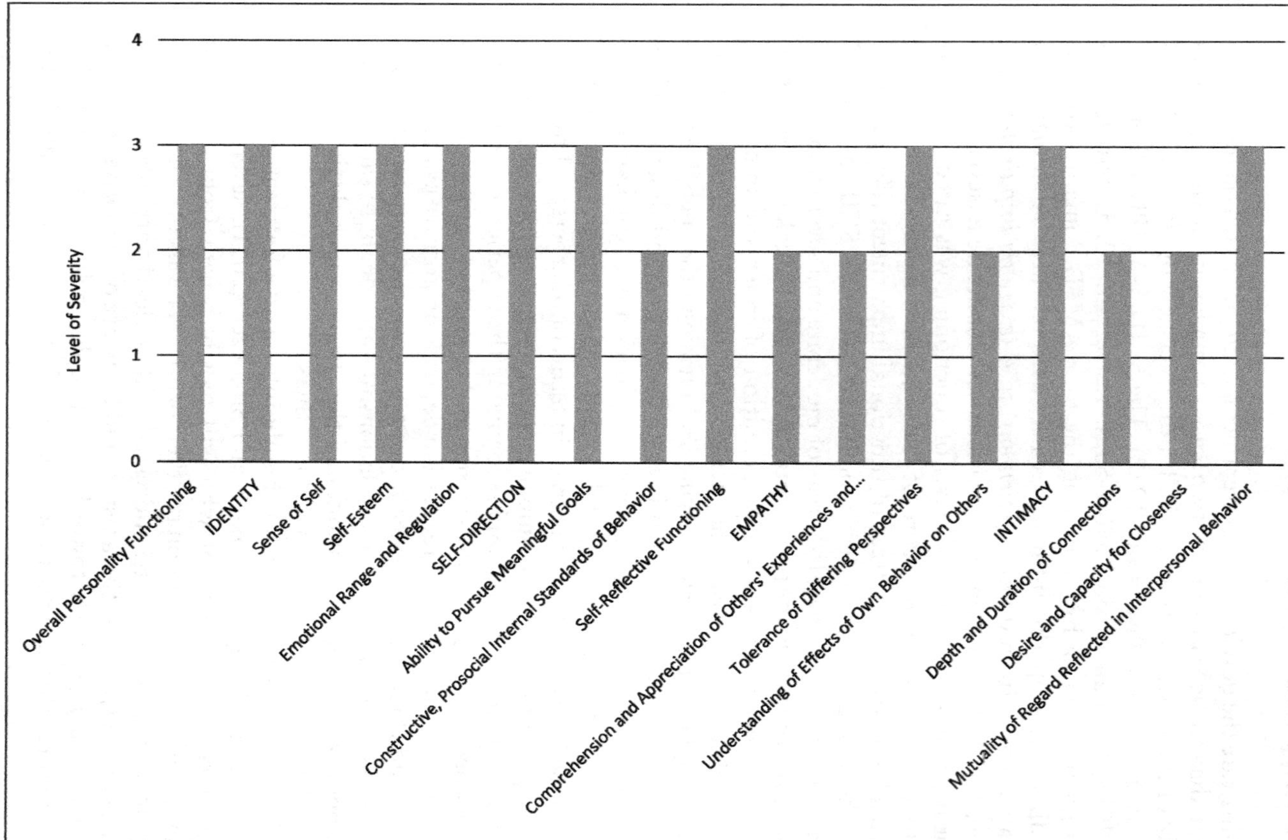

FIGURE 4.1. Dimensional assessment of personality functioning (SCID-5-AMPD-I): Severe impairment.

choosing the main focus. For this patient, the strong impairment in identity and the related difficulties should be addressed in therapy. Underlying splitting processes of the self-image and of relationships should be confronted and changed to build integrated representations. Considering techniques, this can be achieved by using countertransference reactions to detect interpersonal defense mechanisms (e.g., projective processes). As this patient shows very limited capacities to reflect on their own behaviors, an important step would be to help the patient understand the motives of their actions by confronting and interpreting them. Generally speaking, this patient will benefit from the combination of a technically neutral regard with a somewhat confrontative attitude to help them improve their mentalization abilities. From a behavioral therapeutic stance, regulatory skills should be learned and practiced and interpersonal behaviors should be trained. The goals for this patient would be first to stay in treatment and then to significantly improve their capacities to invest (in themselves, society, a job), enhance their abilities to love and have mutually satisfying relationships, and generate a more stable sense of themselves, independent of other people.

Case Example 2 portrays a patient with mild impairment in personality functioning—overall score of 1 (Figure 4.2). The dimensional profile conveys distinct areas of functional impairment. In the foreground are clearly pronounced difficulties in self-esteem regulation, with persistent doubts about their own worth and a strong dependence of self-esteem on feedback from others. In comparison to Patient 1, there are few impairments in empathic abilities and the ability to mentalize. However, in the intimacy dimension, the difficulties in establishing and maintaining enduring relationships and engaging in comparable self-revelation and openness within close relationships are particularly impressive. The therapeutic techniques chosen for this level of personality functioning would differ significantly from those used for Patient 1: The main difficulties lie less in identity pathology but more in the areas of intimacy and rigidity in interpersonal relationships. Here, it is not necessary to place such a strong focus on a fixed framework and contract; instead, the patient can be given more freedom in exploring the underlying internalized relational experiences and current interactions. The rigidity of the self-critical view of the self and the dependence of self-worth on others can be therapeutically addressed through a clarifying approach that confronts the one-sidedness of the self-view. In terms of techniques, this patient may be more likely to benefit from an exploratory approach, as the empathic abilities and the capacity to mentalize are more present. This means that interpretations can also be used to work on the underlying internalized relationship patterns and conflicts, which presumably form the basis of the impeded desire for closeness. Also, this patient may

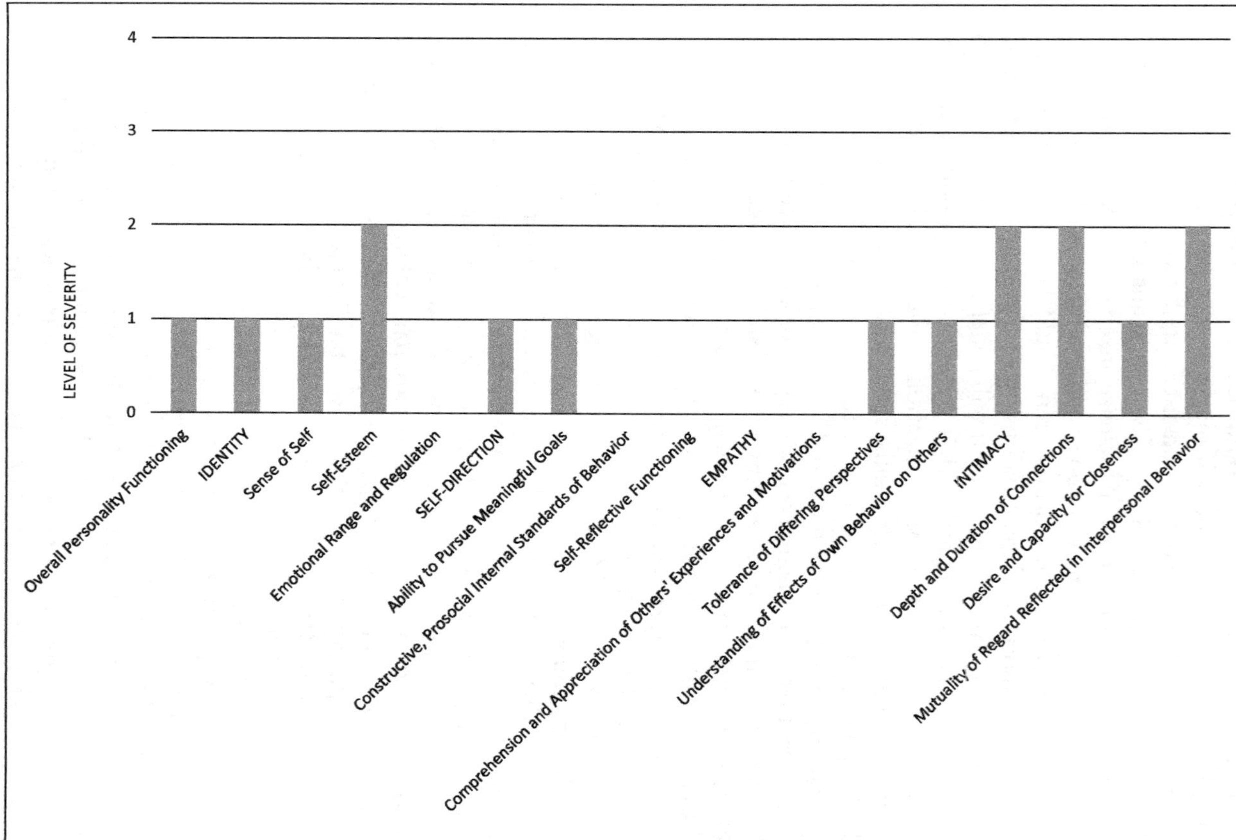

FIGURE 4.2. Dimensional assessment of personality functioning (SCID-5-AMPD-I): Mild impairment.

also benefit from group therapy, whereas Patient 1 should be treated in a dyadic setting (Bach & Simonsen, 2021).

Conclusions

In summary, the therapeutic techniques described for the two patients are based on a dimensional approach that is tailored to the level of severity and results in specific therapeutic interventions and strategies. An example for this kind of psychodynamic approach is TFP (Caligor et al., 2018), but interventions are not specific to that treatment model. Therapists working according to other treatment models (e.g., supportive treatments, cognitive-behavioral treatments) will be able to deduce treatment strategies based on the dimensional assessment of personality functioning and personality profiles and will be able to incorporate them into their therapeutic techniques. By using a dimensional assessment, the clinician can apply different treatment strategies depending on level of personality functioning instead of offering all patients the same treatment. Thus, the assessment of personality functioning can be used for integrative therapeutic procedures that move beyond specific categorical disorders or personality traits.

Clearly, ongoing and future studies will show how and in which order dimensions of personality functioning or dimensional personality traits change over time (Hopwood et al., 2011; Wright et al., 2015; Skodol, 2018) and as a function of which treatment (Kiel et al., 2024). A particularly important future research question is how to systematically develop and evaluate integrative techniques based on current models of severity of personality functioning.

PART I REFERENCES

American Psychiatric Association. (2022). *Diagnostic and statistical manual of mental disorders* (5th ed., text rev.). Author.

Andrews, G. (1996). Comorbidity and the general neurotic syndrome. *British Journal of Psychiatry, 168*(30), 76–84.

Bach, B., & Presnall-Shvorin, J. (2020). Using DSM-5 and ICD-11 personality traits in clinical treatment. In C. W. Lejuez & K. L. Gratz (Eds.), *The Cambridge handbook of personality disorders* (pp. 450–467). Cambridge University Press.

Ball, S. A., Tennen, H., Poling, J. C., Kranzler, H. R., & Rounsaville, B. J. (1997). Personality, temperament, and character dimensions and the DSM-IV personality disorders in substance abusers. *Journal of Abnormal Psychology, 106*(4), 545–553.

Barlow, D. H., Farchione, T. J., Bullis, J. R., Gallagher, M. W., Murray-Latin, H., Sauer-Zavala, S., . . . Cassiello-Robbins, C. (2018). The Unified Protocol for Transdiagnostic Treatment of Emotional Disorders compared with diagnosis-specific protocols for anxiety disorders: A randomized clinical trial. *JAMA Psychiatry, 74*(9), 875–884.

Blashfield, R. K., Keeley, J. W., Flanagan, E. H., & Miles, S. R. (2014). The cycle of classification: DSM-I through DSM-5. *Annual Review of Clinical Psychology, 10*(1), 25–51.

Bleidorn, W., Schwaba, T., Zheng, A., Hopwood, C. J., Sosa, S. S., Roberts, B. W., & Briley, D. A. (2022). Personality stability and change: A meta-analysis of longitudinal studies. *Psychological Bulletin, 148*(7–8), 588.

Bosman, R. C., Ten Have, M., de Graaf, R., Muntingh, A. D., van Balkom, A. J., & Batelaan, N. M. (2019). Prevalence and course of subthreshold anxiety disorder in the general population: A three-year follow-up study. *Journal of Affective Disorders, 247,* 105–113.

Brown, T. A., & Barlow, D. H. (2018). A proposal for a dimensional classification system based on the shared features of the DSM-IV anxiety and mood disorders: Implications for assessment and treatment. *The Neurotic Paradox, 2,* 325–354.

Cassiello-Robbins, C., Southward, M. W., Tirpak, J. W., & Sauer-Zavala, S. (2020). A systematic review of Unified Protocol applications with adult populations: Facilitating widespread dissemination via adaptability. *Clinical Psychology Review, 78,* 101852.

Costa, P. T., & McCrae, R. R. (1990). Personality disorders and the five-factor model of personality. *Journal of Personality Disorders, 4*(4), 362–371.

Hagerty, S. L. (2023). Toward precision characterization and treatment of psychopathology: A path forward and integrative framework of the hierarchical taxonomy of psychopathology and the Research Domain Criteria. *Perspectives on Psychological Science, 18*(1), 91–109.

Hopwood, C. J. (2018). A framework for treating DSM-5 alternative model for personality disorder features. *Personality and Mental Health, 12*(2), 107–125.

Hudson, N. W., Briley, D. A., Chopik, W. J., & Derringer, J. (2019). You have to follow through: Attaining behavioral change goals predicts volitional personality change. *Journal of Personality and Social Psychology, 117*(4), 839–857.

Kazdin, A. E. (2006). Mechanisms of change in psychotherapy: Advances, breakthroughs, and cutting-edge research (Do not yet exist). In R. R. Bootzin & P. E. McKnight (Eds.), *Strengthening research methodology: Psychological measurement and evaluation* (pp. 77–101). American Psychological Association.

Kazdin, A. E. (2009). Understanding how and why psychotherapy leads to change. *Psychotherapy Research, 19*(4–5), 418–428.

Magidson, J. F., Roberts, B. W., Collado-Rodriguez, A., & Lejuez, C. W. (2014). Theory-driven intervention for changing personality: Expectancy value theory, behavioral activation, and conscientiousness. *Developmental Psychology, 50*(5), 1442–1450.

McHugh, R. K., & Barlow, D. H. (2010). The dissemination and implementation of evidence-based psychological treatments. A review of current efforts. *American Psychologist, 65*(2), 73–84.

McHugh, R. K., Murray, H. W., & Barlow, D. H. (2009). Balancing fidelity and adaptation in the dissemination of empirically-supported treatments: The promise of transdiagnostic interventions. *Behaviour Research and Therapy, 47*(11), 946–953.

Mullins-Sweatt, S. N., Hopwood, C. J., Chmielewski, M., Meyer, N. A., Min, J., Helle, A. C., & Walgren, M. D. (2020). Treatment of personality pathology through the lens of the hierarchical taxonomy of psychopathology: Developing a research agenda. *Personality and Mental Health, 14*(1), 123–141.

Roberts, B. W., & DelVecchio, W. F. (2000). The rank-order consistency of personality traits from childhood to old age: A quantitative review of longitudinal studies. *Psychological Bulletin, 126*(1), 3–25.

Roberts, B. W., Luo, J., Briley, D. A., Chow, P. I., Su, R., & Hill, P. L. (2017). A systematic review of personality trait change through intervention. *Psychological Bulletin, 143*(2), 117–141.

Ruggero, C. J., Kotov, R., Hopwood, C. J., First, M., Clark, L. A., Skodol, A. E., . . . Zimmermann, J. (2019). Integrating the hierarchical taxonomy of psychopathology (HiTOP) into clinical practice. *Journal of Consulting and Clinical Psychology, 87*(12), 1069–1084.

Sakiris, N., & Berle, D. (2019). A systematic review and meta-analysis of the Unified Protocol as a transdiagnostic emotion regulation based intervention. *Clinical Psychology Review, 72*, 101751.

Samuel, D. B., & Widiger, T. A. (2006). Clinicians' judgments of clinical utility: A comparison of the DSM-IV and five-factor models. *Journal of Abnormal Psychology, 115*(2), 298–308.

Sauer-Zavala, S., Fournier, J. C., Steele, S. J., Woods, B. K., Wang, M., Farchione, T. J., & Barlow, D. H. (2021). Does the unified protocol really change neuroticism? Results from a randomized trial. *Psychological Medicine, 51*(14), 2378–2387.

Sauer-Zavala, S., Southward, M. W., Fruhbauerova, M., Semcho, S. A., Stumpp, N. E., Hood, C. O., . . . Cravens, L. (2023). BPD compass: A randomized controlled trial of a short-term, personality-based treatment for borderline personality disorder. *Personality Disorders: Theory Research and Treatment, 14*(5), 534–544.

Sauer-Zavala, S., Southward, M. W., & Hood, C. O., (2023). Conceptual development and case data for a modular, personality-based treatment for borderline personality disorder. *Personal Disorders: Theory, Research, & Treatment, 4*(4), 369–380.

Sauer-Zavala, S., Southward, M. W., & Semcho, S. A. (2022). Integrating and differentiating personality and *Journal of Personality, 90*(1), 89–102.

Soto, C. J., John, O. P., Gosling, S. D., & Potter, J. (2011). Age differences in personality traits from 10 to 65: Big Five domains and facets in a large cross-sectional sample. *Journal of Personality and Social Psychology, 100*(2), 330–348.

Steele, S. J., Farchione, T. J., & Cassiello-Robbins, C. (2018). Efficacy of the

Unified Protocol for transdiagnostic treatment of comorbid psychopathology accompanying emotional disorders compared to treatments targeting single disorders. *Journal of Psychiatric Research, 104,* 211–216.

Weisz, J. R., Chorpita, B. F., Palinkas, L. A., Schoenwald, S. K., Miranda, J., Bearman, S. K., . . . Gibbons, R. D. (2012). Testing standard and modular designs for psychotherapy treating depression, anxiety, and conduct problems in youth: A randomized effectiveness trial. *Archives of General Psychiatry, 69*(3), 274–282.

PART II REFERENCES

American Psychiatric Association. (2013). *Diagnostic and statistical manual of mental disorders* (5th ed.). Author.

Bach, B., & Simonsen, S. (2021). How does level of personality functioning inform clinical management and treatment? Implications for ICD-11 classification of personality disorder severity. *Current Opinion in Psychiatry, 34*(1), 54–63.

Bach, B., & Tracy, M. (2022). Clinical utility of the alternative model of personality disorders: A 10th year anniversary review. *Personality Disorders Theory Research and Treatment, 13*(4), 369–379.

Bateman, A., & Fonagy, P. (2004). *Psychotherapy for borderline personality disorder: Mentalization-based treatment.* Oxford University Press.

Bateman, A., Campbell, C., Fonagy, P., Luyten, P., & Debbané, M. (2023). *Cambridge guide to mentalization-based treatment (MBT).* Cambridge University Press.

Bender, D. S., Morey, L. C., & Skodol, A. E. (2011). Toward a model for assessing level of personality functioning in DSM-5, Part I: A review of theory and methods. *Journal of Personality Assessment, 93*(4), 332–346.

Bender, D. S., Skodol, A. E., Oldham, J. M., & First, M. B. (2018). *Structured Clinical Interview for the DSM-5® Alternative Model for Personality Disorders (SCID-5-AMPD) Module I: Level of Personality Functioning Scale.* American Psychiatric Association.

Biberdzic, M., Sowislo, J. F., Cain, N., Meehan, K. B., Preti, E., Di Pierro, R., . . . Clarkin, J. F. (2024). Establishing levels of personality functioning using the Structured Interview of Personality Organization (STIPO-R): A latent profile analysis. *Journal of Personality Assessment, 106*(6), 727–739.

Blüml, V., & Doering, S. (2021). ICD-11 Personality Disorders: A psychodynamic perspective on personality functioning. *Frontiers in Psychiatry, 12,* 654026.

Caligor, E., Kernberg, O. F., Clarkin, J. F., & Yeomans, F. E. (2018). *Psychodynamic therapy for personality pathology: Treating self and interpersonal functioning.* American Psychiatric Publishing.

Clark, L. A., Nuzum, H., & Ro, E. (2018). Manifestations of personality impairment severity: comorbidity, course/prognosis, psychosocial dysfunction, and 'borderline' personality features. *Current Opinion in Psychology, 21,* 117–121.

Clarkin, J. F., Cain, N. M., & Lenzenweger, M. F. (2018). Advances in transference-focused psychotherapy derived from the study of borderline personality disorder: Clinical insights with a focus on mechanism. *Current Opinion in Psychology, 21,* 80–85.

Clarkin, J. F., Caligor, E., & Sowislo, J. (2021). TFP Extended: Development and recent advances. *Psychodynamic Psychiatry, 49*(2), 188–214.

Clarkin, J. F., Levy, K. N., Lenzenweger, M. F., & Kernberg, O. F. (2007). Evaluating three treatments for borderline disorder: A multiwave study. *American Journal of Psychiatry, 164,* 922–928.

Clarkin, J. F., Yeomans, F. E., & Kernberg, O. F. (1999). *Psychotherapy for borderline personality.* Wiley.

Diamond, D., Clarkin, J. F., Levy, K. N., Meehan, K. B., Cain, N. M., Yeomans, F. E., & Kernberg, O. F. (2014). Change in attachment and reflective function in borderline patients with and without comorbid narcissistic personality disorder in transference focused psychotherapy. *Contemporary Psychoanalysis, 50*(1–2), 175–210.

Diamond, D., Keefe, J. R., Hörz-Sagstetter, S., Fischer-Kern, M., Doering, S., & Buchheim, A. (2023). Changes in attachment representation and personality organization in transference-focused psychotherapy. *American Journal of Psychotherapy, 76*(1), 31–38.

Fonagy, P., & Bateman, A. W. (2006). Mechanisms of change in mentalization-based treatment of BPD. *Journal of Clinical Psychology, 62*(4), 411–430.

Hopwood, C. J., Malone, J. C., Ansell, E. B., Sanislow, C. A., Grilo, C. M., McGlashan, T. H., . . . Morey, L. C. (2011). Personality assessment in DSM-5: Empirical support for rating severity, style, and traits. *Journal of Personality Disorders, 25*(3), 305–320.

Hörz, S., Stern, B., Caligor, E., Critchfield, K., Kernberg, O. F., Mertens, W., & Clarkin, J. F. (2009). A prototypical profile of borderline personality organization using the Structured Interview of Personality Organization (STIPO). *Journal of the American Psychoanalytic Association, 57*(6), 1464–1468.

Hörz-Sagstetter, S., Mokros, A., & Zimmermann, J. (2025). *Strukturiertes Klinisches Interview für das DSM-5—Alternatives Modell für Persönlichkeitsstörungen (SCID-5-AMPD).* (German adaptation of the *Structured Clinical Interview for the DSM-5—Alternative model for personality disorders* by Michael B. First, Andrew E. Skodol, Donna S. Bender, and John M. Oldham) Hogrefe.

Hörz-Sagstetter, S., Ohse, L., & Kampe, L. (2021). Three dimensional approaches to personality disorders: A review on personality functioning, personality structure, and personality organization. *Current Psychiatry Reports, 23*(7), 1–16.

Huber, D., Henrich, G., Clarkin, J., & Klug, G. (2013). Psychoanalytic versus psychodynamic therapy for depression: A three-year follow-up study. *Psychiatry: Interpersonal & Biological Processes, 76*(2), 132–149.

Hutsebaut, J. (2023). Isn't criterion A rather than B the language of psychotherapy? Comment on Sauer-Zavala et al. (2022). *Personality Disorders Theory Research and Treatment, 14*(4), 385–387.

Kampe, L., Zimmermann, J., Bender, D., Caligor, E., Borowski, A.-L., Ehrenthal, J. C., . . . Hörz-Sagstetter, S. (2018). Comparison of the Structured DSM-5 Clinical Interview for the Level of Personality Functioning Scale with the Structured Interview of Personality Organization. *Journal of Personality Assessment, 100*(6), 642–649.

Kernberg, O. F. (1967). Borderline personality organization. *Journal of the American Psychoanalytic Association, 15*(3), 641–685.

Kernberg, O. F. (1981). Structural interviewing. *Psychiatric Clinics, 4*(1), 169–195.

Kernberg, O. F. (1984). *Severe personality disorders: Psychotherapeutic strategies*. Yale University Press.

Kiel, L., Hopwood, C. J., & Lind, M. (2024). Changes in personality functioning and pathological personality traits as a function of treatment: A feasibility study. *Journal of Psychopathology and Behavioral Assessment, 46*(3), 695–704.

Kocjan, G. Z., Kavčič, T., & Avsec, A. (2021). Resilience matters: Explaining the association between personality and psychological functioning during the COVID-19 pandemic. *International Journal of Clinical and Health Psychology, 21*(1), Article 100198.

Koelen, J. A., Luyten, P., Eurelings-Bontekoe, L. H. M., Diguer, L., Vermote, R., Lowyck, B., & Bühring, M. E. F. (2012). The impact of level of personality organization on treatment response: A systematic review. *Psychiatry, 75*(4), 355–374.

Levy, K. N., Meehan, K. B., Kelly, K. M., Reynoso, J. S., Weber, M., Clarkin, J. F., & Kernberg, O. F. (2006). Change in attachment patterns and reflective function in a randomized control trial of transference-focused psychotherapy for borderline personality disorder. *Journal of Consulting and Clinical Psychology, 74*(6), 1027.

Luyten, P., Campbell, C., Moser, M., & Fonagy, P. (2024). The role of mentalizing in psychological interventions in adults: Systematic review and recommendations for future research. *Clinical Psychology Review, 108*, 102380.

Ohse, L., Zimmermann, J., Kerber, A., Kampe, L., Mohr, J., Kendlbacher, J., . . . Hörz-Sagstetter, S. (2023). Reliability, structure, and validity of module I (personality functioning) of the Structured Clinical Interview for the alternative DSM–5 model for personality disorders (SCID-5-AMPD-I). *Personality Disorders: Theory, Research, and Treatment, 14*(3), 287.

Ohse, L., Zimmermann, J., Kerber, A., Kampe, L., Mohr, J., Schierz, R., . . . Hörz-Sagstetter, S. (2024). Impairments in cognitive and emotional empathy as markers of general versus specific personality pathology. *Psychopathology, 57*(2), 136–148.

OPD Task Force. (2008). *Operationalized Psychodynamic Diagnosis OPD–2: Manual of diagnosis and treatment planning*. Hogrefe & Huber.

Rentrop, M., Zilker, T., Lederle, A., Birkhofer, A., & Hörz, S. (2014). Psychiatric comorbidity and personality structure in patients with polyvalent addiction. *Psychopathology, 47*(2), 133–140.

Sharp, C., & Wall, K. (2021). DSM-5 level of personality functioning: Refocusing personality disorder on what it means to be human. *Annual Review of Clinical Psychology, 17*(1), 313–337.

Skodol, A. E. (2018). Impact of personality pathology on psychosocial functioning. *Current Opinion in Psychology, 21*, 33–38.

Tyrer, P., Crawford, M., Mulder, R., Blashfield, R., Farnam, A., Fossati, A., . . . Ndetei, D. (2011). The rationale for the reclassification of personality disorder in the 11th revision of the International Classification of Diseases (ICD-11). *Personality and Mental Health, 5*(4), 246–259.

Vierl, L., Wülfing, P., Juen, F., Hörz-Sagstetter, S., Spitzer, C., & Benecke, C. (2024). Unravelling inter-relations within and between psychodynamic constructs and psychopathology using network analysis. *Personality and Mental Health, 18*(4), 323–338.

Waszczuk, M. A., Hopwood, C. J., Luft, B. J., Morey, L. C., Perlman, G., Ruggero, C. J., . . . Kotov, R. (2022). The prognostic utility of personality traits versus past psychiatric diagnoses: Predicting future mental health and functioning. *Clinical Psychological Science, 10*(4), 734–751.

Wendt, L., Klein, E., Benecke, C., Singer, S., Dotzauer, L., Engesser, D., . . . Zimmermann, J. (2024): Clinical utility of the Level of Personality Functioning Scale: A survey of German mental health professionals. *Personality Disorders: Theory, Research, and Treatment, 16*(6), 491–503.

World Health Organization. (2019). *International statistical classification of diseases and related health problems, eleventh revision (ICD-11)*. Author.

Wright, A. G. C., Calabrese, W. R., Rudick, M. M., Yam, W. H., Zelazny, K., Williams, T. F., . . . Simms, L. J. (2015). Stability of the DSM-5 Section III pathological personality traits and their longitudinal associations with psychosocial functioning in personality disordered individuals. *Journal of Abnormal Psychology, 124*(1), 199–207.

Zimmermann, J., Benecke, C., Bender, D. S., Skodol, A. E., Schauenburg, H., Cierpka, M., & Leising, D. (2013). Assessing DSM–5 level of personality functioning from videotaped clinical interviews: A pilot study with untrained and clinically inexperienced students. *Journal of Personality Assessment, 96*(4), 397–409.

CHAPTER 5

What does dimensional diagnosis mean for clinical psychological training?

Shifts in psychiatric taxonomy have a variety of downriver effects, one of the most substantial of which is changes in the training of mental health professionals. The transition to a dimensional model of psychopathology could come with challenges but also opportunities for clinical psychological training. We asked experts to answer three questions about this theme:

What are the main ways that clinical training will need to change to account for the transition to dimensional diagnosis?

Is it possible that the adoption of dimensional diagnosis in the clinic can improve research practice integration in the classroom?

What challenges does the transition to dimensional models of diagnosis represent for training the next generation of clinical psychologists?

Both sets of authors acknowledge significant challenges but also highlight advantages to shifting toward dimensional models. Ruggero and Callahan argue that dimensional models would go hand in hand with a shift to more process-based as opposed to disorder-specific approaches to therapy training, a greater emphasis on common factors, and more routine outcome monitoring, all of which would improve therapy training. At the same time, they recognize the personal and institutional inertia that slows progress and point out certain ways in which educators and students would need to think differently, using hierarchical aspects of dimensional models as an example. Both authors note that the variability in dimensional models currently available might be a barrier to progress. Nelson, Iwanicki, and Wells stress how long it takes for evidence to influence practice and encourage practical implementation strategies to enable a smooth and brisk transition. They emphasize that this might be especially important in training sites such as practica or internships that are external to doctoral training programs where dimensional models may be more popular.

PART I

Dimensional diagnosis will enhance clinical psychological training

CAMILO J. RUGGERO and JENNIFER L. CALLAHAN

The transition from the hegemony of classifying mental illness based on diagnostic categories to the use of dimensional models such as the hierarchical taxonomy of psychopathology (HiTOP; Kotov et al., 2017) has tremendous potential to transform research and treatment of psychopathology (Conway et al., 2019; Ruggero, Kotov, et al., 2019). Yet prevailing nosology reflected in DSM-5 is a *lingua franca* embedded deeply into every aspect of mental health care, so shifting away from this paradigm faces significant barriers and comes at a major cost for training the workforce (Zimmerman, 2021). Here, we focus on what this shift implies for training the next generation of clinical psychologists.

Training Opportunities

A move to a dimensional diagnostic framework portends far-reaching implications for clinical psychology training, from the prosaic to the foundational. Categorical diagnostic systems, intentionally or not, reify artificial boundaries between mental health disorders despite compelling evidence that these boundaries do not reflect the true structure of psychopathology (Kotov et al., 2017). At its core, a move to dimensional frameworks like HiTOP will counter diagnostic silos that often shape training in both clinical research and practice. Most psychopathology textbooks are structured around categorical diagnosis, most assessment texts align measures with categorical frameworks, and even widely used computer-assisted scoring software suggests categorical diagnoses based on patient responses. Likewise, psychotherapy courses and practica in contemporary training programs often emphasize empirically supported treatments predicated on a categorical diagnosis. Training students to conceptualize psychopathology along core symptom dimensions and shared mechanisms will disrupt many of these aspects of clinical training and education, requiring curricular and pedagogical adaptations (Ruggero, Callahan, et al., 2019). Shifting to a dimensional framework will require more explicitly training students to recognize overlapping symptom dimensions, construct treatment plans based on transdiagnostic processes, and develop interventions that address underlying psychological mechanisms rather than discrete disorders (Mullins-Sweatt et al., 2020).

Supervision methods and even the language used in case conceptualization will need to be adapted to align with dimensional frameworks. A significant component of this shift in language and supervision can be facilitated by reviving and expanding the role of process-based therapy, an established approach that despite its deep roots has not always been central to clinical training. Rather than requiring a complete overhaul of existing practices, integrating a dimensional framework can be framed as a natural progression of process-based principles, which have long emphasized psychological mechanisms over disorder-specific treatments (Goldfried, 2019). Over the past 2 decades, psychotherapy training has many times focused on helping students master interventions tailored to individual diagnoses, resulting in a fragmented skill set (Goldfried, 2019; Hayes et al., 2020; Wampold & Imel, 2015). A clinician trained in cognitive-behavioral therapy for panic disorder, for example, might struggle to apply the same principles to trauma-related symptoms despite the shared mechanisms between these conditions. Process-based therapy, in contrast, provides a flexible foundation by focusing on transdiagnostic principles (i.e., cognitive restructuring, exposure techniques, and emotional regulation) that can be applied across symptom spectra.

To further enhance assessment skills, integrating measurement-based care (MBC) into clinical decision making is also essential (Boswell et al., 2023) and aligns with the empirically based foundation of dimensional models. Categorical nosologies can sometimes risk conditioning clinicians to view treatment success in binary terms (e.g., "remission"), whereas symptom change is a continuous phenomenon. Importantly, subsyndromal symptoms may have functional impairments and require care (Noyes et al., 2022), a fact much more easily accommodated by dimensional models of psychopathology that do not reify artificial boundaries. The latter requires students to understand evidence regarding which cutoffs are validated for which functional outcomes versus "one-size-fits-all" cutoffs based on arbitrary, unvalidated thresholds (e.g., 5 of 9 symptoms for depression simply because this is more than half).

Moreover, dimensional frameworks more naturally push trainees to adopt continuous tracking measures, monitoring symptom severity and functional outcomes rather than relying on artificial diagnostic cutoffs. This shift does not require entirely new pedagogical approaches but rather the deliberate application of existing methods, including training in psychometrics, statistical interpretation, and real-time data integration into clinical decision making. These tools are already well established and have been shown to improve clinical outcomes, yet their consistent use in supervision remains uneven (Boswell et al., 2015). Dimensional models of psychopathology can only facilitate their use. By positioning a transition to dimensional models as an evolution rather than a disruption, training programs can build on familiar concepts while gradually shifting toward a more adaptable principle-driven approach to intervention directed at validated outcomes (Hayes et al., 2020).

Alongside process-based principles and MBC, a renewed emphasis on common therapeutic factors can further support this transition in clinical training (Goldfried, 2019). Categorical models, with their rigid adherence to treatment protocols, have sometimes led trainees to prioritize intervention techniques over foundational therapeutic elements; yet decades of research confirms that factors such as therapeutic alliance, empathy, and patient expectations contribute more to treatment outcomes than any disorder-specific intervention does (Wampold & Imel, 2015). A dimensional training model naturally integrates these factors by shifting the focus away from checklist-driven diagnosis and toward individualized case formulation. This not only strengthens students' therapeutic flexibility but also ensures that psychotherapy training fosters clinical judgment rather than a mechanized application of treatment manuals.

Going beyond transdiagnostic awareness, clinical supervision will need to foster deep specialization in specific symptom dimensions to prepare trainees for dimensional models like HiTOP. Just as dimensional diagnosis encourages clinicians to recognize patterns across disorders, it also fosters expertise in distinguishing between more narrow symptom clusters and traits. Under this model, students learn to assess and intervene at the trait level, differentiating between, for instance, impulsivity and emotional dysregulation, even when both are present within a single diagnosis like borderline personality disorder. A clinician trained in categorical models may recognize a patient's impulsivity but struggle to determine whether it stems from sensation seeking (a disinhibition trait) or affective instability (an emotional regulation deficit), a distinction that directly influences treatment decisions. Effective supervision can guide trainees in refining these granular assessment skills to map onto more complex profiles as opposed to categories, allowing for greater precision in intervention. Moreover, this level of granularity promotes development and application of precision-based interventions (Hagerty, 2022).

Beyond changes in clinical training, this shift enhances the quality of research conducted in clinical settings. One of the most significant limitations of categorical diagnosis is that it structures clinical research around DSM-based disorder categories, even when these categories do not accurately reflect symptom presentations in real-world patients (Kotov et al., 2017; Michelini et al., 2021). This issue is particularly evident in clinical trials, where inclusion criteria often exclude individuals with complex comorbidities or additive subsyndromal symptoms, leading to findings that may not generalize to clinical populations (Zimmerman et al., 2005). The result is a gap between research populations and real-world patients, limiting the applicability of evidence-based treatments in practice (Ruggero, Kotov, et al., 2019).

Training Challenges

Many barriers impede the widespread adoption of dimensional models, including faculty reluctance, institutional constraints, curriculum limitations, and accreditation barriers. We agree that these challenges must be addressed for dimensional models to take hold in clinical training settings. However, we also argue that these difficulties are not insurmountable and that there are solutions for each of these obstacles.

One of the most significant barriers is reluctance among faculty and supervisors, many of whom were trained under categorical models and may be hesitant to adopt dimensional frameworks. Given that the DSM and ICD have structured clinical training for decades, shifting away from these familiar systems requires substantial changes to both pedagogy and practice. Many educators may be unwilling to invest time in retraining unless they perceive a clear advantage to dimensional models, particularly if curricular resources and institutional policies remain tied to categorical classification (Zimmerman, 2021). Resistance of this kind is not unique. Similar challenges emerged during past paradigm shifts in clinical psychology, such as the adoption of DSM-III in the 1980s and the push for evidence-based treatments in the 1990s. In both cases, widespread acceptance occurred only after accumulating empirical support and institutional endorsement (Mayes & Horowitz, 2005).

A comparable process will likely be necessary for dimensional diagnosis, requiring both continued research that demonstrates its clinical utility and strategic efforts to facilitate implementation in training programs.

Faculty reluctance is further reinforced by the fact that many professional settings still require categorical diagnoses. Forensic psychology, disability determinations, and health insurance reimbursement all rely on DSM or ICD classifications. Legal systems often mandate DSM-based diagnoses for forensic evaluations, and clinicians may lack familiarity with dimensional alternatives (Mulay et al., 2025). Insurers require ICD codes for billing purposes and may struggle to tie dimensional models to this need (Ruggero, Kotov, et al., 2019). Although crosswalk tools have been developed to translate HiTOP dimensions into DSM or ICD codes, they provide only a partial solution. As a result, clinical training programs must balance teaching dimensional conceptualization with ensuring that students can operate within these professional requirements. Converting a nuanced dimensional profile into a categorical label can obscure clinically relevant information, limiting the potential advantages of dimensional diagnosis in these contexts (Ruggero, Callahan, et al., 2019). Nevertheless, these external constraints will be slow to change and therefore mean that trainees will need to learn to navigate both dimensional and categorical diagnostic models for a substantial period moving forward.

A further challenge in adopting dimensional models in training is the lack of a single dominant framework. Although HiTOP has gained traction, alternative models, such as the DSM-5 alternative model for personality disorders (AMPD; American Psychiatric Association, 2013) and the ICD-11's dimensional system (Clark et al., 2017; Kotov et al., 2017), present competing approaches. This lack of consensus can make it difficult for programs to commit to any one model, as faculty may worry that current frameworks will continue evolving. One way to address this is for training programs to emphasize core transdiagnostic principles, such as shared symptom dimensions and underlying psychological mechanisms rather than aligning with a single diagnostic system (Hopwood et al., 2020; Mullins-Sweatt et al., 2020). This would allow students to apply dimensional approaches flexibly across different clinical settings and adapt to future developments in classification systems.

Another barrier to widespread adoption is the slow pace at which research findings are integrated into training. Despite compelling empirical support for dimensional models (Kotov et al., 2022), they remain secondary to categorical frameworks in most clinical programs. This delay reflects a broader issue in psychology, where new evidence often takes years to reach curricula (Gehlbach & Robinson, 2021). One solution is to establish structured mechanisms for research translation, such as faculty workshops, integration of HiTOP-aligned continuing education, and closer collaboration between researchers and training programs (Boswell et al., 2015; Callahan & Watkins, 2018). Training clinics could also implement routine MBC practices, ensuring that students engage with empirical symptom tracking from the outset of their training (Hagerty, 2022). By actively incorporating new findings, training programs can ensure that students graduate with a conceptual framework that reflects the most current understanding of psychopathology.

Because faculty hesitation and external constraints shape how clinical training is structured, revising curricula to accommodate dimensional models is essential but presents its own set of challenges. Graduate programs in clinical psychology and psychiatry have traditionally organized psychopathology courses around DSM or ICD categories. Textbooks, lectures, and exams are typically structured by diagnostic category, such as a unit on mood disorders or a unit on psychotic disorders. Shifting to a dimensional framework requires a fundamental rethinking of this pedagogy. However, this challenge is not insurmountable. Courses can integrate HiTOP alongside traditional diagnostic instruction, helping students learn to conceptualize "depression" both through DSM criteria and its corresponding dimensional representation. A student might come to understand depression as part of the internalizing spectrum, with high distress subfactor elevations, rather than as a standalone disorder. Prior efforts have demonstrated that integrating HiTOP into coursework is feasible and can be accomplished with minimal disruption while ensuring that students gain proficiency in both categorical and dimensional frameworks (Ruggero, Callahan, et al., 2019).

Closely related to curriculum restructuring are financial and time constraints, which pose significant barriers to implementation. Converting curricula, developing new training materials, and retraining faculty require resources. Many clinical supervisors are unfamiliar with dimensional models, meaning that retraining efforts must extend beyond students to ensure that those overseeing clinical training can provide appropriate guidance (Ruggero, Callahan, et al., 2019). Some concerns about time and cost, however, may be overstated. Many widely used psychological assessments, such as the MMPI and Achenbach System, already function within dimensional frameworks. Because of this, adopting a dimensional nosology like HiTOP may reduce the training burden over time by aligning diagnostic models with assessment tools that trainees already learn (Ruggero, Callahan, et al., 2019; Ruggero, Kotov, et al., 2019). HiTOP may also be more intuitive to learn than DSM, which requires mastery of hundreds of distinct diagnostic categories and complex inclusion or exclusion criteria, with questions about how well clinicians apply its nuances (First et al., 2018). If dimensional training is structured efficiently, it may ultimately prove less cumbersome than DSM training rather than more.

Beyond structural and logistical challenges, transitioning to dimensional models affects treatment planning, requiring a fundamental shift in how students are trained to formulate interventions. Categorical diagnoses provide clear guidelines for intervention selection, making it relatively straightforward for trainees to match specific treatments to specific disorders. In contrast, dimensional models require a more nuanced individualized approach in which clinicians must integrate multiple symptom dimensions and tailor interventions accordingly. This complexity may initially overwhelm trainees, particularly those accustomed to structured protocol-driven treatments. Learning to navigate this flexibility requires additional training and supervision to ensure that clinicians develop confidence in their ability to make data-driven treatment decisions. Without deliberate and systematic training in dimensional approaches, there is a risk that clinicians may either revert to categorical frameworks out of familiarity or apply dimensional models inconsistently, undermining their potential benefits for personalized care.

Although these barriers pose real difficulties, they can be navigated with thoughtful solutions. Successfully transitioning clinical training to a dimensional framework requires overcoming resistance from faculty, navigating external institutional constraints, restructuring curricula, addressing financial concerns, and providing adequate supervision to help trainees adapt to more flexible treatment models. By addressing these barriers proactively, training programs can better prepare clinicians to use empirically grounded flexible diagnostic frameworks, ultimately improving both psychological research and patient care.

Conclusion

Shifting to dimensional diagnosis represents an important transformation in clinical psychology training. This does not simply change how disorders are diagnosed; it redefines how clinical psychologists conceptualize mental health, approach treatment, and integrate scientific findings into practice. There will be major logistical, institutional, and pedagogical barriers, but this shift ultimately may offer a more precise, empirically valid, and clinically useful approach to understanding and treating mental illness. As research increasingly supports dimensional models, training programs can proactively adapt to ensure that clinicians are prepared to apply these frameworks in real-world practice.

PART II

Barriers to integrating dimensional diagnosis into clinical psychology

SHARON M. NELSON, SIERRA A. IWANICKI, and THERESA L. WELLES

Fewer than one in seven evidence-based interventions make their way into real-world settings, and those that do often take nearly 2 decades to get there (Zullig et al., 2024). In academia, research publication output has far outpaced the application of findings to benefit the public (Bauer & Kirchner, 2020). Given this, it's not all that surprising that dimensional models have yet to see widespread adoption within psychological clinical training clinics. Without significant investment in dissemination and implementation efforts, beyond traditional research, dimensional models are unlikely to take hold in clinical training environments.

Dimensional models of psychopathology, such as the AMPD (American Psychiatric Association, 2013) and the hierarchical taxonomy of psychopathology (HiTOP; Kotov et al., 2017), offer significant improvements over categorical approaches in terms of diagnostic precision and treatment planning (Bernstein et al., 2007; Bornstein & Natoli, 2019; Morey & Hopwood, 2019). Despite empirical support, however, these models have seen limited progress in dissemination and implementation. Dissemination refers to spreading research findings to a broader audience, whereas implementation involves integrating these findings into clinical practice (Rubenstein & Purtle, 2020). Without targeted efforts in these areas, even well-supported models often fail to achieve meaningful real-world influence (Davies & Nutley, 2021).

The adoption of a new diagnostic model, particularly one that challenges long-standing paradigms, is inherently disruptive. Shifting to a dimensional framework requires overcoming significant hurdles, including entrenched categorical practices and resistance to change. Nowhere is this more evident than in psychological training clinics where adoption may influence a wide range of stakeholders in psychology training. These include students, clinical faculty, supervisors, undergraduate and graduate instructors, training clinic administrators and staff, billing and insurance agencies, individuals receiving assessment and care, practicum training sites, psychiatrists, clinical social workers, electronic medical record programmers, and textbook publishers. And yet, although empirical support for dimensional models continues to grow, little research has focused on how best to educate and train these diverse groups or how such a shift may influence clinical training operations.

With this in mind and as proponents of dimensional models ourselves, we will use this chapter to examine the real-world barriers to implementing these models in clinical training settings. Specifically, we highlight obstacles that must be addressed before dimensional models can be meaningfully integrated into training clinics and classrooms, preparing the next generation of clinicians and researchers for a conceptual shift that is yet to gain widespread acceptance. This chapter will primarily focus on clinical psychology training; however, the specific challenges to implementing dimensional models will vary (for instance, different barriers could likely be identified with respect to evaluating psychiatric training). Similarly, the authors of this chapter all work in the United States, so barriers and examples provided may not be relevant in all regions.

What Barriers Have Impeded Adoption of Dimensional Diagnosis in Clinical Psychological Training?

The adoption of dimensional diagnostic models in clinical psychological training faces several obstacles that have slowed their acceptance and widespread implementation. The deeply ingrained habits of clinical supervisors are one of the biggest challenges to adopting dimensional diagnostic models in clinical training. Supervisors tend to teach the way they practice, and their clinical methods are often shaped by their own training experiences from decades before. Given that many psychotherapists report that their graduate mentors were among the most significant influences on their professional development (Cook et al., 2009), it follows that diagnostic training is largely an inherited cycle where categorical models persist simply because they are what supervisors know best.

Gaining buy-in from faculty and supervisors is critical, but this requires a shift in institutional culture and a substantial investment in professional development. Many instructors hesitate to adjust established teaching methods, particularly when they already juggle significant demands on their time, supervising students, seeing clients, conducting research, and maintaining administrative duties. Training in dimensional models requires dedicated time, funding, and leadership support, which are often not readily available. To illustrate this challenge, when one of the authors attempted to implement a program for training clinicians to evaluate their own interventions, participants needed to get two different levels of leadership to authorize their taking the time to train, find clinical and supervision coverage, adjust patient scheduling, move meetings, find time to review and study materials, and identify funding to cover the cost of training. Clinicians then needed to do all of this again to schedule time with the individual trainers to tailor what we were teaching to their setting/program and again to participate in follow-up consultation with experts posttraining to address remaining implementation barriers. It is easy to imagine similar needs for faculty to balance supervision, clinical work, teaching, research, and needing to justify any time taken off to learn and apply new models. With many universities tightening budgets (Moody, 2025), supervisors/training clinics may also need to find ways to convince their universities that this is a worthwhile investment or identify and apply for external funding, as even with a fair number of freely accessible materials, implementation of a new model will involve some upfront expense.

Another significant challenge is that most current practitioners were trained in categorical models and continue to use them in their clinical work. Shifting to dimensional models, such as HiTOP, requires a fundamental change in how clinicians conceptualize psychopathology, assess patients, and develop treatment plans. Training clinics would need to overhaul their curricula, moving away from disorder-specific diagnostic categories toward a more symptom-based approach. This is no small task; beyond revising coursework, it requires rethinking assessment measures, case formulations, and supervision strategies. Supervisors, in turn, would need substantial training themselves to competently guide trainees through this transition.

Institutional barriers further complicate the adoption of dimensional models. According to Cook et al. (2009), individuals in institutional settings face 25 times more obstacles in implementing new therapeutic models than do private practitioners. These barriers, such as bureaucratic resistance, curriculum constraints, and limited financial resources, apply just as much to diagnostic frameworks as they do to treatment approaches. Administrators may be reluctant to support such a major shift without clear evidence of improved outcomes, and faculty may lack the autonomy or resources needed to experiment with new approaches.

One particularly pressing issue is the lack of faculty expertise in personality disorders, which are central to many dimensional models. A review by Levy and Ellison (2021) found that of 336 American Psychological Association-accredited programs, only 55 (16.4%) had a faculty member with research interests in personality disorders. This means that many programs lack champions for dimensional models and may struggle to provide adequate training in their application. When faculty who are responsible for teaching personality psychopathology are unfamiliar with dimensional frameworks, they are more likely to stick with traditional methods by default.

Ultimately, adopting dimensional diagnostic models can be challenging for multiple reasons, including ingrained habits, instructor resistance, and institutional barriers. In addition, a lack of faculty expertise and support further slows this transition. Overcoming these barriers will require focused efforts to update training and integrate dimensional diagnostic approaches into clinical psychology training.

What Barriers Make It Difficult to Adopt Dimensional Diagnoses in the Clinic, and How Might That Influence Research–Practice Integration in the Classroom?

Mental health fields, like many disciplines, tend to hold onto familiar tools and frameworks even when newer, research-supported alternatives become available (Gehlbach & Robinson, 2021). This resistance to change is evident in clinical training, where outdated methodologies often persist despite the introduction of improved models. A prime example is the continued use of the MMPI-2 in some training programs, even though the MMPI-2-RF and MMPI-3 have been available for years. Villanueva van den Hurk et al. (2023) found that although nearly all programs (96% in 2021 and 94% in 2022) had incorporated the updated versions in their teachings, a substantial portion (77% in 2021 and 66% in 2022) still included the older MMPI-2 in their curriculum. It is important to note that resistance to transitioning from the MMPI-2 is not just due to institutional inertia; some clinicians and researchers believe the older version has advantages over the updates. This highlights a broader challenge in implementing change: ongoing debates about the effectiveness of new models can slow their adoption, even when they are presented as improvements. If updating something as specific as a psychological test takes time, it is not surprising that a fundamental shift in diagnostic frameworks, such as the adoption of dimensional models, would present even greater challenges.

The sheer logistical challenge of updating training is one of the major barriers to adoption. Faculty already juggle significant demands, including supervision, teaching, research, and administrative responsibilities. Introducing dimensional diagnostic models requires more than just conceptual buy-in; it necessitates a practical overhaul of training materials, including textbooks, lecture slides, and case examples. However, most existing textbooks devote little space to dimensional models, often condensing the topic into a brief section. A quick review of widely used clinical training materials shows that many offer only a paragraph or a few pages on dimensional models, making it difficult for instructors to find comprehensive, easy-to-use teaching resources. The lack of teaching resources creates a cycle where faculty stick to familiar categorical models because they are already in existing materials, perpetuating the continued teaching of traditional categorical models despite growing evidence in favor of dimensional approaches.

Compounding this challenge is a broader lack of consensus on which dimensional model to prioritize. Unlike categorical diagnoses, which have been firmly embedded in training for decades, dimensional models are still evolving, with competing frameworks such as DSM-5's AMPD, HiTOP, and ICD-11's dimensional approach to personality disorders. Although the Research Domain Criteria (RDoC) framework also promotes a dimensional understanding of mental disorders, its integration into clinical practice remains limited. Although ICD-11 has already incorporated a dimensional framework for personality disorders, adoption in the United States remains particularly challenging due to entrenched reliance on the DSM and associated categorical diagnostic structures. Understanding these regional differences is crucial for identifying context-specific implementation strategies. Additionally, the use of different frameworks can cause fragmentation, making training and curricula design more difficult. As a result of such uncertainty, some faculty and clinicians may be hesitant to fully invest in teaching dimensional models, preferring long-standing categorical diagnostic frameworks, worrying that evolving models may become outdated quickly. As a result, dimensional models remain secondary to categorical frameworks, limiting students' exposure to newer, research-backed approaches despite strong evidence supporting their use. However, it is also important to acknowledge that the treatment literature has not yet fully caught up. The widespread emphasis on rigidly applied evidence-based treatments means that until interventions like dialectical behavior therapy (DBT) or mentalization-based therapy (MBT) are empirically validated for AMPD-defined personality pathology, which we assume they will be, training programs may be reluctant to adopt dimensional models for diagnosis.

Another obstacle is the slow translation of research into clinical training and practice (Feifer et al., 2004). Historically, there has been a productive relationship between research and teaching, but the increasing pace and complexity of scientific advancements have widened the gap between discovery and implementation. Research findings take time to disseminate, and publication delays in social science journals have grown from an average of 9 months in 1970 to nearly 24 months by 2000 (Kling & Swygart-Hobaugh, 2002). These delays affect how quickly research findings make their way into textbooks, syllabi, and clinical practice. Even as empirical support for dimensional models grows, categorical models continue to dominate training curricula simply because they are more established in educational materials. For training clinics that accept/bill insurance, this is further complicated. There is a simplicity to categorical diagnosis that insurance companies have traditionally liked, and it is unlikely that faculty have training or time to engage in advocating with insurance companies.

The failure to integrate dimensional models into training has significant consequences for both clinical education and practice. Without exposure to these frameworks in graduate training, students enter practicum and internship settings unprepared to engage with dimensional approaches, reinforcing their underuse in real-world clinical settings. Overcoming these barriers will require more than just advocacy; it will demand the development of accessible training materials, institutional support for updating curricula, and stronger efforts to bridge the research–practice gap. Although challenging, this transition offers the potential for developing more effective approaches to disseminating dimensional models in both university classrooms and clinical training settings.

What Challenges/Barriers Does the Transition to Dimensional Models of Diagnosis Represent for Training the Next Generation of Clinical Psychologists?

Implementing dimensional models in university training clinics is an important step, but it is not enough to bridge the "ivory-tower barrier" that separates academic knowledge from clinical practice. Most clinical psychologists receive training across multiple settings, including external practicums and clinical internships. In many clinical psychology training programs, particularly in North America, doctoral trainees engage in external practica, most complete clinical internships, and some pursue postdoctoral training (APA, 2017). The extent to which students become proficient in the applied use of dimensional models depends not only on their individual graduate programs but also on whether these models are adopted at external training sites. If external settings (including practicum and internship sites) do not integrate dimensional models, or if supervisors are not trained in their application, then the reach of these models will remain limited. Although the structure of training differs across regions, the challenge of integrating dimensional models across academic and applied settings remains a common theme.

Graduate training programs are already under pressure to cover an expanding range of topics despite decreasing resources (Levy, 2022). Research on training costs for implementing cognitive-behavioral therapy in Australian training clinics found direct expenses ranging from $9,000 to $55,000, and significant indirect expenses (e.g., lost billable hours) reveal a considerable financial burden to implement changes (Crome & Baillie, 2016). Integrating dimensional models into curricula requires significant investment, which may not be justified if students subsequently train in settings that do not use these models. This discrepancy between academic training and clinical practice reduces the cost–benefit ratio of including dimensional models in graduate programs. Moreover, trainees who are well-versed in dimensional models may be at a disadvantage when applying to sites that prioritize traditional categorical approaches, further complicating efforts to implement these models in clinical practice.

The challenges extend beyond training clinics to the broader clinical settings where students complete practica and internships. Some specialized settings, such as forensic psychology, rely heavily on categorical diagnoses to meet legal standards (e.g., insanity, competency). Legal systems often require clear diagnostic distinctions (e.g., "present" vs. "absent" diagnoses), which don't fit well within dimensional models. In forensic contexts, where legal decisions might request clear categorizations, mental health professionals must present complex psychological findings in a way that fits legal standards. This creates a dilemma for training programs: If students are trained in models that are not widely applicable, the investment in such training may be perceived as less valuable.

Additionally, multidisciplinary settings, where professionals from various fields collaborate, present unique challenges. The adoption of dimensional models alters how diagnoses are communicated among providers, requiring clear guidelines and training. Successful implementation depends on securing buy-in from multiple disciplines and stakeholders who are involved in psychological training, which adds another layer of complexity (Cook et al., 2009). As previously discussed, training providers in unfamiliar models is resource intensive; the challenge is even greater when a variety of professional groups must be included in the transition.

Cook et al. (2009) identified several training-related barriers in a survey of more than 1,600 North American psychotherapists:

- *Insufficient time (28%)*—The demand for extensive training can overwhelm existing schedules.
- *High cost of training (15%)*—Financial constraints limit access to comprehensive training.
- *Insufficient training/supervision (9%)*—There is a lack of post-training support for skill refinement.
- *Lack of confidence and proficiency (7%)*—Clinicians may feel unprepared to implement new techniques.
- *Lack of accessible local training (7%)*—Limited local training opportunities hinder widespread adoption.

These barriers highlight the complexities of integrating dimensional models into clinical training. Many clinicians are unfamiliar with dimensional approaches, necessitating a substantial retraining effort, one that parallels the shift experienced with the introduction of DSM-III in 1980 (First, 2005; Skodol et al., 1981; Williams et al., 1985). This transition must address both theoretical understanding and practical application to ensure that dimensional models are effectively applied in diverse clinical settings.

In conclusion, although the adoption of dimensional models in clinical training has the potential to improve diagnostic accuracy and treatment outcomes, the transition presents significant challenges. Overcoming these barriers requires a coordinated effort to align academic training with clinical practice, expand the dissemination of dimensional approaches, and provide comprehensive training and support to both trainees and supervisors.

Conclusion

This chapter highlights the significant gap between empirical support for dimensional models and their real-world implementation in mental health practice. Unsurprisingly, fewer than one in seven evidence-based interventions are adopted into practice, and those that are often take decades to do so (Zullig et al., 2024). Despite strong theoretical and empirical support for dimensional models like the AMPD and HiTOP, their adoption in clinical training remains limited. Although personality disorders were among the first areas to adopt dimensional models, these frameworks are now used to understand a wider range of psychopathology. The primary barriers are overwhelmingly practical rather than theoretical, as empirical evidence supports the models but implementation remains difficult. Insufficient training infrastructure such as lack of resources and decreased emphasis on personality training reduce opportunities for students to learn about dimensional models. Additionally, entrenched practices among clinical supervisors, who tend to teach based on their own training experiences, further hinder the adoption of new diagnostic frameworks. Institutional challenges such as rigid curriculum structures and limited faculty expertise also complicate the integration of dimensional models into clinical training.

The chapter underscores the critical need for effective dissemination and implementation strategies to bridge the gap between research and practice. Without these efforts, even well-supported models like AMPD and HiTOP may struggle to achieve widespread use. A shift to dimensional models requires not only changes in curriculum but also broader systemic adjustments across clinical training environments. Strategic rollout methods should be developed in collaboration with all relevant stakeholders, not just researchers but also instructors, supervisors, training clinic administrators, billing and insurance agencies, individuals with lived experience, students, practicum training sites, psychiatrists, clinical social workers, and electronic medical record systems, among others. It is especially important to consider the perspectives of those who may relate strongly to categorical diagnostic models, whether due to personal lived experience, established psychiatric practices, or the logistical constraints of medical charting and billing systems. Without input from these groups, implementation efforts risk being incomplete or ineffective.

In conclusion, although dimensional models have the potential to improve diagnostic accuracy and treatment planning, their successful integration into clinical training is hindered by practical, real-world barriers that are often overlooked by academic researchers. Overcoming these obstacles will require a systemic approach that includes enhancing training resources, securing instructor buy-in, and aligning academic training with clinical practice. By addressing these challenges in a collaborative and inclusive manner, the field can move toward a more clinically useful and scientifically grounded diagnostic system.

PART I REFERENCES

Boswell, J. F., Hepner, K. A., Lysell, K., Rothrock, N. E., Bott, N., Childs, A. W., . . . Bobbitt, B. L. (2023). The need for a measurement-based care professional practice guideline. *Psychotherapy, 60*(1), 1–16.

Boswell, J. F., Kraus, D. R., Miller, S. D., & Lambert, M. J. (2015). Implementing routine outcome monitoring in clinical practice: Benefits, challenges, and solutions. *Psychotherapy Research, 25*(1), 6–19.

Callahan, J. L., & Watkins, C. E. (2018). The science of training III: Supervision, competency, and internship training. *Training and Education in Professional Psychology, 12*(4), 245–261.

Clark, L. A., Cuthbert, B., Lewis-Fernández, R., Narrow, W. E., & Reed, G. M. (2017). Three approaches to understanding and classifying mental disorder: ICD-11, DSM-5, and the National Institute of Mental Health's Research Domain Criteria (RDoC). *Psychological Science in the Public Interest, 18*(2), 72–145.

Conway, C. C., Forbes, M. K., Forbush, K. T., Fried, E. I., Hallquist, M. N., Kotov, R., . . . Eaton, N. R. (2019). A hierarchical taxonomy of psychopathology can transform mental health research. *Perspectives on Psychological Science, 14*(3), 419–436.

First, M. B., Rebello, T. J., Keeley, J. W., Bhargava, R., Dai, Y., Kulygina, M., . . . Reed, G. M. (2018). Do mental health professionals use diagnostic classifications the way we think they do? A global survey. *World Psychiatry,* 17(2), 187–195.

Goldfried, M. R. (2019). Obtaining consensus in psychotherapy: What holds us back? *American Psychologist, 74*(4), 484–496.

Hagerty, G. (2022). Measurement-based care in psychotherapy: The shift from symptom remission to functional wellness. *Journal of Clinical Psychology, 78*(3), 312–328.

Hayes, S. C., Hofmann, S. G., & Ciarrochi, J. (2020). *Process-based CBT: The science and core clinical competencies of cognitive behavioral therapy.* New Harbinger.

Hopwood, C. J., Bagby, R. M., Gralnick, T., Ro, E., Ruggero, C., Mullins-Sweatt, S., & Kotov, R. (2020). Integrating psychotherapy with the hierarchical taxonomy of psychopathology (HiTOP). *Journal of Psychotherapy Integration, 30*(4), 477–497.

Kotov, R., Cicero, D. C., Conway, C. C., DeYoung, C. G., Dombrovski, A., Eaton, N. R., . . . Wright, A. G. (2022). The hierarchical taxonomy of psychopathology (HiTOP) in psychiatric practice and research. *Psychological Medicine*, 52(9), 1666–1678.

Kotov, R., Krueger, R. F., Watson, D., Achenbach, T. M., Althoff, R. R., Bagby, R. M., . . . Zimmerman, M. (2017). The hierarchical taxonomy of psychopathology (HiTOP): A dimensional alternative to traditional nosologies. *Journal of Abnormal Psychology, 126*(4), 454–477.

Mayes, R., & Horwitz, A. V. (2005). DSM-III and the revolution in the classification of mental illness. *Journal of the History of the Behavioral Sciences, 41*(3), 249–267.

Michelini, G., Palumbo, I. M., DeYoung, C. G., Latzman, R. D., & Kotov, R. (2021). Linking RDoC and HiTOP: A new interface for advancing psychiatric nosology and neuroscience. *Clinical Psychology Review, 86,* 102025.

Mulay, A. L., Gottfried, E. D., Ruchensky, J. R., Russell, T., Natoli, A. P., & Hopwood, C. J. (2024). The problem no one is talking about: Forensic evaluators' lack of familiarity with dimensional approaches to personality and psychopathology. *Journal of Personality Assessment, 107*(3), 283–291.

Mullins-Sweatt, S. N., Lengel, G. J., & DeShong, H. L. (2020). Personality pathology and the hierarchical taxonomy of psychopathology (HiTOP): A review of current evidence. *Personality Disorders: Theory, Research, and Treatment, 11*(2), 79–92.

Noyes, B. K., Munoz, D. P., Khalid-Khan, S., Brietzke, E., & Booij, L. (2022). Is subthreshold depression in adolescence clinically relevant? *Journal of Affective Disorders, 309*, 123–130.

Ruggero, C. J., Callahan, J. L., Dornbach-Bender, A., Tackett, J. L., & Kotov, R. (2019). Disquiet in nosology: A primer on an emerging, empirically based approach to classifying mental illness and implications for training. *The Behavior Therapist, 42*(6), 208–211.

Ruggero, C. J., Kotov, R., Hopwood, C. J., First, M., Clark, L. A., Skodol, A. E., . . . Zimmermann, J. (2019). Integrating the hierarchical taxonomy of psychopathology (HiTOP) into clinical practice. *Journal of Consulting and Clinical Psychology, 87*(12), 1069–1084.

Wampold, B. E., & Imel, Z. E. (2015). *The great psychotherapy debate: The evidence for what makes psychotherapy work* (2nd ed.). Routledge.

Zimmerman, M. (2021). Why hierarchical dimensional approaches to classification will fail to transform diagnosis in psychiatry. *World Psychiatry, 20*(1), 70–71.

Zimmerman, M., Chelminski, I., & Posternak, M. A. (2005). Generalizability of antidepressant efficacy trials: Differences between depressed psychiatric outpatients who would or would not qualify for an efficacy trial. *American Journal of Psychiatry, 162*(7), 1370–1372.

PART II REFERENCES

American Psychiatric Association. (2013). *Diagnostic and statistical manual of mental disorders* (5th ed.). Author.

American Psychological Association. (2017). *Standards of accreditation for health service psychology*. American Psychological Association.

Bauer, M. S., & Kirchner, J. (2020). Implementation science: What is it and why should I care? *Psychiatry Research, 283*.

Bernstein, D. P., Iscan, C., & Maser, J. (2007). Opinions of personality disorder experts regarding the DSM-IV personality disorders classification system. *Journal of Personality Disorders, 21*(5), 536–551.

Bornstein, R. F., & Natoli, A. P. (2019). Clinical utility of dimensional models of personality pathology: Five recommendations for advancing the AMPD. *Personality Disorders: Theory, Research, and Treatment, 10*(1), 29–38.

Cook, J. M., Thompson, R., & Schnurr, P. P. (2009). Perceived characteristics of intervention scale: Development and psychometric properties. *Psychological Services, 6*(2), 67–75.

Crome, E., & Baillie, A. J. (2016). Better access and equitable access to clinical psychology services: What do we need to know? *The Medical Journal of Australia, 204*(9), 341–343.

Davies, H. T. O., & Nutley, S. M. (2021). Learning more about how research-based knowledge gets used: Guidance in the development of new empirical research. *Implementation Science, 16*, 56.

Feifer, C., Fifield, J., Ornstein, S., Karson, A. S., Bates, D. W., Jones, K. R., & Vargas, P. A. (2004). From research to daily clinical practice: What are the challenges in "translation"? *Joint Commission Journal on Quality and Safety, 30*(5), 235–245.

First, M. B. (2005). Clinical utility in the revision of the *Diagnostic and Statistical Manual of Mental Disorders* (DSM). *Psychopathology, 38*(4), 197–201.

Gehlbach, H., & Robinson, C. D. (2021). From old school to open science: The implications of new research norms for educational psychology and beyond. *Educational Psychologist, 56*(2), 79–89.

Kling, R., & Swygart-Hobaugh, M. (2002). The internet and the speed of publication: Field differences in publishing practices. *Information Society, 18*(5), 373–386.

Kotov, R., Krueger, R. F., Watson, D., Achenbach, T. M., Althoff, R. R., Bagby, R. M., . . . Zimmerman, M. (2017). The hierarchical taxonomy of psychopathology (HiTOP): A dimensional alternative to traditional nosologies. *Journal of Abnormal Psychology, 126*(4), 454–477.

Levy, K. N. (2022). Personality disorders and graduate training in clinical psychology: Time for a shift. *Journal of Personality Disorders, 36*(2), 150–160.

Levy, K. N., & Ellison, W. D. (2021). The current status and future directions of training in personality disorders. *Personality Disorders: Theory, Research, and Treatment, 12*(1), 1–10.

Moody, J. (2025, February 4). Big state systems were among those announcing cuts in January. *Inside Higher Ed. www.insidehighered.com/news/business/cost-cutting/2025/02/04/big-state-systems-were-among-those-announcing-cuts-january*

Morey, L. C., & Hopwood, C. J. (2019). Expert consensus and evidence-based practice: A critical hybrid approach to personality disorder diagnosis. *Personality Disorders: Theory, Research, and Treatment, 10*(1), 3–12.

Rubenstein, L. V., & Purtle, J. (2020). Dissemination and implementation research: Improving healthcare and public health practice. *Annual Review of Public Health, 41*, 235–252.

Skodol, A. E., Spitzer, R. L., & Williams, J. B. W. (1981). Rethinking the categorical distinction between Axis I and Axis II disorders. *American Journal of Psychiatry, 138*(2), 194–198.

Villanueva van den Hurk, M. C., Sellbom, M., de Ruiter, C., & de Vogel, V. (2023). MMPI-3 and MMPI-2-RF usage in clinical and forensic settings: A survey of practitioners. *Psychological Assessment, 35*(1), 1–14.

Williams, J. B. W., Spitzer, R. L., & Skodol, A. E. (1985). The classification of mental disorders: A reevaluation of the categorical approach. *Psychological Medicine, 15*(2), 467–477.

Zullig, K. J., Matthews, C. E., Robinson, C. T., & Linnan, L. A. (2024). The research-to-practice gap in health behavior change interventions. *Annual Review of Clinical Psychology, 20*, 75–99.

CHAPTER 6

Can dimensional diagnosis of psychopathology help reduce mental health stigma?

Stigma about mental health problems can increase suffering and discourage help-seeking behaviors, and thus it compounds the public and personal health burden of psychopathology. In this section, we asked experts to answer three questions regarding the possibility that moving toward dimensional diagnosis could reduce mental health stigma:

Is dimensional diagnosis less stigmatizing than categorical diagnosis?

Can the transition to dimensional approaches to diagnosis be done in such a way that helps reduce stigma?

Is there potential for dimensional diagnosis to be more stigmatizing (e.g., by implying that the problem lies within the person rather than the disease)?

Both Lahey and Corrigan and Kharbanda argue that by emphasizing the continuity between normal range and maladaptive psychological functioning, dimensional diagnoses have significant potential to reduce mental health stigma in comparison to the medical model approach that has dominated mental health research and practice. Lahey expands the definition of "dimension" beyond that of a mere continuum to suggest the replacement of categorical diagnoses with underlying dimensions that cover individual difference across the full spectrum from typical to atypical. Lahey argues that for such dimensions to help reduce stigma, changes to scientific and clinical practices must be accompanied by focused efforts toward this goal. Corrigan and Kharbanda acknowledge research showing that dimensional approaches to both diagnosis and recovery are less stigmatizing than categorical approaches but also highlight the importance of treating both public and self-stigma as a public health perspective that is not effectively addressed by our typical research approaches. They point out that previous efforts to reduced stigma have not fulfilled their promise and highlight evidence about beneficial strategies such as the value of increasing contact (i.e., incorporating the views of those with lived experience) in addition to education.

PART I

Dimensional assessment and stigma

Benjamin B. Lahey

The editors of this volume set several questions about key aspects of dimensional approaches to psychological problems for the authors of each pair of chapters to address. In this chapter, I attempt to answer the editors' three questions about the implications of shifting from categorical diagnoses of mental disorders to dimensional views of psychological problems for the stigmatization of persons with psychological problems. Our stigmatizing negative attitudes toward mental health problems in ourselves and others multiply the distress and functional impairment that is inherent in psychological problems themselves (Corrigan, 2018; Hinshaw, 2006, 2017; Lahey, 2021). Stigma hurts us in three major ways. First, if we are embarrassed that we feel anxious in the presence of strangers, for example, that embarrassment can make us feel inadequate and foster depression. Second, stigmatizing psychological problems can make it more difficult for parents to seek help for their children when they might benefit from it. Third, the stigma felt by other people about our psychological problems can lead them to treat us as less than fully human, avoid being with us, and create barriers to employment and housing that make our lives far worse.

Since 2021, I have used the term "psychological problems" as a denotative synonym for the term "psychopathology" to avoid the latter term's literal reference to sick mind. I define psychological problems as variations in behavior—broadly construed to include actions, emotions, motivations, and cognitions—that cause distress or impair the individual's life functioning (Lahey, 2021; Lahey et al., 2022).

Are Dimensional Approaches Less Stigmatizing Than Categorical Diagnosis?

There are multiple ways in which dimensional approaches to understanding and measuring psychological problems are more scientifically and practically justifiable than categorical diagnoses, including greater reliability and validity (Krueger & Markon, 2011; Lahey, 2021). Furthermore, dimensional views of psychological problems are inherently less stigmatizing than the categorical view instantiated in the DSMs and ICDs. Categorical views are based on the assumption that one either has a mental disorder or does not. This use of binary categories promotes stigma by suggesting that an individual who exhibits a psychological problem is *qualitatively different* from persons without that problem. In categorical views, a person who has recently met diagnostic criteria for, say, social anxiety disorder is now separate from other human beings because their psychological functioning has supposedly become fundamentally different.

In sharp contrast, the dimensional view portrays people as varying in their psychological functioning by matters of degree. Instead of seeing people with problems as falling into a qualitatively distinct abyss in which normal psychological functioning has been lost, it views people as differing on continua. Many studies reviewed by Lahey (2021) demonstrate that distributions of specific psychological problems ("symptoms" in DSM and ICD) are continuous. Reaching a point on the continuum of psychological functioning that warrants intervention does not mean that a person's humanity has fundamentally changed. They have simply reached a point at which it makes sense to ask for "a little help, please."

Is There Potential for Dimensional Views to Be More Stigmatizing?

The editors of this volume asked the chapter authors to consider the possibility that dimensional views may actually promote stigma by implying that the problem lies within the person rather than being attributable to the "disease." To answer this question, it is necessary to discuss the *medical model of mental disorders* and to distinguish that model from other ways of thinking about biological processes in psychological problems.

Medical Model of Psychological Problems

The medical model asserts that psychological problems are manifestations of diseases of the brain that are best treated by physicians (Guze,

1992). Many scholars argue that the medical model reduces stigma. There is less stigmatization, for example, of a person who is viewed as abusing alcohol because they have a brain disorder than because they have weak moral character (Johnson, 1989; Weiner et al., 1988). Historically, the medical model of psychological problems arose following the truly astonishing discovery by Richard Krafft-Ebing and others that the bacteria that causes syphilis often infect the brain, resulting in the debilitating syndrome of psychosis and dementia known as general paresis. When the treatment of syphilis with penicillin was perfected a hundred years later during World War II, the previously high number of persons with incident cases of general paresis fell to nearly zero in Western countries. Understandably, this electrifying mass alleviation of human suffering led to the optimistic belief that every kind of psychological problem would eventually be found to be caused by germs affecting the brain. This fostered the belief that psychological problems are medical problems and led to the founding of the medical specialty of psychiatry (Guze, 1992). The medical model has persisted even though few other infections that cause psychological problems have been discovered.

Role of Biological Processes in a Dimensional Model

A recent commentary (Hinshaw, 2022) on my earlier writings on the harmfulness of the medical model (Lahey, 2021; Lahey et al., 2022) told me that I had not been clear in distinguishing the disadvantages of the medical model from the value of research on the biology of psychological problems. I was misunderstood as saying that a rejection of the medical model would mean that psychological problems are merely psychological and that biological processes play no part. I actually argued that it would be entirely *incorrect* to understand a rejection of the medical model as a rejection of the role of biological processes in psychological problems.

Psychology and biology are inherently inseparable. Like most scientists, I take a monistic view in which psychological and biological processes are the same phenomena considered at different levels of analysis. One cannot type a word without a corresponding process occurring in the brain. And we can improve our understanding of typing—and all adaptive or maladaptive dimensions of behavior—by studying them at both complementary psychological and biological levels. We most definitely should search for individual differences in biology that are correlated with psychological problems (Lahey et al., 1993, 2024). Everything we learn about variations in biology will help construct a tapestry of evidence that will help us better understand and beneficially modify psychological problems. The issue is how we should think about the biological side of correlations between brain and behavior? It is not only an important question in the philosophy of science (Harden, 2023), it has enormous implications for the stigmatization of psychological problems. There are three facets of this issue:

1. Are relationships between biological variables and psychological problems *deterministic*? Variations brain structure and function, which are influenced to a degree by genetic variation, do not cause psychological problems in any deterministic sense. Rather, they transact with our varying environmental experiences to increase or decrease the likelihood of psychological problems (Lahey, 2021). Genes are not destiny in any sphere of our lives (Plomin, 1986). Even monozygotic twins with identical DNA sequences can differ considerably in their psychological problems (Kato et al., 2005).

2. Does biology have *primacy* in our understanding of psychological problems? No, the association between brain and behavior is bidirectional: Psychological interventions that reduce distressing emotions simultaneously change brain functioning, just as psychoactive medications that change brain functioning also reduce distressing emotions (Nord et al., 2021).

3. When, if ever, is it useful to think of individual differences in brain structure or function as *brain diseases*? If the numbers of postsynaptic receptors for a neurotransmitter are found to have an inverse linear association with increased risk for a specific dimension of psychological problems, should we view lower numbers of this receptor as brain pathology? What about the replicated linear inverse association between global gray matter volume and risk for essentially all dimensions of psychological problems (Durham et al., 2021)? Such linear associations stretch the concept of brain disease, but is it sensible to speak of brain disease for relatively binary conditions such as the presence of a neoplasm, necrotic brain cells following ischemic stroke, or the presence of spirochete bacteria in the brain?

My own conclusion is that viewing individual differences in biology as pathology is sometimes justifiable when medical treatments are available that can solve the specific biological problem, such as antibacterial medication to treat brain infections, but otherwise there seems to be little benefit in terming the variations in biology associated with psychological problems as pathology. There is, of course, every reason to provide medical treatments to persons with treatable infections that cause psychological problems and psychoactive medications that reduce psychological problems even without a clear understanding of the biological targets that may have favorable risk/benefit ratios. Nonetheless, there is a clear downside in viewing individual differences in biology as the disease that causes mental illness when there is no need to do so. We should, for example, make every effort to eschew the view that individual differences in biological processes that accompany the onset of an episode of impairing depression reflect a healthy brain becoming *sick*. There is considerable evidence from experimental studies that this view of psychological problems is harmful. When persons are described as having psychological problems that are attributable to genes and brain dysfunction, that attribution reduces blaming the person for their behavior but increases a perception that the persons is dangerous and unpredictable and increases pessimism regarding improvement (Haslam & Kvaale, 2015; Kvaale et al., 2013; Kvaale & Haslam, 2016; Lebowitz et al., 2013)

The Analogical Medical Model

It is very important to note that the medical model took on a very different and broader meaning when few additional links between germs and psychological problems were discovered by encompassing metaphorical "diseases of the mind"—syndromes of mental "symptoms" without known biological illness (Klerman, 1977). The concept of mental illness has become entrenched among both the public and professionals. Most psychologists and psychiatrists who are active today were trained to believe that they can discern the difference between "normal" and "abnormal" minds and thereby "diagnose mental illnesses." This analogical view has nothing to do with either biology or medicine and should be strictly avoided. Sixty years ago, psychiatrist Thomas Szasz similarly advocated replacing medical model terms such as mental illness with the less judgmental term, "problems in living" (Szasz, 1960, 1974). Szasz has been widely misunderstood as denying the existence of psychological problems. He explicitly did not do so, but he denied the meaningfulness of the concept of mental illnesses based on an analogy to medical illness.

Most of us refer to psychological problems with medical model terms such as "mental illnesses," "mental disorders," or "psychopathology." We generally use these analog medical model terms in caring ways, but they are profoundly stigmatizing terms. They say that our psychological problems are the result of "illness," "disorder," and "pathology." This is an entirely fictional and baseless notion that is toxic to people. Telling people that psychological problems are the result of terrifying change from a normal to an abnormal mind promotes the worst kind of stigma.

Can the Transition to Dimensional Approaches to Diagnosis Be Accomplished in a Way That Helps Reduce Stigma?

Changing the systems that provide care for people with psychological problems to one that is not based on binary medical model diagnoses will require visionary leadership from persons with expertise in the psychological sciences, finance, and politics. Before committing ourselves to this daunting undertaking, we will have to be convinced that such a revolution will have enough benefits to people with problems to warrant and sustain it. Stated differently, we must be certain that the proposed dimensional revolution will do no harm to the persons we are trying to help.

This is to say that we must conduct the relevant research before trying to convince the field and the public that dimensional approaches are better. Two different kinds of research are particularly needed. First, we must conduct better research using large samples of the population to fully describe the distributions of dimensions of psychological problems, how they vary among social groups, and how they change over development. Some important studies have already been conducted, but they have usually used measures that were suitable for categorical diagnoses and not for mapping dimensions. Very importantly, however, these early studies revealed that psychological problems are so *much more common* in the population than we realized (Moffitt et al., 2010). This realization has enormous implications for stigma. When we—both the mental health profession and the general public—understand that the *great majority of us* will experience problems like fear, anxiety, sadness, or cravings for addictive substances at some time in our lives, it will be harder to stigmatize psychological problems. Psychological problems are not rarefied things that are experienced by a few people with diseased minds; they are quite ordinary things that nearly all of us experience.

To illustrate the point, several large longitudinal studies of the general population have been conducted in which the same individuals were asked about their psychological problems multiple times from early adolescence through middle adulthood. These studies (Schaefer et al., 2017) tell us that *80% of people in the general population* met DSM diagnostic criteria for at least one mental disorder at least once during the decades they were studied. Note, too, that these studies only reported the prevalence of meeting *full DSM diagnostic criteria* for a mental disorder. Far more people reported psychological problems that were just below the official DSM threshold for a diagnosis. Therefore, even the remarkable finding that *most* of us will meet full DSM criteria for a mental disorder at some point in our lives understates the ordinariness of psychological problems.

Second, before we commit ourselves to dimensional approaches we must follow the same rules for establishing that any new intervention is evidence based. Although I am personally convinced that moving the practice of providing mental health services based on categorical DSM and ICD diagnoses to the use of empirically based continuous dimensions of psychological problems will improve the lives of people with problems, beginning efforts to provide clinical services based on dimensional approaches (Kotov et al., 2022) is premature until randomized trials have been conducted to compare dimensional approaches to treatment as usual. The history of psychology and psychiatry is littered with ineffective and sometimes harmful treatments that were based on personal views; we must temper our enthusiasm and promulgate evidence-based approaches to human suffering. Fortunately, the author of the chapter on stigma that is paired with this one is one of the leading experts on such intervention research (Corrigan et al., 2017).

PART II

Decreasing stigma with dimensional diagnoses

Does it matter?

Patrick W. Corrigan and Vardha Kharbanda

DSM diagnoses have been viewed as a source of stigma for more than 20 years (Ben-Zeev et al., 2010). Categorical description of people in terms of diagnostic labels enhances the differentness of this group, which is at stigma's core. Dimensional models seem to offer more variability in understanding personal experiences. We begin this chapter with a brief review of the "what" of mental illness stigma, distinguishing public from self-stigma. This will include a summary of research on effective ways to reduce stigma. We then address the three questions posed by the editors about how dimensional perspectives influence public and self-stigma.

What Is the Stigma of Mental Illness?

Researchers have adopted social psychological structures of bigotry to distinguish two types of mental illness stigma: public stigma and self-stigma (Corrigan et al., 2005). These psychological structures include stereotypes (seemingly factual beliefs about a group that present that group poorly; e.g., people with mental illness are dangerous, incompetent, or blameworthy) and prejudice (agreement with the stereotypes leading to negative emotions; e.g., people with mental illness are dangerous and I am afraid of them). Public stigma occurs when the naïve population agrees with stereotypes and acts accordingly. Discrimination is the behavioral result. People who are labeled with mental illness are less able to obtain rightful life opportunities related to education, work, independent living, and good health care because of a stigmatizing public. Self-stigma reflects the harm of internalizing these stigmas on one's self. The discrimination of self-stigma results in the "why try" effect (Corrigan et al., 2016): Why try to get a job when I am not worthy? Why try to live on my own when I am not worth it?

Stigmas are evoked by cues. These cues are obvious for many human conditions including ethnicity (skin color) and gender (body features). However, the stigmatizing condition is mostly hidden for other conditions including sexual orientation, education, and health conditions. Mental illness most often falls in the latter category and is signaled by a label (Link & Phelan, 2001): "That's Harry coming out of the psychiatrist's office. He must be nuts!" (Ben-Zeev et al., 2010). Diagnostic categories have reified an exquisitely complex phenomenon that sorts people and their experiences into good/healthy and bad/sick boxes.

One caveat going forward, especially for chapter readers who are researchers is to beware the esoteric! Stigma is an issue of the population at hand and not highly educated mental health providers. Disentangling the nuance of factor and network analyses that lead to psychiatric dimensions is foreign to the average person who agrees with stereotypes and discriminates against people accordingly. Nor, by the way, is this public likely to be swayed by dimensional arguments. The question here is therefore not so much if dimensional diagnoses are less stigmatizing per se—they may very well be—but whether dimensional diagnoses will change the way mental health workers apply diagnoses.

Are Dimensional Diagnoses Less Stigmatizing Than Categorical Diagnoses?

Significant research has already shown that mental health experiences presented as a continuum show significantly less public stigma than when presented as categories. Categorical perspectives stress the difference between the person with the label and everyone else. The difference is at the heart of stigma because it frames the label as "not like me," and the difference is anchored in disdain (Link & Phelan, 2001). People who vary from the normal are said to be weak, incompetent, or maybe even dangerous. Two case vignettes illustrate the difference.

- Case 1. John is diagnosed with schizophrenia, has hallucinations, and has been hospitalized for his illness.
- Case 2. Mary is diagnosed with schizophrenia and has hallucinatory behaviors, which are experienced by much of the general population, especially related to sleep. Many people receive treatment for mental illness including occasional hospital stays.

The first is about John who is reduced to the categorical diagnosis of schizophrenia with hallucinations and hospitalizations. The label along with what seem to be bizarre experiences—hallucinations—that lead to hospitalizations are viewed by most as foreign and frightening. In the second vignette, Mary's hallucinations and hospitalizations are described from a more fluid perspective. As research shows, hallucinations are not necessarily a black-and-white certainty of severe mental illness. More than 37% of the population reported sleep-related, hypnogogic hallucinations up to twice weekly over the year before a survey (Ohayon et al., 1996). Hospitalization was framed as a possible treatment option for a variety of mental health challenges. Mary's story is on a continuum that places her experiences amid every person. Difference is minimized so stigma is reduced.

Findings from a recent meta-analysis examined what studies have found about continuum beliefs (Peter et al., 2021). Seven studies were cross-sectional, examining correlates to endorsement of continuum beliefs. Higher continuum beliefs were found to be associated with less social distance, fear, anger, dangerousness, and unpredictability. Separate population research showed significant change in continuum beliefs from 2011 to 2020, although the effect varied by diagnosis (Schomerus et al., 2023). Greater continuum beliefs were observed for depression but not for schizophrenia.

The other studies in the meta-analysis examined the use of continuum beliefs as a strategy to decrease stigma. The typical design was randomizing participants to continuum versus categorical manipulations using brief vignettes like those of John and Mary telling their story consistent with categories or continua. All but one of these studies yielded positive results.

Recovery as Continuum

A separate body of research related to recovery also suggests the value of a dimensional (continuum) model. Recovery emerged as the foil to poor prognosis models of serious mental illness such as schizophrenia that dominated psychiatry in the 1900s. Schizophrenia, for example, was thought to result in a progressive downhill course (Kraepelin, 1896). Several long-term follow-up research projects were completed to test this assertion. People with schizophrenia in these studies were typically identified while in a psychiatric hospital and followed from 10 to 30 years. Findings from 10 long-term follow-up studies examined the end state (Corrigan et al., 2024). If Kraepelin was right, we would expect the vast majority of people with schizophrenia still to be symptomatic, dysfunctional, and not working or living independently at follow-up. Findings indicated that roughly half of the participants recovered or significantly improved over the long term, suggesting that remission or recovery is much more common than originally thought. Benign *outcomes* are a reality.

Many scholars, however, argue that recovery as a possible outcome is limiting (van Weeghel et al., 2019). Framing recovery in black-and-white statements about people, such as propositions that people with serious mental illness can be symptom free and obtain personally important life goals, ignores the fact that recovery is a *process*. Despite experiencing recurring symptoms and disabilities, people with serious mental illness should be hopeful and actively pursue their aspirations (Slade et al., 2012). Recovery is a personal journey where treatment may have value but reasonable accommodations are equally necessary. Recovery as a binary outcome may unintentionally exacerbate stigma because people who do not meet the criteria of a positive outcome are somehow not recovered and therefore should consider amending their goals. Recovery as an outcome may be another "categorical" signal leading to negative prognoses. Personal recovery and life journey correspond more clearly with the fluidity of life goals (process). Research, however, shows that stigma and personal recovery as processes are inversely associated (Cunningham & Lucksted, 2017).

Can the Transition to Dimensional Diagnosis Help Reduce Stigma?

Advocates who want to use dimensionality to decrease stigma may consider what research says about how public stigma is best changed. The naïve response is education: prepare webinars or public service announcements where stigma is challenged and opportunity results. Educational approaches contrast myths of mental illness (e.g., people with serious mental illness are unable to obtain meaningful careers) with facts (e.g., people with serious mental illness can achieve even their highest aspirations). Education is often contrasted with contact: stigma is diminished when people with lived experience interact as peers with the general population. Meta-analyses and systematic reviews fairly consistently show that effect sizes for contact are fairly robust, whereas those for education are significantly smaller and may disappear at follow-up (McCullock & Scrivano, 2023).

One study examined how continuum messages interact with education versus contact (Corrigan et al., 2017). Main effects supported expectations: stigma decreased in research participants exposed to contact versus education and continuum versus categorical messaging. Although the interaction—contact and continuum messages—failed to reach significance for measures of stigma, those receiving this combination showed a significant increase in affirming attitudes; namely, people with mental illness recover. Research has elucidated the successful aspects of contact-based stigma change (Corrigan, 2011); people with lived experience lead the anti-stigma effort and others (professionals) are allies. Thus, efforts to strategically use dimensionality to erase stigma must ensure that people with lived experience lead the program.

Might Dimensional Diagnoses Be More Stigmatizing?

Advocates and researchers using dimensional diagnoses need to be vigilant for possible unintended consequences in anti-stigma efforts: efforts that seemingly should decrease stigma but that seem to have little benefit (like education) or that make stigma worse. One approach stands out: calling mental illness a brain disorder. Once a popular tagline, advocates thought framing mental illness in terms of neuroscience would decrease blame toward people with serious mental illness. Similarly, anti-stigma efforts have tried to decrease stigma by framing psychopathology just like any illness. Although medical modeling might reduce blame toward people with serious mental illness, it also decreases recovery beliefs (Loughman & Haslam, 2018).

Replacing categorical diagnoses with continuous dimensions is a clear step away from medical models and the unintended consequences of biologically framing mental illness, which is another reason why dimensional models may diminish stigma. Still, this area of research comes out of a psychopathology paradigm where neuroscience reductionism dominates. Consequently, advocates and scientists who seek to use dimensional diagnosis as a way to reduce stigma should be vigilant to this risk.

Summary and Conclusions

Messages play one part in decreasing the stigma of mental illness. Framing diagnoses as dimensions reflect the power of continuum messages and thus may have value in anti-stigma programs. However, research suggests that the processes of the anti-stigma approach, and in particular increasing contact between people with and without psychiatric diagnoses, have a greater effect than content-based approaches such as educating the public. Therefore, efforts to use dimensionality to decrease stigma must surpass simple education programs and webinars, instead finding ways in which people with lived experience make it part of their anti-stigma stories. Readers of this book are consumers of research on psychopathology and thus oriented to rigorous approaches to science that might gravitate toward educational approaches. Clinical researchers seeking stigma change need to be up to date on the science of stigma change. They need to collaborate with people with lived experience in empirical evaluations of approaches to determine the benefits of approaches as well as unintended consequences.

PART I REFERENCES

Corrigan, P. W. (2018). *The stigma effect: Unintended consequences of mental health campaigns.* Columbia University Press.

Corrigan, P. W., Schmidt, A., Bink, A. B., Nieweglowski, K., Al-Khouja, M. A., Qin, S., & Discont, S. (2017). Changing public stigma with continuum beliefs. *Journal of Mental Health, 26*(5), 411–418.

Durham, E. L., Jeong, H. J., Moore, T. M., Dupont, R. M., Cardenas-Iniguez, C., Cui, Z., . . . Kaczkurkin, A. N. (2021). Association of gray matter volumes with general and specific dimensions of psychopathology in children. *Neuropsychopharmacology, 46*(7), 1333–1339.

Guze, S. B. (1992). *Why psychiatry is a branch of medicine.* Oxford University Press.

Harden, K. P. (2023). Genetic determinism, essentialism and reductionism: Semantic clarity for contested science. *Nature Reviews Genetics, 24*(3), 197–204.

Haslam, N., & Kvaale, E. P. (2015). Biogenetic explanations of mental disorder: The mixed-blessings model. *Current Directions in Psychological Science, 24*(5), 399–404.

Hinshaw, S. P. (2006). *The mark of shame: Stigma of mental illness and an agenda for change.* Oxford University Press.

Hinshaw, S. P. (2017). *Another kind of madness: A journey through the stigma and hope of mental illness.* St. Martin's Press.

Hinshaw, S. P. (2022). Psychological problems, biomedical models, and stigma: A commentary on Lahey et al. (2022). *JCPP Advances, 2*(4), e12119.

Johnson, D. L. (1989). Schizophrenia as a brain disease: Implications for psychologists and families. *American Psychologist, 44,* 553–555.

Kato, T., Iwamoto, K., Kakiuchi, C., Kuratomi, G., & Okazaki, Y. (2005). Genetic or epigenetic difference causing discordance between monozygotic twins as a clue to molecular basis of mental disorders. *Molecular Psychiatry, 10*(7), 622–630.

Klerman, G. L. (1977). Mental illness, medical model, and psychiatry. *Journal of Medicine and Philosophy, 2*(3), 220–243.

Kotov, R., Cicero, D. C., Conway, C. C., DeYoung, C. G., Dombrovski, A., Eaton, N. R., . . . Wright, A. G. C. (2022). The hierarchical taxonomy of psychopathology (HiTOP) in psychiatric practice and research. *Psychological Medicine, 52*(9), 1666–1678.

Krueger, R. F., & Markon, K. E. (2011). A dimensional-spectrum model of psychopathology: Progress and opportunities. *Archives of General Psychiatry, 68,* 10–11.

Kvaale, E. P., Gottdiener, W. H., & Haslam, N. (2013). Biogenetic explanations and stigma: A meta-analytic review of associations among laypeople. *Social Science & Medicine, 96,* 95–103.

Kvaale, E. P., & Haslam, N. (2016). Motivational orientations and psychiatric stigma: Social motives influence how causal explanations relate to stigmatizing attitudes. *Personality and Individual Differences, 89,* 111–116.

Lahey, B. B. (2021). *Dimensions of psychological problems: Replacing diagnostic categories with a more science-based and less stigmatizing alternative.* Oxford University Press.

Lahey, B. B., Durham, E. L., Brislin, S. J., Barr, P. B., Dick, D. M., Moore, T. M., . . . Kaczkurkin, A. N. (2024). Mapping potential pathways from polygenic liability through brain structure to psychological problems across the transition to adolescence. *Journal of Child Psychology and Psychiatry, 65*(8), 1047–1060.

Lahey, B. B., Hart, E. L., Pliszka, S., Applegate, B., & McBurnett, K. (1993). Neuropsychological correlates of conduct disorder: A rationale and review of research. *Journal of Clinical Child Psychology, 22*(2), 141–153.

Lahey, B. B., Tiemeier, H., & Krueger, R. F. (2022). Seven reasons why binary diagnostic categories should be replaced with empirically sounder and less stigmatizing dimensions. *JCPP Advances, 2,* e12108.

Lebowitz, M. S., Ahn, W. K., & Nolen-Hoeksema, S. (2013). Fixable or fate? Perceptions of the biology of depression. *Journal of Consulting and Clinical Psychology, 81*(3), 518–527.

Moffitt, T. E., Caspi, A., Taylor, A., Kokaua, J., Milne, B. J., Polanczyk, G., & Poulton, R. (2010). How common are common mental disorders? Evidence that lifetime prevalence rates are doubled by prospective versus retrospective ascertainment. *Psychological Medicine, 40,* 899–909.

Nord, C. L., Barrett, L. F., Lindquist, K. A., Ma, Y. N., Marwood, L., Satpute, A. B., & Dalgleish, T. (2021). Neural effects of antidepressant medication and psychological treatments: a quantitative synthesis across three meta-analyses. *British Journal of Psychiatry, 219*(4), 546–550.

Plomin, R. (1986). *Development, genetics and psychology.* Erlbaum.

Schaefer, J. D., Caspi, A., Belsky, D. W., Harrington, H., Houts, R., Horwood, L. J., . . . Moffitt, T. E. (2017). Enduring mental health: prevalence and prediction. *Journal of Abnormal Psychology, 126*(2), 212–224.

Szasz, T. S. (1960). The myth of mental illness. *American Psychologist, 15*(2), 113–118.

Szasz, T. S. (1974). *Myth of mental illness: Foundations of a theory of personal conduct.* Harper.

Weiner, B., Perry, R. P., & Magnusson, J. (1988). An attributional analysis of reactions to stigmas. *Journal of Personality and Social Psychology, 55,* 738–748.

PART II REFERENCES

Ben-Zeev, D., Young, M. A., & Corrigan, P. W. (2010). DSM-V and the stigma of mental illness. *Journal of Mental Health, 19*(4), 318–327.

Corrigan, P. W. (2011). Best practices: Strategic stigma change (SSC): Five principles for social marketing campaigns to reduce stigma. *Psychiatric Services, 62*(8), 824–826.

Corrigan, P. W., Bink, A. B., Schmidt, A., Jones, N., & Rüsch, N. (2016). What is the impact of self-stigma? Loss of self-respect and the "why try" effect. *Journal of Mental Health, 25*(1), 10–15.

Corrigan, P. W., Kerr, A., & Knudsen, L. (2005). The stigma of mental illness: Explanatory models and methods for change. *Applied and Preventive Psychology, 11*(3), 179–190.

Corrigan, P. W., Rüsch, N., Watson, A. C., Kosyluk, K., & Sheehan, L. (2024). *Principles and practice of psychiatric rehabilitation: Promoting recovery and self-determination* (3rd ed.). Guilford Press.

Corrigan, P. W., Schmidt, A., Bink, A. B., Nieweglowski, K., Al-Khouja, M. A., Qin, S., & Discont, S. (2017). Changing public stigma with continuum beliefs. *Journal of Mental Health, 26*(5), 411–418.

Cunningham, K. C., & Lucksted, A. (2017). Social cognition, internalized stigma, and recovery orientation among adults with serious mental illness. *Psychiatric Rehabilitation Journal, 40*(4), 409–411.

Kraepelin, E. (1896). *Psychiatrie: Ein Lehrbuch fur Studirende und Aerzte. https://search.worldcat.org/title/68264358*

Link, B. G., & Phelan, J. C. (2001). Conceptualizing stigma. *Annual Review of Sociology, 27*(1), 363–385.

Loughman, A., & Haslam, N. (2018). Neuroscientific explanations and the stigma of mental disorder: A meta-analytic study. *Cognitive Research: Principles and Implications, 3*(1), 43.

McCullock, S. P., & Scrivano, R. M. (2023). The effectiveness of mental illness stigma-reduction interventions: A systematic meta-review of meta-analyses. *Clinical Psychology Review, 100,* 102242.

Ohayon, M. M., Priest, R. G., Caulet, M., & Guilleminault, C. (1996). Hypnagogic and hypnopompic hallucinations: Pathological phenomena? *British Journal of Psychiatry, 169*(4), 459–467.

Peter, S. C., Horn, T. L., McPhail, A., Meyers, A. W., & Whelan, J. P. (2021). Frequent gamblers' reasons for and against completing a problem gambling screener. *Journal of Gambling Studies, 37*(4), 1335–1346.

Schomerus, G., Schindler, S., Baumann, E., & Angermeyer, M. C. (2023). Changes in continuum beliefs for depression and schizophrenia in the general population 2011–2020: A widening gap. *Social Psychiatry and Psychiatric Epidemiology, 58*(1), 17–23.

Slade, M., Leamy, M., Bacon, F., Janosik, M., Le Boutillier, C., Williams, J., & Bird, V. (2012). International differences in understanding recovery: A systematic review. *Epidemiology and Psychiatric Sciences, 21*(4), 353–364.

Van Weeghel, J., Van Zelst, C., Boertien, D., & Hasson-Ohayon, I. (2019). Conceptualizations, assessments, and implications of personal recovery in mental illness: A scoping review of systematic reviews and meta-analyses. *Psychiatric Rehabilitation Journal, 42*(2), 169–181.

CHAPTER 7

What is the intersection between dimensional diagnosis and diversity, equity, and inclusion?

Issues of diversity, equity, and inclusion have come into increasing focus in mental health during the last decade, coincident with the momentum toward dimensional diagnosis. Shifts in diagnostic models offer opportunities to address systemic injustice in mental health care but may also create new challenges. In this section, we asked experts to answer three questions regarding the intersection between dimensional diagnosis and diversity, equity, and inclusion:

Does dimensional diagnosis have the potential to make mental health care more inclusive?

Can it make mental health training more inclusive?

How can the transition to dimensional diagnosis be done in a way that would be more forward-thinking about DEI issues?

Asadi et al. argue that dimensional models have the potential to make mental health care more inclusive by their multidimensional nature and because they are more conducive to psychometric study but note that so far dimensional models have mostly adopted the universalist decontextualized assumptions of categorical models. They argue that the incorporation of intersectional theories in diagnosis, psychopathology research, and training have the potential to advance a more contextualized approach to mental health. Pedersen et al.

assert that by focusing on the whole person, dimensional models have greater potential than categorical models do to place people's problems in their sociocultural context. At the same time, they note that research methods used to derive dimensional models typically do not incorporate context and do not account for mechanisms that can address the role of context. They emphasize the importance of centering psychopathology research on the lived experience of diverse people to move forward.

PART I

Integrating dimensions of context within dimensional diagnosis

SHAYAN ASADI, SIENNA NIELSEN, and CRAIG RODRIGUEZ-SEIJAS

Dimensional diagnosis[1] has the potential to improve both the science and practice of clinical assessment, diagnosis, and intervention. The purpose of this chapter, however, is to discuss some issues pertaining to dimensional diagnosis and diversity, equity, and inclusion considerations. Our major focus for this chapter will be on how dimensional diagnostic/classification models of psychopathology integrate sociocontextual factors within their remit. As it stands, sociocontextual factors are underresearched and underintegrated in *all* nosologies—be they dimensional or categorical. The urgency of integrating sociocontextual factors is underscored by evidence of mental health disparities in minoritized populations (Langwerden et al., 2021). One step to ameliorating health disparities is to implement dimensional assessment (Eaton et al., 2021) because dimensional classifications systems—like the hierarchical taxonomy of psychopathology (HiTOP)—can capture psychopathology with improved validity and reliability relative to categorical paradigms (Kotov et al., 2017). The next step, and most pertinent to this chapter, is integrating sociocontextual factors within dimensions of psychopathology.

We use the language of sociocontextual factors in this discussion. For our purposes, we use sociocontextual factors as a catch-all for the myriad factors *outside* of the individual that can affect the mental health and well-being *within* the person. Sociocontextual factors refer

[1] We use the term "diagnosis" here to refer to the identification of a psychological problem that can route an individual to intervention.

to aspects of the environment that stretch beyond—yet fundamentally affect—inter- and intrapersonal factors. Yet, they are not often the levels of focus in mainstream psychopathology theory and research. They include the political and social climates in which individuals exist. They are particularly important to understand and incorporate when considering the psychosocial health of individuals from diverse, underrepresented, and epistemically excluded (Settles et al., 2020) populations. In mainstream psychopathology theory, research, and practice, sociocontextual factors are typically operationalized as categorical demographic proxies for the ways structural and societal level factors shape how individuals interact with their worlds and vice versa.

Does Dimensional Diagnosis Have the Potential to Make Mental Health Care More Inclusive

Potentially. Dimensional diagnosis can make mental health care more inclusive, contingent on how well sociocontextual factors are integrated into the dimensional model.

How Are Sociocontextual Factors Integrated in Traditional Categorical Diagnosis?

DSM-5 instantiates sociocontextual processes through the language and definitions of "culture." DSM-5's working definition of "culture" refers to the "language, religion and spirituality, family structures, life-cycle stages, ceremonial rituals, and customs, as well as moral and legal systems" (American Psychiatric Association, 2013, p. 14). We see parallels with "moral and legal systems" and our focus of sociocontextual factors, with particular emphasis on social norms, systems, and structures that influence individual behavior. Thus, a focus on sociocontextual considerations is indeed compatible with the traditional categorical nosology. However, other inherent limitations of the traditional categorical approach, in our opinions, present difficulties in the practical incorporation of sociocontextual factors.

For instance, categorical disorders and their constituent criteria are thought to be universal across groups and sociocultural contexts. Thus, culture-related diagnostic issues are—arguably—conceptualized as glitches within a universal diagnostic system. Integrating sociocontextual issues can fundamentally contradict assumptions that polythetic behavioral indicators of an assumedly static underlying categorical psychiatric disorder apply universally. Identity disturbance as a diagnostic criterion for borderline personality disorder, for instance, is more frequently endorsed among sexual and gender minority individuals (Goldhammer et al., 2019; Rodriguez-Seijas et al., 2021). However, without critical understanding of the sociocontextual factors (i.e., minority stress processes) that sexual and gender minority individuals experience, behaviors related to identity experiences among gender-diverse individuals in the face of cissexism and heterosexism can become misconstrued as evidence for a borderline personality disorder diagnosis (Goldhammer et al., 2019; Rodriguez-Seijas, Rogers, et al., 2023) rather than recognizing that these behaviors are affected by minority stress processes that are a fundamental part of the sociocontextual experiences of individuals with sexual and gender minority identities—that is, normatively expectable (e.g., Nielsen et al., 2024).

How Are Sociocontextual Factors Integrated in Dimensional Systems?

Dimensional psychopathology models improve on myriad limitations of the traditional categorical classification system—high comorbidity, poor construct validity, limited reliability, artificial discontinuity (Kotov et al., 2017). One advantage that we consider particularly relevant for the incorporation of sociocontextual factors within the dimensional framework is the relative plurality of psychopathology dimensions; individuals vary across multiple dimensions instead of having/not having a specific disorder. In addition, the relative ease with which empirical evidence can drive modification and adjustment of dimensional models (e.g., HiTOP structural revisions; Forbes et al., 2024) would suggest that dimensional psychopathology models can theoretically accommodate a plurality of associations between behaviors and underlying psychopathology dimensions by virtue of the influence of various sociocontextual factors.

As behavioral indicators reflect underlying dimensions, one can incorporate differential functioning of specific behaviors into dimensional psychopathology models. For instance, understanding that due to sociocontextual factors, engaging in casual sexual behavior is a more normative behavior among some sexual minority populations as a part of positive identity and sexual development in the face of chronic stigma (Hanna-Walker et al., 2023) can be used to explicitly test how sexual behaviors differentially relate to underlying psychopathology dimensions. Casual sexual behavior and substance use during sex might be more strongly related to dimensions of impulsivity and disinhibition among sexual majority rather than sexual minority individuals (Asadi et al., 2025; Rodriguez-Seijas et al., 2024). And a plurality of indicators can be explicitly integrated within dimensional models like HiTOP

(Rodriguez-Seijas, Li, et al., 2023), making them particularly relevant for better capturing the influence of sociocontextual processes that are relevant for diverse and marginalized populations (Eaton et al., 2021).

What the above illustration demonstrates, however, is that the use of sociocontextual factors to guide research often remains at the identity-grouping level. The focus for understanding mental health among underrepresented and marginalized populations remains at the level of the proxy identity variable, as it remains in research using categorical domains. At this time, dimensional psychopathology models remain overwhelmingly decontextualized, with sociocultural context relegated to the fringes. Indeed, we have previously outlined how the philosophy of dimensional psychopathology models like HiTOP reflect epistemologies that are similar to those of the dominant categorical approaches, much to the detriment of underrepresented, marginalized, and epistemically excluded populations (Rodriguez-Seijas, Li, et al., 2023). We have also outlined how the social decontextualization affects other dimensional models like the alternative model for personality disorders (AMPD; Rodriguez-Seijas, Rogers, et al., 2023). Similarly, the environment is ill-integrated into the National Institute of Mental Health's Research Domain Criteria (RDoC). Environment is included in the model as a determinant of psychopathology (Cuthbert, 2022) but is not meaningfully integrated within the model as either a domain that can shape psychopathology or as a unit of analysis that can be used to understand psychopathology. So, dimensional models of psychopathology are not *inherently* more inclusive.

How Can the Transition to Dimensional Diagnosis Be Done in a Way That Would Be More Forward-Thinking about Diversity, Equity, and Inclusivity Issues?

Intersectionality Theory to Inform Dimensions of Context

Intersectionality theory (Cole, 2009; Crenshaw, 1991) lays down a useful foundation for understanding social context via systems of power, privilege, and disadvantage. Intersectionality is not a testable theory per se. Rather, it reflects an "analytic sensibility" (Cho et al., 2013), or a way of thinking that can inform the analyses that one conducts. In that vein, we can draw from psychological theories that are intersectionally informed to guide testable hypotheses about how social contexts affect dimensions of psychopathology. In intersectional frameworks, aspects of an individual's identity (e.g., race, sex/gender, sexual orientation) are tied to the social power and disadvantage associated with them.

Psychological Theories Bridge Intersectionality and Psychopathology Research

Sociocontextual factors interact with dimensions of psychopathology in ways that are nonlinear and nonadditive, with components that are both nomothetic and idiographic. And so, no one theory alone can link context to psychopathology for all individuals. Understanding sociocontextual factors as described in critical intersectionality-based theories—such as minority stress theory (Meyer, 2003), racial identity frameworks (Sellers et al., 1998), and adversity frameworks (Hyde et al., 2022; McLaughlin et al., 2014)—can inform the assessment and integration of sociocontextual factors within dimensional psychopathology literature to the benefit of underrepresented populations. Furthermore, their incorporation can help stakeholders to focus beyond the individual and sidestep mistakes of assuming essentialist conclusions based on identity groupings. Sociocontextual factors determine the identity variables and not the other way around.

For example, sexual and gender minority stress theories focus on how heterosexism and cissexism create different levels of stigma that increase vulnerability for psychopathology in sexual and gender minority individuals (Meyer, 2003; Tan et al., 2020). Similarly, theories of ethnic identity—like the multidimensional theory of Black identity (Sellers et al., 1998)—highlight how identity salience, centrality, regard, and ideology are dimensions of Black Americans' identities that influence their well-being and stress (Pascoe & Smart Richman, 2009). Racial socialization theories focus on how individuals learn about their ethnic/cultural identities and which messages about ethnicity/race are internalized, with implications for psychological well-being (Neblett et al., 2008). The dimensions outlined in Black identity frameworks are individual-level dimensions that originate from the experiences of being an African American person in the United States. They are descended from a critical understanding of policies and societal perspectives that historically disadvantage Black Americans. Theories of racial and ethnic development also integrate traumatic historical experiences as determinants of psychopathology, such as slavery and Jim Crow-era laws in the United States (Murry et al., 2018) and residential schools for indigenous populations in North America (Gone, 2023). Thus, critical understanding of how power and privilege underlie sociocontextual factors is fundamental in understanding psychopathology and psychiatric disparities.

Sociocontextual factors also operate outside of the individual and span factors that are broader than the immediate interpersonal sphere of that individual (Bronfenbrenner, 1977). One example is socioeconomic status, which has long been studied as an environmental determinant of health and development. Components of socioeconomic status (e.g., parental education, receipt of public income) are related to psychopathology in children (Peverill et al., 2021). However, socioeconomic status operates on multiple levels, including at the neighborhood level, where differential exposure to environmental toxins in more deprived neighborhoods may reduce resources for cognitive development in children (Hyde et al., 2022). These external factors differentially affect specific populations based on historical sociopolitical processes. For instance, redlining—where denial of loans to Black residents led to divestment in primarily Black neighborhoods in the United States (Bailey et al., 2021)—is one determinant of poorer neighborhood socioeconomic status and, in-turn, poverty. One study found that neighborhood poverty is associated with trauma-related psychopathology in primarily lower income Black women when controlling for racial discrimination (Ravi et al., 2023). Another study found no direct relationship with low versus high redlining and anxiety in Black adults in Detroit, Michigan, but found an indirect relationship between redlining status and higher anxiety through higher experiences of discrimination (Pearson et al., 2023). Thus, understanding sociocontextual processes becomes important for understanding psychiatric health and well-being in marginalized populations.

Just as intersectionality theory explains, structures of power and (dis)advantage combine in ways that are difficult to separate. The inseparability of power and privilege is inherent in the examples illustrated above—individuals from minoritized backgrounds who grow up in poorer neighborhoods that were systematically underfunded due to structural racism may be more likely to experience adversity, and, in-turn, psychopathology. For instance, that sexual minority adults aggregate in more economically deprived neighborhoods relative to heterosexual individuals is likely a function of more the precarious labor opportunities and poverty that result from the manifestation of sociocontextual factors of heterosexism (Kinitz et al., 2024). Dimensional psychopathology scholarship must draw from such theoretical frameworks to develop research questions rooted in understanding privilege, power, and psychopathology rather than exclusively focusing on individual characteristics and demographic groupings as proxies of such.

Can Dimensional Diagnosis Make Mental Health Training More Inclusive?

Potentially. Dimensional diagnosis does not inherently make mental health training more inclusive. What would make it more inclusive is the comprehensive and systematic integration of sociocontextual factors in the science of diagnosis and intervention. We see advantages for pedagogy as a downstream consequence of integrating dimensions of context with dimensional diagnosis. As we consider training the current (and future) generation of clinicians and clinician-scientists, we provide some recommendations for future research on dimensional psychopathology.

Looking toward the Future: Barriers and Solutions

Research that considers both sociocontextual and psychopathology dimensions is rare (Rodriguez-Seijas, Li, et al., 2023). Yet is it deeply important to advance the study of dimensional psychopathology and the increased pertinence of these models to understanding psychosocial health of marginalized populations. One difficulty in achieving this integration is that dimensional psychopathology and sociocontextually focused science operate almost totally independently. Studies of mental illness that adequately assess sociocontextual factors often use truncated symptom measures; research focused squarely on the breadth of psychopathology often omits the measurement of sociocontextual factors beyond demographic identity proxies. Another reason for the paucity of this work is the epistemic exclusion of minority scholars and scholarship in mainstream psychiatric science (Rodriguez-Seijas, McClendon, et al., 2023; Settles et al., 2020) and specifically within dimensional psychopathology research (Rodriguez-Seijas, Li, et al., 2023). Scholarship on minority issues is relegated to speciality journals (Settles et al., 2020), which deliberately pushes the study of sociocontextual factors—and scholars from minoritized backgrounds themselves—into the scientific fringes. Methods and approaches that scholars with such a focus may use to account for the nuance of participants' experiences of power and marginalization (e.g., qualitative/mixed methods, community-based approaches) are considered less objective than quantitative methods (Settles et al., 2020). Qualitative methods are seldom used in dimensional psychopathology research; indeed, research on the dimensional HiTOP model is currently based exclusively on quantitative study. However, we see an important opening for qualitative methods as a complement to quantitative methods, particularly when examining psychopathology in minoritized populations (Causadias, 2013).

We must consider dimensions of context in tandem and phenotype the *context* of our samples accordingly. There is no extant integrative theory of all domains of context and their influences on psychopathology dimensions, and there likely never will be. Just as there are concerns with ignoring the range of psychopathology in categorical paradigms, there are concerns with ignoring the richness of how social contextual factors shape psychopathology. The consequences of ignoring sociocontextual factors include misattributing reactions to the environment as pathological (Rodriguez-Seijas, Rogers, et al., 2023) and losing important information for understanding the etiology and maintenance of psychopathology. Although dimensional psychopathology classification models hold numerous benefits when compared with traditional categorical models, scholars in this field must critically contend with the generalizability of their models to underrepresented, marginalized, and epistemically excluded populations.

PART II

Possibilities and challenges for enhancing equity and inclusivity through dimensional models of psychopathology[2]

Sarah L. Pedersen, Frances Wang,
Rachel A. Vaughn-Coaxum, Paula Marie Powe,
and Cassandra L. Boness

There has been a justified shift to dimensional models of psychopathology, whereby psychological problems are conceptualized as existing on a continuum of frequency, severity, distress, and impairment rather than categorically as "normal" versus "abnormal." This shift presents an important opportunity to advance equity and inclusivity and decrease stigma. In this chapter, we briefly describe how categorical approaches may exacerbate misdiagnosis of psychiatric disorders for individuals with minoritized identities (e.g., racial, ethnic, LGBTQIA+) and have bias in diagnosis across gender and age. Then, we outline possibilities and challenges for dimensional frameworks to improve equity and inclusivity in mental health treatment and outcomes. Last, we provide examples demonstrating the importance of centering voices of individuals who have been historically excluded from mental health research.

Categorical Diagnoses Differ in Accuracy across Subpopulations

Research has shown over- *and* underdiagnosis of psychiatric disorders as well as the accurate identification of specific symptoms for individuals

[2]We would like to acknowledge our community partners for their feedback and participation in the examples we provide in this chapter as well as their responses during focus groups where we asked members to define "psychiatric illness." These contributions contributed to our decisions on how to focus this chapter.

from minoritized racial or ethnic groups (Vickers-Smith et al., 2023), LGBTQIA+ individuals (Rodriguez-Seijas et al., 2021), and across gender and age (Garb, 2021). For example, rates of conduct disorder have been shown to be higher among urban, low-income African American and Latine youth relative to non-Latine White youth (Fadus et al., 2020). This may owe in part to the symptoms of the disorder, which do not account for how factors related to the environment shape behaviors. Behavior such as using a violent weapon in an interpersonal interaction or stealing from others could be instead understood as responses to chronic violence exposure or to impoverishment (Mizock & Harkins, 2011). Additionally, major depressive disorder is significantly less likely to be diagnosed among individuals with minoritized racial and ethnic identities, including African American, Latine, and Asian individuals, relative to non-Latine White individuals (Shao et al., 2016). Differences in the clinical presentation of major depressive disorder across these groups may partially account for disparities across groups, with individuals from minoritized racial and ethnic groups often presenting with predominantly somatic and neurovegetative symptoms and less with mood or cognitive symptoms (Shao et al., 2016). Similarly, somatic complaints may be central to trauma-related disorders in many groups but are not included in the criteria for posttraumatic stress disorder (Hinton & Lewis-Fernández, 2011). A lack of symptoms that accurately represent psychological problems across different groups or the pathologizing of behaviors that have a normative function in certain environments will inevitably lead to misdiagnosis. This is especially concerning given that structural, interpersonal, and vicarious discrimination increase trauma and stress exposure (Kirkinis et al., 2021) and ultimately risk for certain psychological problems, which exacerbates the need for accurate and early identification of psychological problems for individuals with minoritized identities.

Possibilities for Dimensional Approaches to Advance Equity and Inclusivity Relative to Traditional Categorical Approaches

Comprehensive Assessments

Although we recognize that a lack of valid symptoms can affect dimensional as well as categorical approaches, dimensional approaches often assess a broader range of signs, symptoms, and indicators of functioning that can capture a variety of psychological problems that are not reflected well by the more restricted indicators used currently in categorical diagnostic approaches (Hinton & Lewis-Fernández, 2011). This limitation of categorical approaches may also be compounded by endorsement of symptoms at "subthreshold" levels that have restricted response options (absent, subthreshold, present) and can not only miss people experiencing impairment but limit what we know about the severity of those who get labeled as having the "disorder" (Brown & Barlow, 2009). Assuming that dimensional models mean broader assessments, the inclusion of more items and a wider range of response options may also mitigate the influence of individual items or indicators that differentially function or hold bias across subpopulations, improving their accuracy with respect to individuals with minoritized identities.

More Reliable and Less Biased Thresholds

An increasing body of research shows that psychological problems are dimensional, with symptoms experienced on a spectrum (Haslam et al., 2020). Viewing impairment on a continuum rather than as categorical (present or absent) can improve outcomes by broadening the likelihood that those who might otherwise be considered "subthreshold" by binary thresholds receive care (Lahey et al., 2022). Indeed, dimensions are more reliable than categories and are also stronger predictors of outcomes than categorical diagnoses (Lahey et al., 2022). Separately, experimental research has shown that there is implicit clinician bias in the application of diagnostic thresholds, especially when diagnosing individuals based on perceived or known identities. For example, in a sample of medical students and psychiatrists, participants more quickly paired Black (vs. White) faces with psychosis (vs. mood disorders), patient noncompliance (vs. compliance), and antipsychotic medication (vs. antidepressants; Londono Tobon et al., 2021) during three implicit associations tests. These biases were most pronounced for White participants with higher levels of training (e.g., psychiatrists relative to medical students). The use of a dimensional approach that recognizes impairment and distress on a continuum may be even more important for increasing reliability for minoritized individuals by reducing opportunities for bias in the determination and application of categorical diagnostic criteria and thresholds.

Reduced Stigma

Stigma toward individuals with psychiatric problems is prevalent and more pronounced for minoritized racial and ethnic communities in the United States (Misra et al., 2021). The shift toward dimensional models of psychological problems has the potential to reduce stigma in several ways. For example, dimensional models move away from reifying people with psychological problems as fundamentally different from others and instead reframes them as existing on a continuum that ranges from low to high across the entire population (Lahey et al., 2022). This, in turn, can normalize the experience of psychological problems at the societal level, reducing the potential for "othering" individuals as inherently flawed. This shift is important because research suggests that viewing psychological problems on a continuum, rather than as categorical, can support individual problem recognition, which may lead to treatment seeking and improved outcomes (Peter et al., 2021).

Inclusion of History and Context

Research suggests that consideration of the deleterious effects of discrimination in relation to psychological problems and on underlying transdiagnostic mechanisms can identify points of intervention (Eaton, 2020). Advocates of dimensional models note how the integration of culture and context into systems for understanding psychological problems, functioning, and impairment may be more easily embedded in these approaches relative to categorical approaches (Lahey et al., 2021). It is important to note that attempts have been made to include culture in categorical diagnoses. For example, the Cultural Formulation Interview (CFI) was designed to capture an individual's experience and perspective on their symptoms to inform diagnosis, case conceptualization, and treatment planning (Aggarwal & Lewis-Fernández, 2015) for DSM-5. However, quantitative research showing how information from the CFI gets integrated into making a diagnosis is largely lacking (Aggarwal et al., 2020).

Precision Medicine and Clinical Benefits of a Dimensional Approach

Given that dimensional models can support a more holistic and precise conceptualization of psychological problems for a given person, including their unique profile of symptoms and how these are influenced by context, they naturally align with precision medicine approaches. Precision medicine seeks to match treatments to an individual's unique profile of problems, with the goal of improving outcomes for that specific person (Litten et al., 2012). This may be particularly important for people with minoritized identities given that the most commonly used treatment approaches have been developed and tested in homogenous samples that lack representation of individuals with minoritized identities (Bernal & Adames, 2022). Dimensional models can allow for the assessment of an individual's profile of symptoms with greater nuance than categorical diagnoses, which can then support the identification of a treatment or treatments (as well as other supports) that would best reduce such symptoms and impairment and thus result in the best treatment outcomes (Boness & Witkiewitz, 2023). This approach could also lead to individuals from minoritized populations feeling better acknowledged and understood by mental health professionals (Sewell, 2016). Offering a menu of treatments that might be appropriate for a given person can support a person's autonomy in choosing a treatment approach that is best for them based on their unique beliefs, traditions, culture, strengths, needs, and preferences.

Dimensional Models Still Have Limitations That Reduce Equity and Inclusivity

Although we hold the belief that a dimensional approach advances equity and inclusivity over a categorical framework, existing limitations hamper this potential. For example, some research shows that dimensional approaches can more easily include context but other work has noted a lack of consensus on the type of statistical model to be used in dimensional taxonomies that incorporate context (Lahey et al., 2021). Indeed, researchers have acknowledged that the range of results that can be obtained from certain models (e.g., factor-analytic models) suggests that dimensional models may not be inherently applicable to individuals across cultural groups and that many components of dimensional models still need to be evaluated cross-culturally to ensure that culture and context are not simply included as an afterthought (Conway et al., 2023). In this way, dimensional and categorical approaches may be limited in similar ways with respect to their potential to truly advance mental health equity.

Another ongoing challenge for dimensional models is their focus on clinical description of signs, symptoms, traits, and maladaptive behaviors rather than mechanisms (i.e., the processes that cause and maintain maladaptive behaviors). The focus on signs and symptoms is potentially problematic given that they are contextually influenced nonspecific markers of psychological problems. For example, the experience of psychosocial problems because of substance use is one symptom underlying substance use disorder that could be caused by one's propensity toward interpersonal or occupational problems in the first place rather than by problematic substance use itself. Accordingly, symptom indicators may also be vulnerable to more restricted perspectives (e.g., Western perspectives or majority-White cultures) of what psychological problems are and are not (Verona, 2022). Because signs and symptoms don't focus on fundamental features (e.g., mechanisms) of psychological problems, they are less informative for treatment planning purposes, which may lead to suboptimal treatment outcomes.

Mental health research, including examination of dimensional taxonomies, has historically been conducted "on" people as opposed to "with" people. Community-engaged research, such as community-based participatory research (CBPR), which includes an ongoing partnership among scientists, people with lived experience, and other partners (e.g., providers) throughout the life cycle of a study, can increase the positive influence of classification research and treatment development for individuals with lived experience of psychological problems (Corrigan & Oppenheim, 2024). However, CBPR for mental health research or measure development is infrequently used (Jones et al., 2020). For example, a review of CBPR research studies conducted in partnership with individuals with a psychiatric illness from 2000 to 2020 resulted in locating only 31 articles and most of these were qualitative (Nieweglowski et al., 2024). Consistent with this, a separate review found 29 articles that used mixed-methods research (e.g., qualitative and quantitative approaches) and CBPR in studies on mental health. Continuing to view researchers as the sole "experts" will continue to limit the inclusivity, equity, and influence of dimensional approaches to psychological problems.

There may also be challenges with the utility and implementation of dimensional approaches in clinical care, and these may disproportionately affect minoritized individuals. Individuals with minoritized identities experience barriers to mental health care (e.g., access, culturally informed treatment; Cheng, 2021), and as dimensional models are implemented into clinical practice, this may raise further challenges. For example, there may be a need for longer and more detailed assessments to ensure a comprehensive understanding of presenting symptoms and to appropriately monitor treatment response and psychoeducation efforts to increase knowledge about when to seek treatment.

Ways to Strengthen Both Categorical and Dimensional Approaches

Although conceptualization and classification decisions for psychological problems are based on empirical evidence, they are also influenced by a host of nonempirical factors including sociopolitical influences and changes in what is considered "normative" in specific societies over time (Boness, Votaw, et al., 2023; van de Water et al., 2016). However, the voices influencing change in diagnostic criteria have been relatively homogenous and have not historically included those with lived experience (Boness, Votaw, et al., 2023). The historical and current issues related to equity and sociopolitical power within health sciences governing psychiatric health and services are pivotal for informing the inclusion of culture and context in dimensional models of psychological problems. It is critical that the individuals and groups that govern the advancement of dimensional models heed these lessons moving forward (Verona, 2022).

In considering the advancement of categorical and dimensional models, the conceptualization and operationalization of relevant psychological problems (e.g., signs and symptoms) is critical. To date, the decisions about what signs and symptoms are relevant have been derived from "expert" consensus as well as empirical evidence, especially in the case of categorical models of psychological problems. Although dimensional models are often driven by structural analyses (e.g., factor analysis), the selection of indicators is often still determined by "experts." We argue that people with lived (and living) experience of psychological problems can make critical contributions to the identification and operationalization of such problems as well as the selection of indicators to include in structural analyses and the ensuring appropriateness, comprehensiveness, and relevance of such indicators (Boness et al., 2025).

We present examples from our work to demonstrate the possibility of these approaches. As one example, the craving criteria in DSM-5 is "wanted a drink so badly you couldn't think of anything else." Many of the self-report measures for craving similarly focus on thinking or feeling a strong desire to drink. However, when one of us (S. L. P.) asked community members who were currently in treatment for alcohol use disorder to describe craving, they provided very different descriptions. Specifically, they described physical sensations such as "Feels like I want to crawl out of my skin. That nothing will be OK until I get that drink"; "Like when you are really hungry. I feel it from my stomach to head"; "A crippling pain that takes over my whole body." These examples highlight how current conceptualizations of craving might not accurately capture this construct in the populations for whom they were intended. Furthermore, they suggest that reconceptualizing craving to include the voices of people with lived experience could result in improved measurement, clinical utility, treatment targets, and needed differentiation from other criteria for alcohol use disorder (Boness et al., 2025). Consistent with this, we have shown that community consultation via community advisory boards and cognitive interviews is critical for highlighting problems with self-report indicators of alcohol use disorder and related constructs (Boness et al., 2022).

In a separate example with young adults classified as regular drinkers recruited from the community, one of us (C. L. B.) conducted cognitive interviews on interpretations about a widely used item to assess tolerance to alcohol: "In the past 12 months, did you find that your usual number of drinks had much less effect on you than it once did?" The time frame for comparison (i.e., "than it once did") varied markedly. For example, some respondents reported that they were comparing the number of drinks needed currently relative to when they first started drinking. Others reported they were comparing currently needed numbers of drinks to a wide range of earlier experiences including their freshmen year of college, to the beginning of the current year, to 12 months ago, and to the start of the school year (i.e., last semester). One respondent, who self-reported having a "drinking problem" 2 years prior to the interview reported they were comparing the current number of drinks needed relative to that period. As can been seen, clarity about the intended time frame is important and varies widely in interpretation. When developing measures, seeking and including feedback from individuals who have the greatest potential to benefit from the measure can significantly advance understanding, equity, and inclusivity.

Conclusion

In summary, we believe there are several important areas of relative strength for dimensional taxonomies that could advance equity and inclusivity relative to categorical diagnoses. These include more nuanced capability to include contextual and cultural factors, reducing stigma and bias, and building a framework for personalizing profiles of symptoms and functioning on a continuum. We have also laid out areas of growth that, if not addressed, are likely to perpetuate existing problems despite any shifts toward dimensional approaches. Our primary assertion is that to accurately reflect psychological problems and impairments, decrease stigma, and improve treatment outcomes, it is necessary to center the voices of people with lived experiences across a diversity of identities and backgrounds in the development and refinement of categorical *and* dimensional models of psychological problems.

PART I REFERENCES

American Psychiatric Association. (2013). *Diagnostic and statistical manual of mental disorders* (5th ed.). Author.

Asadi, S., Suzuki, T., & Rodriguez-Seijas, C. (2025). Investigating differential item functioning among borderline personality disorder diagnostic criteria and internalizing/externalizing domains based on sexual orientation. *Journal of Psychopathology and Clinical Science, 134,* 97–111.

Bailey, Z. D., Feldman, J. M., & Bassett, M. T. (2021). How Structural racism works—Racist policies as a root cause of U.S. racial health inequities. *New England Journal of Medicine, 384*(8), 768–773.

Bronfenbrenner, U. (1977). Toward an experimental ecology of human development. *American Psychologist, 32*(7), 513–531.

Causadias, J. M. (2013). A roadmap for the integration of culture into developmental psychopathology. *Development and Psychopathology, 25*(4pt2), 1375–1398.

Cho, S., Crenshaw, K. W., & McCall, L. (2013). Toward a Field of Intersectionality Studies: Theory, Applications, and Praxis. *Signs: Journal of Women in Culture and Society, 38*(4), 785–810.

Cole, E. R. (2009). Intersectionality and research in psychology. *American Psychologist, 64*(3), 170–180.

Crenshaw, K. (1991). Demarginalizing the intersection of race and sex: A black feminist critique of antidiscrimination doctrine, feminist theory, and antiracist politics [1989]. In K. T. Bartlett & R. Kennedy (Eds.), *Feminist legal theory: Readings in law and gender.* Routledge.

Cuthbert, B. N. (2022). Research Domain Criteria (RDoC): Progress and potential. *Current Directions in Psychological Science, 31*(2), 107–114.

Eaton, N. R., Rodriguez-Seijas, C., & Pachankis, J. E. (2021). Transdiagnostic approaches to sexual- and gender-minority mental health. *Current Directions in Psychological Science, 30*(6), 510–518.

Forbes, M. K., Ringwald, W. R., Allen, T., Cicero, D. C., Clark, L. A., DeYoung, C. G., . . . Wright, A. G. C. (2024). Principles and procedures for revising the hierarchical taxonomy of psychopathology. *Journal of Psychopathology and Clinical Science, 133*(1), 4–19.

Goldhammer, H., Crall, C., & Keuroghlian, A. S. (2019). Distinguishing and addressing gender minority stress and borderline personality symptoms. *Harvard Review of Psychiatry, 27*(5), 317–325.

Gone, J. P. (2023). Community mental health services for American Indians and Alaska Natives: Reconciling evidence-based practice and alter-native psyence. *Annual Review of Clinical Psychology, 19,* 23–49.

Hanna-Walker, V., Snapp, S., Campos, E. B., Saldana, X., & Watson, R. J. (2023). "This is real, this is the way that things are": Hooking up as a pathway for sexual identity development among SGM emerging adults. *Emerging Adulthood, 11*(1), 110–120.

Hyde, L. W., Gard, A. M., Tomlinson, R. C., Suarez, G. L., & Westerman, H. B. (2022). Parents, neighborhoods, and the developing brain. *Child Development Perspectives, 16*(3), 148–156.

Kinitz, D. J., Shahidi, F. V., Kia, H., MacKinnon, K., MacEachen, E., Gesink, D., & Ross, L. E. (2025). Precarious employment: A neglected issue among lesbian, gay, bisexual, and transgender workers. *Sexuality Research and Social Policy, 22,* 376–392.

Kotov, R., Krueger, R. F., Watson, D., Achenbach, T. M., Althoff, R. R., Bagby, R. M., . . . Zimmerman, M. (2017). The hierarchical taxonomy of psychopathology (HiTOP): A dimensional alternative to traditional nosologies. *Journal of Abnormal Psychology, 126*(4), 454–477.

Langwerden, R. J., Thompson, M. G., & Wagner, E. F. (2021). Multidimensional conceptualization of identity and psychopathology: Assessing mental health disparities from an intersectional and dimensional framework. *Personality and Mental Health, 15*(4), 293–308.

McLaughlin, K. A., Sheridan, M. A., & Lambert, H. K. (2014). Childhood adversity and neural development: Deprivation and threat as distinct dimensions of early experience. *Neuroscience & Biobehavioral Reviews, 47*, 578–591.

Meyer, I. H. (2003). Prejudice, social stress, and mental health in lesbian, gay, and bisexual populations: Conceptual issues and research evidence. *Psychological Bulletin, 129*(5), 674–697.

Murry, V. M., Butler-Barnes, S. T., Mayo-Gamble, T. L., & Inniss-Thompson, M. N. (2018). Excavating New constructs for family stress theories in the context of everyday life experiences of Black American families. *Journal of Family Theory & Review, 10*(2), 384–405.

Neblett, E. W., White, R. L., Ford, K. R., Philip, C. L., Nguyên, H. X., & Sellers, R. M. (2008). Patterns of racial socialization and psychological adjustment: Can parental communications about race reduce the impact of racial discrimination? *Journal of Research on Adolescence, 18*(3), 477–515.

Nielsen, S., R., Rodriguez-Seijas, C., Choukas-Bradly, S., & Wright, A. G. C. (2023, September). *Sexual and gender minority (SGM) stress and personality processes in daily life.* Paper presented at the meeting of the Society for Research in Psychopathology.

Pascoe, E. A., & Smart Richman, L. (2009). Perceived discrimination and health: A meta-analytic review. *Psychological Bulletin, 135*(4), 531–554.

Pearson, A. L., Zhou, Y., Buxton, R. T., Horton, T. H., Pfeiffer, K. A., & Beyer, K. M. M. (2023). The effects of contemporary redlining on the mental health of Black residents. *SSM - Population Health, 23*, 101462.

Peverill, M., Dirks, M. A., Narvaja, T., Herts, K. L., Comer, J. S., & McLaughlin, K. A. (2021). Socioeconomic status and child psychopathology in the United States: A meta-analysis of population-based studies. *Clinical Psychology Review, 83*, 101933.

Ravi, M., Mekawi, Y., Blevins, E. J., Michopoulos, V., Stevens, J., Carter, S., & Powers, A. (2023). Intersections of oppression: Examining the interactive effect of racial discrimination and neighborhood poverty on PTSD symptoms in Black women. *Journal of Psychopathology and Clinical Science, 132*(5), 567–576.

Rodriguez-Seijas, C., Li, J. J., Balling, C., Brandes, C., Bernat, E., Boness, C. L., . . . Eaton, N. R. (2023). Diversity and the hierarchical taxonomy of psychopathology (HiTOP). *Nature Reviews Psychology, 2*(8), Article 8.

Rodriguez-Seijas, C., McClendon, J., Wendt, D. C., Novacek, D. M., Ebalu, T., Hallion, L. S., . . . Mekawi, Y. (2023). The next generation of clinical psychological science: Moving toward antiracism. *Clinical Psychological Science, 12*(3), 526–546.

Rodriguez-Seijas, C., Morgan, T. A., & Zimmerman, M. (2021). A population-based examination of criterion-level disparities in the diagnosis of borderline personality disorder among sexual minority adults. *Assessment, 28*(4), 1097–1109.

Rodriguez-Seijas, C., Rogers, B. G., & Asadi, S. (2023). Personality disorders research and social decontextualization: What it means to be a minoritized human. *Personality Disorders: Theory, Research, and Treatment, 14*(1), 29–38.

Rodriguez-Seijas, C., Rogers, B. G., Harkness, A., Safren, S. A., & Pachankis,

J. E. (2024). ParTy 'n' Play: Associations between sex-related substance use and the disinhibited externalizing spectrum among gay and bisexual men. *Clinical Psychological Science, 12*(1), 83–97.

Sellers, R. M., Smith, M. A., Shelton, J. N., Rowley, S. A. J., & Chavous, T. M. (1998). Multidimensional model of racial identity: A reconceptualization of African American racial identity. *Personality and Social Psychology Review, 2*(1), 18–39.

Settles, I. H., Warner, L. R., Buchanan, N. T., & Jones, M. K. (2020). Understanding psychology's resistance to intersectionality theory using a framework of epistemic exclusion and invisibility. *Journal of Social Issues, 76*(4), 796–813.

Tan, K. K. H., Treharne, G. J., Ellis, S. J., Schmidt, J. M., & Veale, J. F. (2020). Gender minority stress: A critical review. *Journal of Homosexuality, 67*(10), 1471–1489.

PART II REFERENCES

Aggarwal, N. K., Jarvis, G. E., Gómez-Carrillo, A., Kirmayer, L. J., & Lewis-Fernández, R. (2020). The Cultural Formulation Interview since DSM-5: Prospects for training, research, and clinical practice. *Transcultural Psychiatry, 57*(4), 496–514.

Aggarwal, N. K., & Lewis-Fernández, R. (2015). An introduction to the Cultural Formulation Interview. *Focus, 13*(4), 426–431.

Bernal, G., & Adames, C. (2022). Cultural adaptations: Tools for evidence-based practice with diverse populations. In M. A. Gallo & G. Bernal (Eds.), *Culturally adapted interventions: A guide to improving effectiveness with diverse populations*. American Psychological Association.

Boness, C. L., Gatten, N., Treece, M. K., & Miller, M. B. (2022). A mixed-methods approach to improve the measurement of alcohol-induced blackouts: ABOM-2. *Alcohol Clinical and Experimental Research, 46*(8), 1497–1514.

Boness, C. L., Hebden, H., Lardier, D. T., Spurgeon, L., Timmons, A., Simms, L. J., . . . Witkiewitz K. (2025). Engaging people with lived experience of psychological disorders: Current research and future directions for community-engaged measure development in psychological science. *Clinical Psychological Science, 13*(4), 720–739.

Boness, C. L., Votaw, V. R., Francis, M. W., Watts, A. L., Sperry, S. H., Kleva, C. S., . . . Witkiewitz, K. (2023). Alcohol use disorder conceptualizations and diagnoses reflect their sociopolitical context. *Addiction Research and Theory, 31*(5), 307–312.

Boness, C. L., & Witkiewitz, K. (2023). Precision medicine in alcohol use disorder: Mapping etiologic and maintenance mechanisms to mechanisms of behavior change to improve patient outcomes. *Experimental Clinical Psychopharmacology, 31*(4), 769–779.

Brown, T. A., & Barlow, D. H. (2009). A proposal for a dimensional classification system based on the shared features of the DSM-IV anxiety and mood disorders: Implications for assessment and treatment. *Psychological Assessment, 21*(3), 256–271.

Cheng, H. G., Kohn, R., & Levav, I. (2021). Barriers to mental health care among racial and ethnic minority groups in the United States: Current challenges and future directions. *Current Psychiatry Reports, 29*(9), 61.

Conway, C. C., Kotov, R., Krueger, R. F., & Caspi, A. (2023). Translating the hierarchical taxonomy of psychopathology (HiTOP) from potential to practice: Ten research questions. *American Psychologist, 78*(7), 873–885.

Corrigan, P. W., & Oppenheim, M. (2024). The power of community-based participatory research (CBPR). *Psychiatric Rehabilitation Journal, 47*(1), 2–8.

Eaton, N. R. (2020). Measurement and mental health disparities: Psychopathology classification and identity assessment. *Personality and Mental Health, 14*(1), 76–87.

Fadus, M. C., Ginsburg, K. R., Sobowale, K., Halliday-Boykins, C. A., Bryant, B. E., . . . Squeglia, L. M. (2020). Unconscious bias and the diagnosis of disruptive behavior disorders and ADHD in African American and Hispanic youth. *Academic Psychiatry, 44*(1), 95–102.

Garb, H. N. (2021). Race bias and gender bias in the diagnosis of psychological disorders. *Clinical Psychology Review, 90,* 102087.

Haslam, N., McGrath, M. J., Viechtbauer, W., & Kuppens, P. (2020). Dimensions over categories: A meta-analysis of taxometric research. *Psychological Medicine, 50*(9), 1418–1432.

Hinton, D. E., & Lewis-Fernández, R. (2011). The cross-cultural validity of posttraumatic stress disorder: Implications for DSM-5. *Depression and Anxiety, 28*(9), 783–801.

Jones, D. E., Lindquist-Grantz, R., & DeJonckheere, M. (2020). A review of mixed methods community-based participatory research applications in mental health. *Journal of Social, Behavioral, and Health Sciences, 14,* 254–288.

Kirkinis, K., Pieterse, A. L., Martin, C., Agiliga, A., & Brownell, A. (2021). Racism, racial discrimination, and trauma: A systematic review of the social science literature. *Ethnicity & Health, 26*(3), 392–412.

Lahey, B. B., Moore, T. M., Kaczkurkin, A. N., & Zald, D. H. (2021). Hierarchical models of psychopathology: Empirical support, implications, and remaining issues. *World Psychiatry, 20*(1), 57–63.

Lahey, B. B., Tiemeier, H., & Krueger, R. F. (2022). Seven reasons why binary diagnostic categories should be replaced with empirically sounder and less stigmatizing dimensions. *JCPP Advances,* 2(4), e12108.

Litten, R. Z., Egli, M., Heilig, M., Cui, C., Fertig, J. B., Ryan, M. L., . . . Noronha, A. (2012). Medications development to treat alcohol dependence: a vision for the next decade. *Addiction Biology, 17*(3), 513–527.

Londono Tobon, A., Flores, J. M., Taylor, J. H., Johnson, I., Landeros-Weisenberger, A., Aboiralor, O., . . . Bloch, M. H. (2021). Racial implicit associations in psychiatric diagnosis, treatment, and compliance expectations. *Academic Psychiatry, 45*(1), 23–33.

Misra, S., Jackson, V. W., Chong, J., Choe, K., Tay, C., Wong, J., & Yang, L. H.

(2021). Systematic review of cultural aspects of stigma and mental illness among racial and ethnic minority groups in the United States: Implications for interventions. *American Journal of Community Psychology, 68*(3–4), 486–512.

Mizock, L., & Harkins, D. (2011). Diagnostic bias and conduct disorder: Improving culturally sensitive diagnosis. *Child & Youth Services, 32*(3), 243–253.

Nieweglowski, K., Sheehan, L., & Deshpande, A. (2024). A systematic review of community-based participatory research studies involving individuals with mental illness. *Psychiatric Rehabilitation Journal, 47*(1), 9–21.

Peter, L.-J., Schindler, S., Sander, C., Schmidt, S., Muehlan, H., McLaren, T., . . . Schomerus, G. (2021). Continuum beliefs and mental illness stigma: A systematic review and meta-analysis of correlation and intervention studies. *Psychological Medicine, 51*(5), 716–726.

Rodriguez-Seijas, C., Morgan, T. A., & Zimmerman, M. (2021). Is there a bias in the diagnosis of borderline personality disorder among lesbian, gay, and bisexual patients? *Assessment, 28*(3), 724–738.

Sewell, A. A. (2016). The racism-race reification process: A mesolevel political economic framework for understanding racial health disparities. *Sociology of Race and Ethnicity, 2*(4), 402–432.

Shao, Z., Richie, W. D., & Bailey, R. K. (2016). Racial and ethnic disparity in major depressive disorder. *Journal of Racial and Ethnic Health Disparities, 3*(4), 692–705.

van de Water, T., Suliman, S., & Seedat, S. (2016). Gender and cultural issues in psychiatric nosological classification systems. *CNS Spectrum, 21*(4), 33–340.

Verona, E. (2022). Assessment of HiTOP constructs across the population: A commentary on the HiTOP Measure Development Project. *Assessment, 29*(1), 88–92.

Vickers-Smith, R., Justice, A. C., Becker, W. C., Rentsch, C. T., Curtis, B., Fernander, A., . . . Kranzler, H. R. (2023). Racial and ethnic bias in the diagnosis of alcohol use disorder in veterans. *American Journal of Psychiatry, 180*(6), 426–436.

CHAPTER 8

How does dimensional diagnosis change psychopathology research?

When mental health problems are assumed to be categorical, a natural approach in experimental psychopathology is to distinguish people with different diagnoses from controls to identify the mechanisms underlying their problems. However, if mental health problems are assumed to be dimensional in terms of distinguishing both clinical from nonclinical ranges of functioning and different kinds of problems, how valid is this approach? In this section, we asked experts to answer three questions:

What is the role of case-control studies in psychopathology?

How does dimensional diagnosis affect the way we sample participants for psychopathology research?

How will research methods change in the era of dimensional diagnosis?

Conway advocates for a clean departure from approaches to psychopathology research based on the categorical model and in favor of approaches based on a hierarchical dimensional model. He is critical of case-control studies, emphasizes the advantages of using hierarchical models to sample based on the specificity of research questions, and argues that reformulating psychopathology theories based on syndromes would improve research. Baskin-Sommers and colleagues take a more conservative position, highlighting how statistical covariance models can be used to arrange psychopathology indicators into dimensions, categories, or combinations of the two. They reserve room for the utility of case-control designs and argue that research designs vary across but can be appropriate for either categorical or dimensional approaches. They also draw attention to broader issues in sampling for clinical research, such as the importance of increasing generalizability by recruiting participants from broader, more representative, and more diverse samples.

PART I

Dimensional diagnosis can improve theory building and testing in psychopathology research

CHRISTOPHER C. CONWAY

My goal in this chapter is to describe how multidimensional diagnostic systems, particularly the hierarchical taxonomy of psychopathology (HiTOP; Kotov et al., 2021), *function as research frameworks* and enable new insights into the origins and outcomes of mental health problems.

Two distinctive properties of the HiTOP model account for its utility as a research tool: hierarchy and dimensionality. HiTOP is hierarchical because, much like accepted models of personality and cognitive ability domains, it organizes mental health conditions at different levels of breadth (Figure 8.1). All levels, ranging from broad to specific, are equally valid representations of psychopathology. For instance, sleep difficulties could be understood by referring to narrow homogeneous constructs near the base of the hierarchy (e.g., "early morning awakening" is located at the symptom level, where the various basic units of psychopathology are too numerous to list in Figure 8.1; "insomnia" is a symptom component that aggregates various specific expressions of insomnia, including early morning awakening), intermediate constructs ("vegetative depression" syndrome, "distress" subfactor), or broad, heterogeneous constructs near the top of the hierarchy ("internalizing spectrum," "general-factor superspectrum").

HiTOP is dimensional because it recognizes that, according to the available data, individual differences on virtually all psychopathology constructs are a matter of degree, not kind (Haslam et al., 2020). Therefore, the model attempts to locate people at some level of, say, the insomnia dimension rather than positing separate populations of people who do versus do not have clinically significant insomnia.

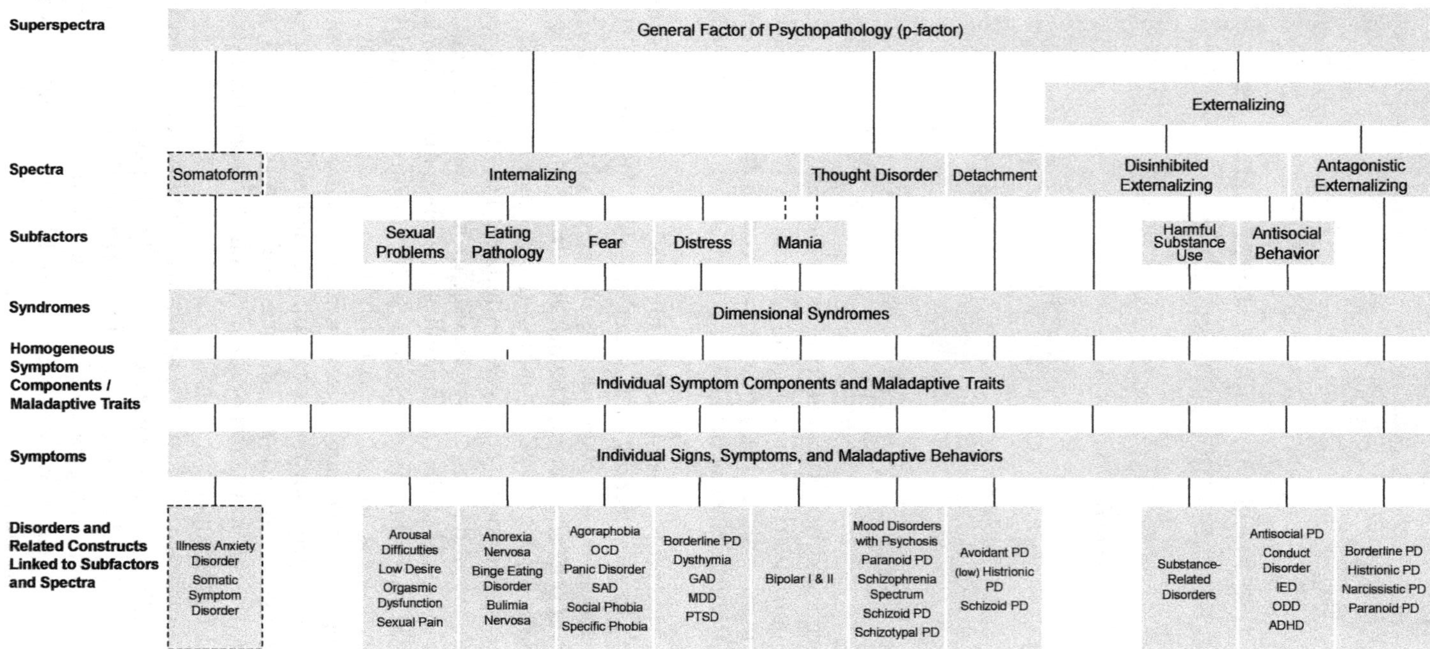

FIGURE 8.1. HiTOP model. Dashed lines indicate dimensions included as provisional aspects of the framework. Abbreviations: ADHD, attention-deficit/hyperactivity disorder; GAD, generalized anxiety disorder; IED, intermittent explosive disorder; MDD, major depressive disorder; OCD, obsessive–compulsive disorder; ODD, oppositional defiant disorder; PD, personality disorder; PTSD, posttraumatic stress disorder; SAD, separation anxiety disorder.

Below I address the implications of a hierarchical dimensional conceptualization of psychopathology for prominent questions in mental health research.

What Is the Role of Case-Control Studies in Psychopathology?

There are a few ways in which frameworks like HiTOP are out of sync with a case-control design. First, if psychological problems are continuously distributed in the population, then imposing a dividing line between cases and controls binarizes what is naturally continuous information. I am unaware of robust evidence for a categorical (or categorical–dimensional hybrid) model for any mental health problem. Whereas one can always fit a categorical model to observed symptom data and often get interpretable results, this is not evidence that the categorical model is a better representation of the symptoms (on conceptual or empirical grounds) than a dimensional model.

Assuming a dimensional structure to psychopathology, creating binary diagnoses essentially discards information, which usually dilutes a construct's "signal" in relation to the outcome of interest (MacCallum et al., 2002). For example, there are almost always meaningful differences among cases in disorder severity. We can probably all think of clinical examples of people who were especially extreme cases of some diagnosis. But analysis of case-control data assumes that all cases have the same degree of disorder (e.g., all cases are coded as 1 in the dataset, and all controls as 0). Along these same lines, the case-control design misses the fact that there will be cases who have more in common with the typical control than they have in common with the typical case.

Second, whereas HiTOP attempts to model comorbidity (i.e., diagnostic co-occurrence) with higher level dimensions near the top of the hierarchy, case-control studies generally ignore comorbidity. But this comes at an interpretative cost. Comorbidity means that in a study of generalized anxiety disorder (GAD) cases who are compared with healthy (i.e., no GAD diagnosis) controls, other diagnoses might account for GAD's effects. Panic disorder, social phobia, and many other conditions tend to co-occur with GAD (e.g., Brown et al., 2001). Any of these might be driving the observed effects. This threat of confounding makes it almost impossible to draw clear conclusions.

Some studies have tried to sidestep the problem by recruiting samples of cases with only one disorder and comparing them with healthy controls. But these "pure" cases are not representative of the general population or patient populations. Again, comorbidity is ubiquitous.

Therefore, this workaround generally does not improve the quality of inferences in case-control designs.

Third, case-control studies overlook heterogeneity within categorical diagnoses. Virtually all categorical diagnoses are multidimensional in the sense that they comprise lower level components that are meaningfully different. Borderline personality disorder, for example, includes symptoms that reflect concerns ranging from identity disturbance to affective instability to recklessness. In theory, these different narrow features have distinct patterns of association with clinical outcomes. Yet the case-control design collapses them into a single binary concept, obscuring the reason(s) for any observed case-control differences.

How Does Dimensional Diagnosis Affect the Way We Sample Participants for Psychopathology Research?

One implication of a hierarchical perspective on psychopathology is that investigators can recruit participants based on their standing on broad, intermediate, or narrow psychopathology dimensions. Thinking about sampling this way enforces extra precision in a researcher's theory of the etiological factor or outcome they intend to study. For example, if you plan to study the correlates of sleep difficulties, you could sample people based on early insomnia; a composite of early, middle, and late insomnia; distress; or internalizing. This decision-making process will presumably help you clarify the exact component(s) of categorical disorders that theoretically generates associations with the outcomes under study.

I present two illustrative examples. First, Edershile and Wright (2021) sampled adults with respect to vulnerable narcissism, a lower-level characteristic of the externalizing domain. They planned to study interpersonal dynamics among people who tend to have exaggerated affective responses to perceived criticism and slights, which are part of the clinical profile in vulnerable narcissism. Therefore, enriching the sample for this condition increased the chances of capturing the sorts of problematic interpersonal patterns they were targeting.

Second, Craske et al. (2019) created a psychotherapy meant to address low positive affect (anhedonia), a feature primarily associated in categorical nosologies with major depressive disorder (MDD), social phobia, posttraumatic stress disorder (PTSD), and schizophrenia-spectrum disorders. They recruited participants who were very low on positive affect because this was the psychological problem they intended their treatment to reach. They could have recruited based on a categorical MDD, but this group would probably have included people who were not especially low on positive affect. (Again, categorical diagnoses are multidimensional and anhedonia is not required for a DSM depression diagnosis.) Their clinical theory operated at this lower order level, and sampling on the anhedonia dimension ensured their study design was a good match to their theory.

How Will Research Methods Change in the Era of Dimensional Diagnosis?

If we do enter an era of dimensional diagnosis, the biggest change I expect for applied research is that we will realize that examining the validity (with respect to causes, correlates, and outcomes) of any one syndrome (categorically or dimensionally defined) in isolation is unnecessarily limiting. The bivariate correlation between syndrome and outcome collapses a lot of information that we could separate, if we considered the syndrome's location within a hierarchy of psychopathology dimensions.

As mentioned, syndromes are multifaceted, and normally we are unaware which facets are contributing most to the correlation between syndrome and outcome. Syndromes represent variance from higher-order dimensions in the hierarchy, too. It could be that a syndrome's correlation with some outcome primarily reflects the relationship that some higher-order dimension has with the outcome. Deconstructing traditional syndromes into constituent dimensions across levels of the hierarchy will help to discover from where in the hierarchy predictive information (i.e., validity) comes (Conway et al., 2019). This approach will pinpoint what part or parts of a mental health condition matter most in a given research context. It may be the case that for some outcomes in some research settings, "traditional" syndromes (e.g., MDD, PTSD) will be the optimal level of analysis. The main point is that we will be able to empirically test that idea instead of just assuming it as we do now when working with categorical disorders.

One implication of this perspective is that virtually any theory of psychopathology that is based on a categorical diagnosis can—and maybe should—be reformulated through a hierarchical dimensional lens. For the past few decades, many theories of the origins, outcomes, and treatment of psychopathology have been framed by categorical DSM entities. One example from my own research field involves the concept of "stress generation." The original theory behind stress generation was oriented around MDD (Hammen, 1991). The idea was that people who were diagnosed with MDD were more likely than those who were not to encounter future stressful life events, particularly those that they had a hand in creating. The theory calls this sort of event "dependent stress."

For example, the theory holds that people with an MDD diagnosis are more likely than their peers to get fired from work because of absenteeism, break up with romantic partners over major disagreements, and get suspended from school for disciplinary problems.

The theory was formulated around MDD because this was considered by most investigators at the time (and probably still is) to be the most valid way of describing people who struggle with depressed mood and associated cognitive, physical, and interpersonal problems. However, as you can see in Figure 8.1, MDD is a heterogeneous mixture of internalizing problems. Dimensional systems like HiTOP urge researchers to consider which aspects of the condition—at higher and lower levels of granularity—are most closely linked with the target outcome.

With some coworkers, I attempted an expanded test of the stress generation phenomenon in a group of 800 young adults, many of whom were at high risk for depression due to maternal history of depression (Conway et al., 2012). All respondents completed interview assessments of psychopathology and stressors at ages 15 and 20. MDD did indeed have a prospective link, on a bivariate level, to dependent stressors. So, the traditional stress generation hypothesis was supported. Then, we used a latent-variable model to parse the pathology that was common to all the emotional disorders we assessed (i.e., a higher-order dimension) from the pathology that was unique to each of the disorders in our study (i.e., a lower order dimension). We found that the broad internalizing dimension had a moderate prospective association with dependent stress. We also saw that the unique part of MDD had an independent association, albeit a relatively small one, with dependent stress. Also, the unique part of panic disorder had an *inverse* relation to dependent stress, an effect we named "stress inhibition" to contrast with stress generation.

We used these findings to reformulate the stress generation theory from a dimensional diagnosis perspective. We argued that stress generation is not best conceptualized as an outcome of MDD per se. The pattern of results was not that simple. Instead, it seems that between-person variation on the dimension that cuts across all emotional disorders is the strongest predictor of who encounters more dependent stressors. And the unique pieces of MDD and panic disorder—which were not measured directly in this study so remain unknown—contribute too in different ways. In other words, we learned that the original theory is incomplete and that the predictive validity is distributed across relatively broad and narrow levels of the internalizing domain, at least in this population.

In conclusion, I think the major lesson from this one study is that all theories can become more refined and more versatile if rethought from a hierarchical dimensional perspective. With enough testing along these lines, investigators will be able to home in on the psychopathology dimensions that should take center stage in their theories. And, if there is compelling evidence that a dimensional perspective enhances theories' utility (e.g., better prediction, more complete explanation), people will be motivated to generate new theories that are oriented around psychopathology dimensions rather than categories.

This perspective is progressive, and there may be a cost here in terms of continuity with prior research guided by categorical diagnoses (sacrificing "replication and extension"). But I see this as a healthy paradigm shift that is unequivocally worth exploring. A multidimensional research framework, like HiTOP, takes what we know about the organization of psychopathology symptoms and sets up a more informative theory-advancing approach to studying mental disorders.

PART II

Exploring the strengths and weaknesses of different models used in psychopathology classification

ARIELLE BASKIN-SOMMERS, BRENDAN LAM,
and SAMUEL PASKEWITZ

In recent years, there has been a growing tension in clinical psychology regarding the appropriate ways to classify psychopathology. On the one hand, proponents of categorical classification suggest that there are distinct groups that separate people based on levels of psychopathology (e.g., *Diagnostic Statistical Manual of Mental Disorders* [DSM] diagnosis vs. no diagnosis, Zachar, 2000). However, critics suggest that there is little empirical evidence for discrete cutoffs between people who have or do not have psychopathology (Haslam et al., 2020). On the other hand, proponents of dimensional classification believe that psychopathology is reflected in continuously distributed symptoms (Conway et al., 2019). However, the dimensional approach has been criticized for not having been compared with more data-driven categorical models (Van Dam et al., 2017) and for having substantial practical limitations in real-world clinics (Haeffel et al., 2022; Weinberger et al., 2015). Here, we suggest that the tension can be resolved by improving the accuracy and transparency of methods used in this area. We provide a brief primer on the strengths and weaknesses of different statistical models: factor-analytic (which identify dimensions), latent-class (which identify categories), and factor mixture models (which identify categories and dimensions). We highlight examples of appropriate applications and potential misapplications of these models, which has muddied the waters in terms of identifying accurate classifications of psychopathology. Based on the extant research, we do not believe that the tension has been resolved: some studies support hybrid dimensional–categorical models (e.g., Muthén, 2006), whereas others support dimensions (e.g., McBride et al., 2011).

We then discuss other methodological considerations including whether to treat psychopathology as a categorical or dimensional variable, sampling, and case-control design for research on psychopathology classification. We believe that research methods in this area should balance efforts to replicate effects, leverage inclusive sampling approaches, and select a design that reflects the literature and addresses the core research question.

A Brief Primer on Relevant Statistical Methods

Dimensional, Categorical, and Hybrid Latent Variable Models

Two of the most common types of models used in research on the classification of psychopathology are factor analysis and latent class analysis. Factor analysis is a purely dimensional model and is the main method used in the hierarchical taxonomy of psychopathology (HiTOP) system (Waszczuk et al., 2017). Factor analysis explains symptoms using latent variables (factors) that are distributed continuously throughout the population, and each factor reflects a subset of correlated symptoms. In contrast, latent class analysis is a purely categorical model. It divides people into categories (latent classes), and each latent class has a different set of symptom probabilities. These two methods have different limitations in representing symptom correlations: factor analysis assumes that correlations are uniform across the population, whereas latent class analysis explains the correlations among symptoms solely in terms of classes differences, where symptoms are not correlated within each latent class.

Factor mixture models (Clark et al., 2013; Muthén, 2006) are a hybrid of dimensional and categorical models. Like factor analysis, symptom probabilities are determined by continuous latent factors (dimensions). However, individuals also belong to latent classes (categories) and specific parameters vary across latent classes (which parameters vary depends on the type of model, see Clark et al., 2013). We will focus on what we term "proper" factor mixture models—that is, those that allow individuals in the same latent class to have different factor scores. Proper factor mixture models have two primary properties: (1) symptoms are correlated within latent classes (unlike latent class analysis), and (2) symptom correlations differ across the population (unlike factor analysis).

Before concluding this section, we want to comment on latent class factor analysis (Muthén, 2006). This model can be viewed as a factor mixture model in which everyone in a latent-classes class has the exact same factor score (Clark et al., 2013). However, this is distinct from the proper factor mixture models, which allow within-class variation in factor scores. Thus, mathematically, latent class factor analysis is merely a more parsimonious reparameterization of latent class analysis: both models (unlike proper factor mixtures) assume that symptoms are uncorrelated within each latent class. Latent class factor analysis, then, is not an accurate representation of a hybrid model (e.g., Conway et al., 2012).

Deciding among Dimensional, Categorical, and Hybrid Models

There are two main methods for deciding among dimensional, categorical, and hybrid models of psychopathology: (1) comparing latent variable models using fit statistics (e.g., Bayesian Information Criterion; Clark et al., 2013; Muthén, 2006), and (2) taxometric analysis (Meehl, 1992). The advantage of the former approach is that multiple dimensions of symptoms (factor analysis), multiple categories with different symptom patterns (latent class analysis), and different patterns of correlation within categories (proper factor mixture models) can be compared. However, this approach requires distributional assumptions (e.g., normality). The advantage of the latter approach is that it uses nonparametric methods to compare highly categorical and dimensional models. However, it assumes that there are at most only two categories (e.g., depressed and not depressed) and that all indicator variables (symptoms) represent the same type of psychopathology (i.e., all symptoms are higher in one category than in the other if the categorical hypothesis is true or are all positively correlated if the dimensional hypothesis is true). In some simulations, reviewing fit statistics for latent variable model comparison performs better than taxometric analysis in detecting categorical structure and correctly assigning participants to latent profiles (Lubke & Tueller, 2010). Thus, at this time researchers may want to start with using fit statistics to compare latent variable models and perhaps use taxometric methods as a secondary analysis.

Evidence for Dimensional, Categorical, and Hybrid Models of Psychopathology

The findings from comparing models of psychopathology symptoms are equivocal. Studies using taxometric analysis show that many forms of psychopathology are dimensional (Haslam et al., 2020). That being said, given the limitations of the method noted above, we should be cautious in viewing the tension between dimensional and categorical classifications as resolved. Other studies that use fit statistics to compare latent variable models show mixed support for different models: Muthén

(2006) found that a proper factor mixture model (hybrid) provided the best description of alcohol use disorder symptoms, but McBride et al. (2011) reported that a factor analysis model (dimensional) provided the best fit. Conflicting results also have been reported in other areas of psychopathology, including depression (Lubke & Tueller, 2010; Sunderland et al., 2013) and borderline personality disorder (Conway et al., 2012; Johnson & Levy, 2020). Thus, given the mixed evidence we believe that whether various forms of psychopathology are purely dimensional or include categories is still an open question.

Research Methods Considerations

Whether one views psychopathology as dimensional or categorical influences various aspects of research methods. Advocates of dimensional diagnosis argue that psychopathology should only be treated as a continuous rather than discrete variable in statistical analyses, that it is imperative to use less restrictive criteria for sampling participants, and that the case-control design should be abandoned (Conway et al., 2019). Based on the extant literature, we do not believe that the dimensional-versus-categorical question has been definitively settled and worry about prescribing all the shifts in methods encouraged by proponents of the dimensional approach. We do not believe sufficient data supports a move to always analyze psychopathology as a continuous variable or to not use case-control designs; however, we certainly agree that inclusive sampling is critical.

Treating Psychopathology as a Discrete or Continuous Variable

Consider research on the relationship between delay discounting (represented as a continuous variable) and attention-deficit/hyperactivity disorder (ADHD). A categorical analysis would first sort participants into discrete groups based on ADHD symptoms and then look for group differences in delay discounting. A dimensional analysis would use regression to relate delay discounting to a continuous measure of ADHD symptoms. Which is the correct approach?

As noted above, some (but not all) studies support a hybrid model with both categories and dimensions for certain forms of psychopathology (e.g., Clark et al., 2013; Muthén, 2006). Additionally, in the ADHD example much of the literature on ADHD and delay discounting uses DSM diagnoses (e.g., Jackson & MacKillop, 2016), providing a pragmatic reason to do similar analyses for the sake of comparison. Thus, there are at least two cases where researchers could treat psychopathology as categorical: (1) when analysis of symptom data supports data-driven categories and (2) when using DSM diagnoses is needed for replication and extension from previous research. This does not preclude the use of dimensional analyses, but the rationale should be stated (or better yet, tested) rather than presumed.

Sampling

Sampling is a fundamental aspect of the research process. To date, sampling strategies are often too restrictive in terms of eligible target populations and comorbidities. Historically, there have been many reasons given for restrictions in sampling. Often, researchers have excluded particular individuals to either reduce the effects of confounding from other variables or because it was not practical to recruit a diverse sample (Ellard-Gray et al., 2015). However, it is important that the sample include a wide range of individuals with diverse backgrounds and levels of psychopathology (Haeffel et al., 2022; Kaiser & Weaver, 2019).

One way in which samples have been restricted is through the excess use of exclusion criteria (Charlson & Wells, 2022; Newman et al., 1998). To illustrate the point, we look at some research on substance use disorders. Many studies on alcohol treatment exclude people with neurological impairment and problems with drugs (Monahan & Finney, 1996). However, approximately 50–80% of those with alcohol use disorder show neurological impairments (Maillard et al., 2020; Oscar-Berman et al., 2014) and approximately 38% have another comorbid substance disorder (Saha et al., 2018). Furthermore, Humphreys and Weisner (2000) found that common exclusion criteria (e.g., serious medical problems, neurological impairment, other substance use problems) result in samples that miss those with more severe alcohol use whose backgrounds and experiences may hold significant clues as to the efficacy of treatment and to the factors related to initiation, maintenance, or desistance from alcohol misuse. In research on the classification of psychopathology, which ultimately seeks to identify the true structure of and relationships among symptoms, it therefore becomes imperative to have a sample that represents the characteristics of the population with these symptoms (Haeffel et al., 2022; Humphreys & Weisner, 2000; Shen et al., 2011; Steinley & Brusco, 2008). Almost any restriction due to exclusion criteria undermines external validity and runs the risk of studying participants whose etiopathogenesis and symptom structure differ from those of the population of interest.

It also is crucial to consider the range of psychopathology severity in a sample. Clinical scientists continue to overrely on college students and other samples of convenience (Roberts & Ilardi, 2008). Although this may allow for larger sample sizes, these samples often do not include a sufficiently broad range of severity levels of psychopathology and do not resemble the clinical population of interest.

As a result, researchers may not be able to distinguish between categories and dimensions reliably and the factor loading estimation in factor analysis may be biased (Franco-Martínez et al., 2023). For example, Steppan et al. (2014) found that including versus excluding people with at least one criterion for alcohol abuse and dependence (from DSM-IV) changed the dimensionality of factor-analytic models. As another example, sampling on the low range of alcohol use resulted in a dimensional structure when, in reality, high levels of alcohol increased the likelihood of other symptoms (e.g., use of other substances), which then resulted in different symptoms and a different structure of high alcohol use (Helle et al., 2020). Thus, who, how, and, where participants are sampled from can affect the levels of observed severity, which can influence findings on the structure of psychopathology.

Design

Some researchers who advocate for dimensions suggest that case-control designs no longer have a place in research (Conway et al., 2019). However, as we have argued, categories may play an important role in understanding the structure of psychopathology as well as other clinically relevant features (e.g., biological sex, race/ethnicity, or specific experiences [e.g., combat trauma vs. other types of traumas]). Some research supports the existence of categories in certain forms of psychopathology (e.g., Clark et al., 2013), which allows for the comparison of different groups in a case-control design. In a study on anxiety sensitivity, Volarov and colleagues (2020) identified a three-class structure, and if this research is replicated, then a case-control design based on anxiety sensitivity levels may be appropriate. Of note, factor mixture models typically require large sample sizes (Wang et al., 2021), making it difficult to test whether groups should be formed in a specific study. Thus, researchers may have to rely on previous research that has extracted latent categories of psychopathology to decide whether a case-control design is appropriate for a given research question.

Case-control designs may also be justified when participants can be divided into groups based on a clinically relevant categorical variable. For instance, Galovski and colleagues (2013) were interested in whether biological males and females with posttraumatic stress disorder differed in their response to cognitive-processing therapy. Therefore, a case-control design with groups stratified by biological sex was appropriate. Case-control designs can also be used to test theories that posit the existence of discrete groups. For example, Moffitt (1993) hypothesized that there are two trajectories of antisocial behavior in youth: (1) an "adolescent-limited" group in which antisocial behavior occurs in teenage years and decreases afterwards and (2) a "life-course persistent" in which antisocial behavior starts early in life and persists into adulthood. To adequately test and understand this developmental taxonomy, researchers need to categorize youth into these two groups and assess the extent to which they differ on other variables (e.g., family interactions, brain structure) or even the structure of their symptoms. Ultimately, the choice of a research design should be decided by the research question and no design should be eliminated solely based on its use of categories.

Summary

We urge researchers to be open-minded about the use of both categories and dimensions as classifications of psychopathology. Rather than assuming one model of psychopathology is incorrect, we think there are many opportunities to uncover the structure of psychopathology with appropriate statistical and research methods while keeping in mind practical considerations and the people affected by psychopathology.

PART I REFERENCES

Brown, T. A., Campbell, L. A., Lehman, C. L., Grisham, J. R., & Mancill, R. B. (2001). Current and lifetime comorbidity of the DSM-IV anxiety and mood disorders in a large clinical sample. *Journal of Abnormal Psychology, 110*(4), 585.

Conway, C. C., Forbes, M. K., Forbush, K. T., Fried, E. I., Hallquist, M. N., Kotov, R., . . . Eaton, N. R. (2019). A hierarchical taxonomy of psychopathology can transform mental health research. *Perspectives on Psychological Science, 14,* 419–436.

Conway, C. C., Hammen, C., & Brennan, P. A. (2012). Expanding stress generation theory: Test of a transdiagnostic model. *Journal of Abnormal Psychology, 121,* 754–766.

Craske, M. G., Meuret, A. E., Ritz, T., Treanor, M., Dour, H., & Rosenfield, D. (2019). Positive affect treatment for depression and anxiety: A randomized clinical trial for a core feature of anhedonia. *Journal of Consulting and Clinical Psychology, 87*(5), 457–471.

Edershile, E. A., & Wright, A. G. C. (2021). Fluctuations in grandiose and vulnerable narcissistic states: A momentary perspective. *Journal of Personality and Social Psychology, 120*(5), 1386–1414.

Ellard-Gray, A., Jeffrey, N. K., Choubak, M., & Crann, S. E. (2015). Finding the hidden participant: Solutions for recruiting hidden, hard-to-reach, and

vulnerable populations. *International Journal of Qualitative Methods, 14*(5), 1609406915621420.
Hammen, C. (1991). Generation of stress in the course of unipolar depression. *Journal of Abnormal Psychology, 100*(4), 555.
Haslam, N., McGrath, M. J., Viechtbauer, W., & Kuppens, P. (2020). Dimensions over categories: A meta-analysis of taxometric research. *Psychological Medicine, 50*(9), 1418–1432.
Kotov, R., Krueger, R. F., Watson, D., Cicero, D. C., Conway, C. C., DeYoung, C. G., . . . Wright, A. G. (2021). The hierarchical taxonomy of psychopathology (HiTOP): A quantitative nosology based on consensus of evidence. *Annual Review of Clinical Psychology, 17,* 83–108.
MacCallum, R. C., Zhang, S., Preacher, K. J., & Rucker, D. D. (2002). On the practice of dichotomization of quantitative variables. *Psychological Methods, 7*(1), 19.

PART II REFERENCES

Charlson, M. E., & Wells, M. T. (2022). Comorbidity: From a confounder in longitudinal clinical research to the main issue in population management. *Psychotherapy and Psychosomatics, 91*(3), 145–151.
Clark, S. L., Muthén, B., Kaprio, J., D'Onofrio, B. M., Viken, R., & Rose, R. J. (2013). Models and strategies for factor mixture analysis: An example concerning the structure underlying psychological disorders. *Structural Equation Modeling: A Multidisciplinary Journal, 20*(4), 681–703.
Conway, C. C., Forbes, M. K., Forbush, K. T., Fried, E. I., Hallquist, M. N., Kotov, R., . . . Eaton, N. R. (2019). A hierarchical taxonomy of psychopathology can transform mental health research. *Perspectives on Psychological Science, 14*(3), 419–436.
Conway, C. C., Hammen, C., & Brennan, P. (2012). A Comparison of latent class, latent trait, and factor mixture models of *DSM-IV* borderline personality disorder criteria in a community setting: Implications for *DSM-5*. *Journal of Personality Disorders, 26*(5), 793–803.
Franco-Martínez, A., Alvarado, J. M., & Sorrel, M. A. (2023). Range restriction affects factor analysis: Normality, estimation, fit, loadings, and reliability. *Educational and Psychological Measurement, 83*(2), 262–293.
Galovski, T. E., Blain, L. M., Chappuis, C., & Fletcher, T. (2013). Sex differences in recovery from PTSD in male and female interpersonal assault survivors. *Behaviour Research and Therapy, 51*(6), 247–255.
Haeffel, G. J., Jeronimus, B. F., Kaiser, B. N., Weaver, L. J., Soyster, P. D., Fisher, A. J., . . . Lu, W. (2022). Folk classification and factor rotations: Whales, sharks, and the problems with the hierarchical taxonomy of psychopathology (HiTOP). *Clinical Psychological Science, 10*(2), 259–278.
Haslam, N., McGrath, M. J., Viechtbauer, W., & Kuppens, P. (2020). Dimensions over categories: A meta-analysis of taxometric research. *Psychological Medicine, 50*(9), 1418–1432.
Helle, A. C., Trull, T. J., Watts, A. L., McDowell, Y., & Sher, K. J. (2020).

Psychiatric comorbidity as a function of severity: DSM-5 alcohol use disorder and HiTOP classification of mental disorders. *Alcoholism: Clinical and Experimental Research, 44*(3), 632–644.

Humphreys, K., & Weisner, C. (2000). Use of exclusion criteria in selecting research subjects and its effect on the generalizability of alcohol treatment outcome studies. *American Journal of Psychiatry, 157*(4), 588–594.

Jackson, J. N. S., & MacKillop, J. (2016). Attention-deficit/hyperactivity disorder and monetary delay discounting: A meta-analysis of case-control studies. *Biological Psychiatry: Cognitive Neuroscience and Neuroimaging, 1*(4), 316–325.

Johnson, B. N., & Levy, K. N. (2020). Identifying unstable and empty phenotypes of borderline personality through factor mixture modeling in a large nonclinical sample. *Personality Disorders: Theory, Research, and Treatment, 11*(2), 141.

Kaiser, B. N., & Weaver, L. (2019). Culture-bound syndromes, idioms of distress, and cultural concepts of distress: New directions for an old concept in psychological anthropology. *Transcultural Psychiatry, 56*(4), 589–598.

Lubke, G., & Tueller, S. (2010). Latent class detection and class assignment: A comparison of the MAXEIG taxometric procedure and factor mixture modeling approaches. *Structural Equation Modeling: A Multidisciplinary Journal, 17*(4), 605–628.

Maillard, A., Cabé, N., Viader, F., & Pitel, A. L. (2020). Neuropsychological deficits in alcohol use disorder: Impact on treatment. In A. Verdejo-Garcia (Ed.), *Cognition and Addiction* (pp. 103–128). Academic Press.

McBride, O., Teesson, M., Baillie, A., & Slade, T. (2011). Assessing the dimensionality of lifetime DSM-IV alcohol use disorders and a quantity-frequency alcohol use criterion in the Australian population: A factor mixture modelling approach. *Alcohol and Alcoholism, 46*(3), 333–341.

Meehl, P. E. (1992). Factors and taxa, traits and types, differences of degree and differences in kind. *Journal of Personality, 60*(1), 117–174.

Moffitt, T. E. (1993). A developmental taxonomy. *Psychological Review, 100*(4), 674–701.

Monahan, S. C., & Finney, J. W. (1996). Explaining abstinence rates following treatment for alcohol abuse: a quantitative synthesis of patient, research design and treatment effects. *Addiction, 91*(6), 787–805.

Muthén, B. (2006). Should substance use disorders be considered as categorical or dimensional? *Addiction, 101*(1), 6–16.

Newman, D. L., Moffitt, T. E., Caspi, A., & Silva, P. A. (1998). Comorbid mental disorders: Implications for treatment and sample selection. *Journal of Abnormal Psychology, 107*(2), 305–311.

Oscar-Berman, M., Valmas, M. M., Sawyer, K. S., Ruiz, S. M., Luhar, R. B., & Gravitz, Z. R. (2014). Profiles of impaired, spared, and recovered neuropsychological processes in alcoholism. *Handbook of Clinical Neurology, 125*, 183–210.

Roberts, M. C., & Ilardi, S. S. (2008). *Handbook of research methods in clinical psychology*. John Wiley & Sons.

Saha, T. D., Grant, B. F., Chou, S. P., Kerridge, B. T., Pickering, R. P., & Ruan,

W. J. (2018). Concurrent use of alcohol with other drugs and DSM-5 alcohol use disorder comorbid with other drug use disorders: Sociodemographic characteristics, severity, and psychopathology. *Drug and Alcohol Dependence, 187,* 261–269.

Shen, W., Kiger, T. B., Davies, S. E., Rasch, R. L., Simon, K. M., & Ones, D. S. (2011). Samples in applied psychology: over a decade of research in review. *Journal of Applied Psychology, 96*(5), 1055.

Steinley, D., & Brusco, M. J. (2008). Selection of variables in cluster analysis: An empirical comparison of eight procedures. *Psychometrika, 73*(1), 125–144.

Steppan, M., Piontek, D., & Kraus, L. (2014). The effect of sample selection on the distinction between alcohol abuse and dependence. *International Journal of Alcohol and Drug Research, 3*(2), 2.

Sunderland, M., Carragher, N., Wong, N., & Andrews, G. (2013). Factor mixture analysis of DSM-IV symptoms of major depression in a treatment seeking clinical population. *Comprehensive Psychiatry, 54*(5), 474–483.

Van Dam, N. T., O'Connor, D., Marcelle, E. T., Ho, E. J., Cameron Craddock, R., Tobe, R. H., . . . Milham, M. P. (2017). Data-driven phenotypic categorization for neurobiological analyses: Beyond DSM-5 labels. *Biological Psychiatry, 81*(6), 484–494.

Volarov, M., Allan, N. P., & Mihić, L. (2020). Factor mixture modeling of anxiety sensitivity: Support for the three-class solution in a Serbian sample. *Psychological Assessment, 32*(10), 915.

Wang, Y., Hsu, H.-Y., & Kim, E. (2021). Investigating the impact of covariate inclusion on sample size requirements of factor mixture modeling: A Monte Carlo simulation study. *Structural Equation Modeling: A Multidisciplinary Journal, 28*(5), 716–724.

Waszczuk, M. A., Kotov, R., Ruggero, C., Gamez, W., & Watson, D. (2017). Hierarchical structure of emotional disorders: From individual symptoms to the spectrum. *Journal of Abnormal Psychology, 126*(5), 613–634.

Weinberger, D. R., Glick, I. D., & Klein, D. F. (2015). Whither Research Domain Criteria (RDoC)? The good, the bad, and the ugly. *JAMA Psychiatry, 72*(12), 1161–1162.

Zachar, P. (2000). Psychiatric disorders are not natural kinds. *Philosophy, Psychiatry, & Psychology, 7*(3), 167–182.

CHAPTER 9

How can developmental processes help us understand the similarities and differences between personality and psychopathology?

Although most psychopathology research is done using cross-sectional data and often different methods are used to study people at different ages, theories of personality and psychopathology emphasize the importance of developmental processes. It stands to reason that development could also help articulate differences between personality and psychopathology. In this chapter, we asked experts to answer three questions:

Does developmental psychology support a personality-based conception of psychopathology?

What does developmental research say about how personality and psychopathology reflect the same phenomena?

How can developmental methods help distinguish personality from psychopathology?

Lahey takes a trait disposition approach to these questions and emphasizes that largely orthogonal personality dimensions provide a framework for understanding both the personological foundations of psychopathology and differences between kinds. Correlations between traits and psychopathology support a personality-based conception of psychopathology, but the fact that traits are mostly orthogonal, whereas psychopathology constructs are strongly correlated suggests that there are different causal influences. From his perspective, different kinds of studies are needed to better understand these causal mechanisms. In contrast, Zell and Sharp take an identity-based approach to argue that traits are not sufficient to understand the development of psychopathology. Although they acknowledge a close correspondence between personality traits and psychopathology constructs, they emphasize and illustrate with selected developmental findings that psychopathology, and personality disorder in particular, is also a result of failures to integrate different features of the self into a coherent identity during the transition to adulthood.

PART I

A developmental perspective on personality and psychological problems

Benjamin B. Lahey

I address the use of dispositions to interrogate the causal mechanisms of psychological problems. The term dispositions is a synonym for temperament, but without the theoretical baggage attached to that term (Mischel, 2004). Psychological problems is a synonym for psychopathology, without the stigmatizing implication that psychological problems are "pathological" (Lahey, 2021, 2024).

Differentiating Dispositions and Psychological Problems

The distinction between dispositions and psychological problems is fuzzy (DeYoung et al., 2022), but we have proposed a pragmatic distinction to open a window on the causal mechanisms of psychological problems (Lahey et al., 2017). Like others (Cuthbert & Insel, 2013), I suspect that urgent questions about the nature of psychological problems are intractable without using dispositions to pry apart the overlapping causal mechanisms of psychological problems (Lahey, 2024; Lahey et al., 2017). Unlike the *highly correlated* dimensions of psychological problems, the dispositional dimensions discussed in this chapter are *essentially orthogonal.* This stark difference in correlational structures distinguishes dispositions and psychological problems. This is key because, if they are reliably measured, it is unlikely that uncorrelated dispositional dimensions share the same causal mechanisms. If they did, they would be correlated. Thus, unlike the correlated dimensions of psychological problems, each dispositional dimension is likely to be associated with relatively unique causal mechanisms (Lahey, Applegate, et al., 2008; Lahey et al., 2010, 2017). In this brief chapter, I mostly refer to the measure of dispositions in children and adolescents termed the Child and Adolescent Dispositions Scale (CADS; Lahey, Applegate, et al., 2008; Lahey et al., 2010). Because our specific goal was to study relationships between dispositions and psychological problems, the item pool for the CADS *did not include synonyms or antonyms of items that define psychological problems.* This avoids spurious correlations between dispositions and psychological problems due to item overlap (Lahey, 2004). The exclusion of items similar to symptoms of psychopathology means that some temperament dimensions identified in general-use measures are not included in the CADS. For example, the trait of "effortful control" is not measured in the CADS because it is mostly defined by antonyms of symptoms of attention-deficit/hyperactivity disorder (ADHD).

Children who are high on CADS "negative emotionality" respond frequently and intensely with negative emotions to loss, threat, and frustration (Lahey et al., 2010). The particular negative emotions evoked depend on the nature of the stressor, the circumstances, and other characteristics of the individual (Compas et al., 2004). This dimension is essentially neuroticism (Barbaranelli et al., 2003; Lahey, 2009), but without the synonyms of symptoms of mental disorders included in measures of neuroticism. Many studies have identified a dimension of caring about the well-being of others, attempting to help and please others, and enjoying the company of others (Flook et al., 2019; Spinrad & Eisenberg, 2014), termed "prosociality" in the CADS (Lahey, Applegate, et al., 2008; Lahey et al., 2010). Children who are low on CADS "daring" avoid danger, whereas children high on daring find intense and risky situations to be attractive and rewarding. Daring overlaps with the concepts of sensation seeking (Mann et al., 2017) at one end of the continuum and behavioral inhibition (Schwartz et al., 1996) and risk intolerance (Karlsson Linnér et al., 2019) at the other end. Individual differences in cognitive skills constitute another dispositional dimension related to psychological problems not measured in the CADS. More research is needed to parse the roles of general intelligence, language development, and executive functioning and how they are related to psychological problems (Lahey et al., 2017).

How Are Dispositional Traits Related to the Development of Psychological Problems?

Measures of temperament in infancy through adolescence predict psychological problems later in life (Del Giudice et al., 2020; Keenan, 2000; Lahey, 2004, 2009; Ormel et al., 2013; Sanson et al., 2004). Each CADS dimension is concurrently associated with multiple dimensions of psychological problems (Lahey, Applegate, et al., 2008; Lahey et al., 2010; Taylor et al., 2013) and higher CADS negative emotionality, higher daring, and lower prosociality in early adolescence prospectively predict antisocial behavior in later adolescence (Trentacosta et al., 2009). Indeed, these CADS dimensions rated by parents during childhood and adolescence predicted self-reported antisocial behavior 12 years later (Lahey et al., 2018) and predicted the variance common to a broad range of adult psychological problems (i.e., the general factor of psychological problems) during early adulthood (Class et al., 2019).

If we are to use dispositions to understand psychological problems, we must know why they are correlated. CADS dispositions and psychological problems substantially share the same genetic and family influences (Hink et al., 2013; Mikolajewski et al., 2013; Tackett et al., 2013). It is likely that this sharing arises largely through transactional processes. Dispositional dimensions are hypothesized to transact with the environment to influence the development of psychological problems. Gene–environment correlations arise when genetically influenced dispositional behavior selects and alters the child's environment and influences how the environment changes the child's behavior (Lahey, 2021; Plomin et al., 1977). Specifically, the CADS dimension of negative emotionality is hypothesized to transact with the environment in ways that foster the development of psychological problems in two ways. First, negative emotionality provides the diffuse child emotions that our experiences shape into specific psychological problems such as depression and oppositional behavior. Second, negative emotional behavior influences the ways in which others in the environment respond to the individual, often in ways that foster maladaptive behavior (Snyder et al., 2003). In addition, persons high in negative emotionality learn fears more easily (Servaas et al., 2013). In addition, when children who are high in prosociality behave in ways that upset others, the natural consequences of their behaviors on others are hypothesized to be punishing. Furthermore, children who are high in prosociality care about the opinions of other people and are hypothesized to be more responsive to social rewards, fostering the learning of adaptive behavior (Lahey & Waldman, 2012). At the other end of the continuum, children low in prosociality are not motivated to please others and likely find the adverse consequences that their behavior has on others—such as making another child cry—to be neutral or even reinforcing (Frick & Viding, 2009). The rough and tumble of fighting, the intense stimulation of vandalism, and the risk of being caught when shoplifting are attractive and positively reinforcing to highly daring children and likely teach them to be antisocial. In contrast, these same consequences would be aversive to children who are high in daring and discourage their antisocial behavior.

Can Dispositions Be Used to Disaggregate Cross-Cutting Causal Mechanisms of Psychological Problems?

Two high barriers to discovering the causal mechanisms of psychological problems are that all dimensions are both highly correlated with one another—and therefore share causal mechanisms—and likely to be heterogeneous—the same psychological problems arise in different persons through different mechanisms (Cuthbert & Insel, 2013; Lahey, 2021, 2024; Lahey et al., 2011, 2017). Fortunately, we can use orthogonal dispositional traits to parse the causal influences and mechanisms underlying psychological problems. The lack of correlations among the CADS dispositions is critical here because it is unlikely that uncorrelated dimensions share the same causes and mechanisms. If they did, they would be correlated.

Something approaching a *paradigm shift* in our research strategies will be needed, however (Cuthbert & Insel, 2013; Lahey et al., 2017). We can easily discover the causes and mechanisms of orthogonal dispositional dimensions if we conduct the right kinds of large-scale studies of dispositions—which we are not currently conducting—and then determine how the causal mechanisms of dispositions contribute to psychological problems. There is already growing evidence that dispositional dimensions are associated with the correlated problem dimensions in a *cross-cutting* fashion (Lahey et al., 2017). This means that each disposition is related to more than one problem dimension and each problem dimension is associated with more than one dispositional dimension. To illustrate this, I estimated cross-cutting associations by regressing 10 illustrative dimensions of psychological problems on the three CADS dimensions in separate multiple regression analyses using data from the Tennessee Twin Study (Lahey, Rathouz, et al., 2008) adjusting for age, sex, and race/ethnicity and taking the clustering within twin pairs into account (Lahey, 2024). Figure 9.1 shows that each parent-rated psychological problem dimension was significantly associated with at least one parent-rated CADS dispositional dimension after controlling for multiple testing but that every dimension of psychological problems differed from the others in terms of the magnitudes, and sometimes the directions, of their associations with the dispositions.

Notably, *every* dimension of psychological problems is positively associated with CADS negative emotionality. This implies that the

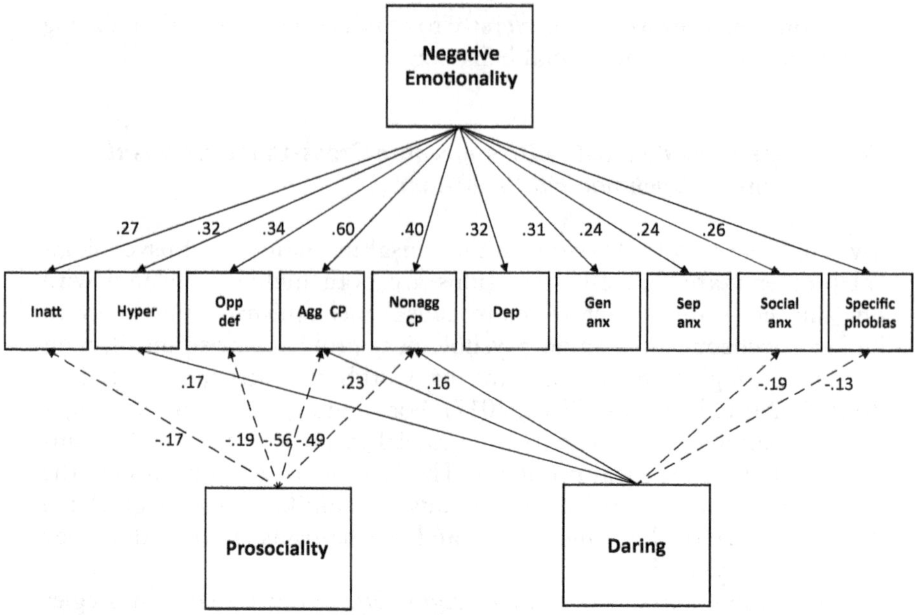

FIGURE 9.1. Standardized regression coefficients for concurrent cross-cutting associations between three dispositions measured using the CADS in children and adolescents in the Tennessee Twins Study (Lahey, 2024). Dashed lines indicate inverse associations. Only significant coefficients (≥.10) are shown.

causes of individual differences in negative emotionality increase the likelihood of every dimension of psychological problems and contribute to the ubiquitous positive correlations among them. Negative emotionality is associated with each dimension of psychological problems to varying degrees, however. For example, parent-rated negative emotionality accounted for 36.0% of the variance in aggressive conduct problems, 11.4% of the variance in oppositional defiant problems, 10.2% of the variance in depression, and 4.8% of the variance in specific fears. These marked variations in the magnitudes of associations of negative emotionality with each dimension of psychological problems suggest that the various dimensions of psychological problems are differentiated to a degree partly because they are associated with negative emotionality to varying extents. In addition, every dimension of psychological problems is associated to varying degrees with prosociality and daring. For example, inverse associations with parent-rated prosociality accounted for 31.4% of the variance in aggression and 2.9% of the variance in inattention. The positive association with daring accounted for 4.8%

of the variance in aggression, whereas *inverse* associations with daring accounted for 3.6% of the variance in social anxiety and 4.0% of the variance in fears.

The cross-cutting associations of dispositions with psychological problems should provide a way to address the problem of heterogeneity in causal mechanisms of psychological problems. For example, some youth with high levels of conduct problems are likely to be high on negative emotionality and daring and low on prosociality. Other youth with high levels of conduct problems will be high on only one or both dispositions. Each dimension of psychological problems is likely to have additional causes and mechanisms that are unique to that dimension (Lahey et al., 2011, 2017). Furthermore, the particular problems developed by each individual are not determined only by dispositions. Transactions of children with similar dispositional profiles in different environments will result in different problems. Orthogonal dispositional traits provide an important starting point for etiologic and mechanistic research, however.

PART II

Developmental personality–psychopathology spectrum approaches

Are traits enough?

CHARLOTTE S. ZELL and CARLA SHARP

Personality–psychopathology spectrum approaches began to emerge in the literature in the early 1990s and focused initially on adult personality and psychopathology. The spectrum model conceptualizes personality traits and psychopathology as lying on a continuum, with psychopathology representing extreme manifestations of personality dimensions that cause impairment in functioning. In support of this model, a substantial body of research links personality traits and psychopathology to shared etiological factors and demonstrates that personality traits map onto internalizing, externalizing, and psychotic spectra dimensions of psychopathology (e.g., Kotov et al., 2021).

Following the principles of developmental psychopathology however, one cannot assume a perfect match between models and frameworks used to explain phenomenology in adults and its downward extension to children and adolescents. Using a developmental psychopathology framework, several developmentalists therefore evaluated the developmental fit of adult models to explain relations between personality and psychopathology from a developmental point of view (e.g., De Clercq et al., 2006). Broadly speaking, personality–psychopathology spectrum approaches were shown to extend downward to children and adolescents, thereby providing a framework for understanding the early emergence of psychopathology in youth. However, arguing from a basic science point of view, McAdams (e.g., 2015) has promoted the idea that traits are not enough to fully capture the nature and function of personality. If this is so, there may be limitations to the ability of the personality–psychopathology spectrum approach to explain the onset and development of psychopathology. In this chapter, we use personality disorder as a prime example of how traits may be insufficient to explain the onset and development of psychopathology. We rely on the work of McAdams and Sharp (e.g., Sharp, 2020; Sharp & Wall, 2021) to answer three questions that the editors asked us to focus on in service of shedding light on the broader topic of dimensional diagnosis that seeks to integrate personality and psychopathology: Does developmental psychology support a personality-based conception of psychopathology? What does developmental research say about how personality and psychopathology reflect the same phenomena? How can developmental methods help distinguish personality from psychopathology? By using personality disorder as an example to illustrate problems in trait-only conceptualizations, the difficulties in equating personality with internalizing–externalizing–psychotic-spectra psychopathology are elucidated. In short, the answers to the questions posed to us are that developmental psychology supports a personality-based conception of psychopathology but that a trait-only conceptualization of personality, and by extension, personality disorder is inadequate to fulfill this function. We argue that to facilitate dimensional diagnosis of personality disorder (and potentially all psychopathology) in adolescents (and adults), a more comprehensive understanding of personality, also including the intrapersonal (or self) functions of personality, is necessary. Whether this argument elevates personality pathology as a special case of psychopathology that is not accounted for by traits or pertains to all psychopathology remains an open question, one that we return to briefly throughout the chapter.

Does Developmental Psychology Support a Personality-Based Conception of Psychopathology?

Personality traits can be understood as outward expansions of temperament (biologically based early individual differences in reactivity and regulation) that develop as children gain new skills and capacities that allow them to experience and respond to their environment in increasingly complex ways (Tackett, 2006). As shown in Figure 9.2, temperamental traits interact with the early environmental context to produce a child's basic personality trait profile, which can be organized into the Big Five dimensions of Extraversion, Neuroticism, Conscientiousness, Agreeableness, and Openness/Intellect as early as the preschool period. The temperament dimension of positive emotionality typically develops into the broader personality trait of extraversion in childhood, whereas negative emotionality is the temperamental precursor to neuroticism. Effortful control, a third dimension of temperament, maps onto childhood conscientiousness and influences extraversion and agreeableness. Early childhood personality traits and life experiences continue to exert reciprocal influence throughout childhood and adolescence to produce adult personality traits that can be measured along the same basic dimensions. Extreme, maladaptive variants of the Big Five also emerge in childhood; show moderate to high stability over time; and exhibit a similar structure in children, adolescents, and adults (De Clercq et al., 2006).

Research investigating the hierarchical structure of temperament and childhood personality traits as well as child mental health symptoms shows that all three are explained by the same higher-order internalizing and externalizing spectra (see Figure 9.2 for a visual summary). That traits and mental health symptoms are accounted for by the same dimensions (across development) has allowed for the reorganization of psychopathology in models like the hierarchical taxonomy of psychopathology (HiTOP; Kotov et al., 2021), with five of HiTOP's six major spectra dimensions mapping onto maladaptive variants of the Big Five personality traits (Negative Affectivity, Psychoticism, Disinhibition, Antagonism, and Detachment). According to this model then, personality traits subserve almost all forms of psychopathology.

What Does Developmental Research Say about How Personality and Psychopathology Reflect the Same Phenomena?

Although developmental research clearly supports a personality–psychopathology spectrum, by equating (or conflating) personality and psychopathology, however, it renders one or the other of these constructs obsolete. Put differently, if personality simply represents internalizing, externalizing, and psychotic spectra, we could simply do away with the concept of personality and, by extension, personality disorder. As

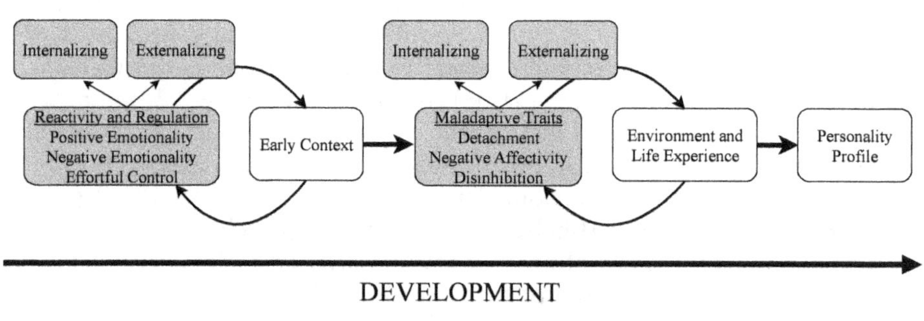

FIGURE 9.2. The codevelopment of personality, temperament, and psychopathology according to the personality–psychopathology spectrum approach.

we discuss below, however, doing so poses a significant challenge to explaining the onset of psychopathology. We illustrate this with reference to the onset of personality disorder.

Proponents of the spectrum approach have contended that elevated traits do account for the adolescent onset of personality disorder, as the specific developmental demands of this period become impossible to navigate for a young person with elevated maladaptive traits. Although we agree that the environmental demands of adolescence are critical to understanding the onset of personality disorder, the mechanism by which the adolescent fails to adapt to life demands is still not explained by the personality–psychopathology spectrum approach. Moreover, the environmental demands associated with other developmental periods (e.g., going to school at age 5/6) are equally difficult to manage for children with elevated traits yet do not signal the onset of personality disorder during these periods. We have argued that instead we must turn to developmental research beyond traits to help us identify the mechanisms by which elevated traits turn into disorder during adolescence.

A more comprehensive framework for personality development, drawing on decades of developmental research and encompassing goals, values, and narrative identity in addition to traits, was put forth by Dan McAdams (2015). Within this model, dispositional traits represent just the first layer of personality, or "self as actor." A second layer of personality, "self as agent," develops around ages 5–7 years, as increasing cognitive and social abilities allow children to establish and work toward goals and link motives to behaviors in both self and others. Critically, it is not until adolescence that more advanced metacognitive capacities facilitate the emergence of the third layer of personality, self as author, which involves the integration of personal past, present, and future into a cohesive life story and self-narrative. It is this process of meaning making that binds personality and gives the self a sense of coherence and purpose. We argue that it is not elevated traits alone but rather the failure or delay to integrate the different layers of personality into a coherent whole that explains the onset of personality disorder. In contrast, other forms of psychopathology may not need the second and third layers of personality to onset. For instance, major depressive disorder could simply be viewed as severe enough negative affectivity or neuroticism to impair general functioning.

How Can Developmental Methods Help Distinguish Personality from Psychopathology?

Developmental psychopathology research on the onset of personality disorder shows us that personality disorder, especially borderline personality disorder, can be reliably assessed and is diagnosable in adolescence. Despite the continuity of personality traits across development, the same is not true in preadolescence. Why? Because, as outlined above, a core piece of personality—an integrated sense of self—is not developmentally deployed until adolescence. We argue here that for the diagnosis of personality disorder, but not other psychopathology, this piece of personality needs to be in place.

To elaborate, as McAdams's (e.g., 2015) model of personality development lays out, traits provide only the initial building blocks for personality functioning. We can imagine two young people with high trait emotional lability. As they advance through adolescence, one learns to channel their emotions to excel in creative pursuits, creating a narrative of themselves as deeply sensitive, in touch with the world around them, and able to convey intense feeling in music and art. The other feels overwhelmed and confused by their emotions, experiencing themselves as unstable, defective, and burdensome to others. This example illustrates that personality involves an active process of directing our dispositional traits toward values and goals and ultimately making sense of ourselves and our relationships, a view that aligns with level of personality functioning (LPF) within the alternative model of personality disorders (AMPD). LPF, conceptualized as the core of personality disorder, is defined as self (identity and self-direction) and interpersonal (empathy and intimacy) functioning, or the capacity (and process) of understanding and managing the self in the context of interpersonal relationships to fulfill adult role functions (Sharp & Wall, 2021). The self as the core of personality and its pathology is not a new idea; early conceptualizations of personality also emphasized the active construction of a representation of self (Freud, 1923; James, 1892; Mead, 1934).

We have argued that a particularly critical process or mechanism facilitating progression through the layers of personality development, and ultimately the formation of a coherent sense of self, is the development of mentalizing (Sharp & Wall, 2021). This process begins in infancy with social referencing, where infants observe caregivers' emotional reactions to guide their own responses, laying the foundation for a shared understanding of the world. Caregivers also play a critical role in mediating infants' experiences through labeling, including of the infant's own emotions and behaviors. As infants gain language skills, they begin naming their own feelings and actions. At around 2 years of age, toddlers begin to engage in pretend play, marking the initial recognition of the content of their mind as separate from reality. By age 4, children develop basic theory of mind, enabling them to infer others' thoughts, a precursor to more complex mentalizing. Between ages 6 and 8, children begin reflecting on their own thoughts and those of others, with the continued support of caregivers in mediating their inner experience. In middle childhood, perspective-taking skills advance significantly, enabling children to navigate complex social interactions, experience more self-conscious emotions like shame and pride, and develop a more defined self-concept. It is not until adolescence, however, that metacognitive abilities mature sufficiently for individuals to integrate multiple abstract ideas about the self in relation to others into a cohesive narrative identity, with decreasing reliance on caregiver mediation (Ferrer-Wreder & Kroger, 2019).

When mentalizing development is disrupted, individuals may be unable to achieve successful binding of personality at each stage and construct an integrated representation of self (Sharp, 2020). Without a coherent and flexible sense of self, including the ability to merge with others while maintaining one's own identity, close relationships also become difficult to form and maintain. Healthy, close relationships, in turn, are critical for the further development of self-understanding. Thus, self- and interpersonal functioning exert reciprocal influence and become intractably linked, forming a unidimensional severity continuum (i.e., personality functioning).

Throughout the development of mentalization and binding of personality, traits remain fairly stable (De Clercq et al., 2009). Traits can pave the way for greater difficulty with moving through the layers of personality development (e.g., by evoking less sensitive responses from caregivers, which in turn disrupts the development of mentalization) and shape the specific manifestation of personality pathology should it emerge. Indeed, longitudinal work has shown that childhood maladaptive traits are associated with poor social functioning in early adolescence and difficulties in self-functioning in early adulthood (Vanwoerden et al., 2022). Although traits may be an important early risk marker and may be sufficient to explain internalizing–externalizing-spectra symptomology, it is ultimately other qualitative (and thus discontinuous) developmental shifts facilitated by more advanced mentalizing abilities that explain the emergence of personality disorder (Sharp, 2020). We cannot reliably assess personality disorder until adolescence because the domains of LPF—which coalesce around the representation of self—are not developmentally deployed until adolescence.

Empirical support for our application of McAdams' theory of personality development to the emergence of personal disorder is growing. Space does not allow a full discussion of this work, but readers are referred to (1) longitudinal research supporting the idea that identity formation is an important developmental task of adolescence (e.g., Bogaerts et al., 2021; Eggermont et al., 2023) and (2) research linking personality pathology with identity disturbance (e.g., Sharp et al.,

2021; Balzen et al., 2024; Lind et al., 2019, 2020, 2022; Penner et al., 2019). Another important line of evidence shows that LPF is distinct from general psychiatric severity and maladaptive traits (Criterion B of the AMPD) in adolescents—in other words, that it is not accounted for by internalizing–externalizing–psychotic spectra (or the higher-order p-factor; e.g., Sharp & Cervantes, 2023; Barkauskiene et al., 2022) as well as general psychosocial disability (Sharp et al., 2022).

Conclusion

In this chapter, we have argued that the personality–psychopathology spectrum model, although useful in understanding the relationship between personality traits and internalizing, externalizing, and psychotic disorders, does not adequately capture personality or personality disorder. For dimensional diagnosis to reach its full potential specifically as it relates to personality disorder, theories and diagnostic models of personality must go beyond traits; specifically, they must maintain a central focus on self and interpersonal impairment, the unique core of personality and personality disorder. The implication of this line of reasoning is that although personality (traits) can explain general internalizing–externalizing-spectra disorders, ironically, personality (traits) are insufficient to explain personality disorder. Another potential contender to illustrate the insufficiency of traits may be schizophrenia-spectrum disorder—a topic we do not have space for here but that warrants further elaboration. Regardless, a developmental perspective shows us that it is through the additional layers of personality, and in particular self-functioning, that we can distinguish personality from psychopathology, understand diverging personality trajectories, and explain the onset of personality disorder in adolescence.

PART I REFERENCES

Barbaranelli, C., Caprara, G. V., Rabasca, A., & Pastorelli, C. (2003). A questionnaire for measuring the Big Five in late childhood. *Personality and Individual Differences, 34,* 645–664.

Class, Q. A., Rathouz, P. J., Van Hulle, C. A., Applegate, B., Waldman, I. D., Zald, D. H., & Lahey, B. B. (2019). Socioemotional dispositions of children and adolescents predict general and specific second-order factors of psychopathology in early adulthood across informants: A 12-year prospective study. *Journal of Abnormal Psychology, 128,* 574–584.

Compas, B. E., Connor-Smith, J., & Jaser, S. S. (2004). Temperament, stress reactivity, and coping: Implications for depression in childhood and adolescence. *Journal of Clinical Child and Adolescent Psychology, 33*(1), 21–31.

Cuthbert, B. N., & Insel, T. R. (2013). Toward the future of psychiatric diagnosis: The seven pillars of RDoC. *Bmc Medicine, 11,* Article 126.

Del Giudice, T., Tervoort, J., Hautmann, C., Walter, D., & Döpfner, M. (2020). Cross-cultural validity of the child and adolescent dispositions model in a clinical sample of children with externalizing behavior problems. *Frontiers in Psychology, 11,* 641.

DeYoung, C. G., Chmielewski, M., Clark, L. A., Condon, D. M., Kotov, R., Krueger, R. F., . . . Mullins-Sweatt, S. N. (2022). The distinction between symptoms and traits in the hierarchical taxonomy of psychopathology (HiTOP). *Journal of Personality, 90*(1), 20–33.

Flook, L., Zahn-Waxler, C., & Davidson, R. J. (2019). Developmental differences in prosocial behavior between preschool and late elementary school. *Frontiers in Psychology, 10,* Article 876.

Frick, P. J., & Viding, E. (2009). Antisocial behavior from a developmental psychopathology perspective. *Development and Psychopathology, 21,* 1111–1131.

Hink, L. K., Rhee, S. H., Corley, R. P., Cosgrove, V. E., Hewitt, J. K., Schulz-Heik, R. J., . . . Waldman, I. D. (2013). Personality dimensions as common and broadband-specific features for internalizing and externalizing disorders. *Journal of Abnormal Child Psychology, 41,* 939–957.

Karlsson Linnér, R., Biroli, P., Kong, E., Meddens, S. F. W., Wedow, R., Fontana, M. A., . . . Beauchamp, J. P. (2019). Genome-wide association analyses of risk tolerance and risky behaviors in over 1 million individuals identify hundreds of loci and shared genetic influences. *Nature Genetics, 51*(2), 245–257.

Keenan, K. (2000). Emotion dysregulation as a risk factor for child psychopathology. *Clinical Psychology-Science and Practice, 7,* 418–434.

Lahey, B. B. (2004). Commentary: Role of temperament in developmental models of psychopathology. *Journal of Clinical Child and Adolescent Psychology, 33*(1), 88–93.

Lahey, B. B. (2009). Public health significance of neuroticism. *American Psychologist, 64,* 241–256.

Lahey, B. B. (2021). *Dimensions of psychological problems: Replacing diagnostic categories with a more science-based and less stigmatizing alternative.* Oxford University Press.

Lahey, B. B. (2024). Using dispositions to understand otherwise intractable causal pathways to psychological problems during childhood and adolescence. *Journal of Clinical Child and Adolescent Psychology, 53*(2), 328–341.

Lahey, B. B., Applegate, B., Chronis, A. M., Jones, H. A., Williams, S. H., Loney, J., & Waldman, I. D. (2008). Psychometric characteristics of a measure of emotional dispositions developed to test a developmental propensity model of conduct disorder. *Journal of Clinical Child and Adolescent Psychology, 37,* 794–807.

Lahey, B. B., Class, Q. A., Zald, D. H., Rathouz, P. J., Applegate, B., &

Waldman, I. D. (2018). Prospective test of the developmental propensity model of antisocial behavior: from childhood and adolescence into early adulthood. *Journal of Child Psychology and Psychiatry, 59,* 676–683.

Lahey, B. B., Krueger, R. F., Rathouz, P. J., Waldman, I. D., & Zald, D. H. (2017). A hierarchical causal taxonomy of psychopathology across the life span. *Psychological Bulletin, 143,* 142–186.

Lahey, B. B., Rathouz, P. J., Applegate, B., Tackett, J. L., & Waldman, I. D. (2010). Psychometrics of a self-report version of the child and adolescent dispositions scale. *Journal of Clinical Child and Adolescent Psychology, 39,* 351–361.

Lahey, B. B., Rathouz, P. J., Applegate, B., Van Hulle, C., Garriock, H. A., Urbano, R. C., . . . Waldman, I. D. (2008). Testing structural models of DSM-IV symptoms of common forms of child and adolescent psychopathology. *Journal of Abnormal Child Psychology, 36,* 187–206.

Lahey, B. B., Van Hulle, C. A., Singh, A. L., Waldman, I. D., & Rathouz, P. J. (2011). Higher-order genetic and environmental structure of prevalent forms of child and adolescent psychopathology. *Archives of General Psychiatry, 68,* 181–189.

Lahey, B. B., & Waldman, I. D. (2012). Annual research review: Phenotypic and causal structure of conduct disorder in the broader context of prevalent forms of psychopathology. *Journal of Child Psychology and Psychiatry, 53,* 536–557.

Mann, F. D., Engelhardt, L., Briley, D. A., Grotzinger, A. D., Patterson, M. W., Tackett, J. L., . . . Harden, K. P. (2017). Sensation seeking and impulsive traits as personality endophenotypes for antisocial behavior: Evidence from two independent samples. *Personality and Individual Differences, 105,* 30–39.

Mikolajewski, A. J., Allan, N. P., Hart, S. A., Lonigan, C. J., & Taylor, J. (2013). Negative affect shares genetic and environmental influences with symptoms of childhood internalizing and externalizing disorders. *Journal of Abnormal Child Psychology, 41,* 411–423.

Mischel, W. (2004). Toward an integrative science of the person. *Annual Review of Psychology, 55,* 1–22.

Ormel, J., Jeronimus, B. F., Kotov, R., Riese, H., Bos, E. H., Hankin, B., . . . Oldehinkel, A. J. (2013). Neuroticism and common mental disorders: Meaning and utility of a complex relationship. *Clinical Psychology Review, 33,* 686–697.

Plomin, R., DeFries, J. C., & Loehlin, J. C. (1977). Genotype–environment interaction and correlation in the analysis of human behavior. *Psychological Bulletin, 84,* 309–322.

Sanson, A., Hemphill, S. A., & Smart, D. (2004). Connections between temperament and social development: A review. *Social Development, 13,* 142–170.

Schwartz, C. E., Snidman, N., & Kagan, J. (1996). Early childhood temperament as a determinant of externalizing behavior in adolescence. *Development and Psychopathology, 8*(3), 527–537.

Servaas, M. N., van der Velde, J., Costafreda, S. G., Horton, P., Ormel, J., Riese, H., & Aleman, A. (2013). Neuroticism and the brain: A quantitative meta-analysis of neuroimaging studies investigating emotion processing. *Neuroscience and Biobehavioral Reviews, 37,* 1518–1529.

Snyder, J., Reid, J. B., & Patterson, G. R. (2003). A social learning model of child and adolescent antisocial behavior. In B. B. Lahey, T. E. Moffitt, & A. Caspi (Eds.), *Causes of conduct disorder and juvenile delinquency* (pp. 27–48). Guilford Press.

Spinrad, T. L., & Eisenberg, N. (2014). Empathy, prosocial behavior, and positive development in schools. In M. J. Furlong, R. Gilman, & E. S. Huebner (Eds.), *Handbook of positive psychology in schools* (pp. 82–98). Routledge/Taylor & Francis Group.

Tackett, J. L., Lahey, B. B., Van Hulle, C. A., Waldman, I. D., Krueger, R. F., & Rathouz, P. J. (2013). Common genetic influences on negative emotionality and a general psychopathology factor in childhood and adolescence. *Journal of Abnormal Psychology, 122,* 1142–1153.

Taylor, J., Allan, N., Mikolajewski, A. J., & Hart, S. A. (2013). Common genetic and nonshared environmental factors contribute to the association between socioemotional dispositions and the externalizing factor in children. *Journal of Child Psychology and Psychiatry, 54,* 67–76.

Trentacosta, C. J., Hyde, L. W., Shaw, D. S., & Cheong, J. W. (2009). Adolescent dispositions for antisocial behavior in context: The roles of neighborhood dangerousness and parental knowledge. *Journal of Abnormal Psychology, 118,* 564–575.

PART II REFERENCES

Balzen, K. M., Blacutt, M., Lind, M., Penner, F., & Sharp, C. (2024). Awareness of Narrative Identity Questionnaire (ANIQ) in early adolescents: Psychometric evaluation and association with features of personality disorder. *Journal of Personality Assessment, 106*(3), 337–346.

Barkauskiene, R., Gaudiesiute, E., Adler, A., Gervinskaite-Paulaitiene, L., Laurinavicius, A., & Skabeikyte-Norkiene, G. (2022). Criteria A and B of the alternative DSM-5 model for personality disorders (AMPD) capture borderline personality features among adolescents. *Frontiers in Psychiatry, 13,* 828301.

Bogaerts, A., Claes, L., Buelens, T., Verschueren, M., Palmeroni, N., Bastiaens, T., & Luyckx, K. (2021). Identity synthesis and confusion in early to late adolescents: Age trends, gender differences, and associations with depressive symptoms. *Journal of Adolescence, 87,* 106–116.

De Clercq, B., De Fruyt, F., Van Leeuwen, K., & Mervielde, I. (2006). The structure of maladaptive personality traits in childhood: A step toward an integrative developmental perspective for *DSM-V. Journal of Abnormal Psychology, 115*(4), 639–657.

Eggermont, K., Raymaekers, K., Claes, L., Buelens, T., Bogaerts, A., & Luyckx,

K. (2023). Impairment in personality functioning throughout adolescence and co-development with personality traits, emotion regulation strategies, and psychopathology. *Journal of Research in Personality, 104,* 104380.

Ferrer-Wreder, L., & Kroger, J. (2019). *Identity in adolescence: The balance between self and other.* Routledge.

Freud, S. (1923). *The ego and the id.* Hogarth.

James, W. (1892). The self. In *Psychology* (pp. 176–216). Fawcett.

Kotov, R., Krueger, R. F., Watson, D., Cicero, D. C., Conway, C. C., DeYoung, C. G., . . . Wright, A. G. C. (2021). The hierarchical taxonomy of psychopathology (HiTOP): A quantitative nosology based on consensus of evidence. *Annual Review of Clinical Psychology, 17,* 83–108.

Lind, M., Vanwoerden, S., Bo, S., & Sharp, C. (2022). Borderline personality disorder in adolescence: The role of narrative identity in the intrapsychic reasoning system. *Personality Disorders, 13*(5), 451–459.

Lind, M., Vanwoerden, S., Penner, F., & Sharp, C. (2019). Inpatient adolescents with borderline personality disorder features: Identity diffusion and narrative incoherence. *Personality Disorders, 10*(4), 389–393.

Lind, M., Vanwoerden, S., Penner, F., & Sharp, C. (2020). Narrative coherence in adolescence: Relations with attachment, mentalization, and psychopathology. *Journal of Personality Assessment, 102*(3), 380–389.

McAdams, D. P. (2015). *The art and science of personality development.* Guilford Press.

Mead, G. H. (1934). *Mind, self, and society from the standpoint of a social behaviorist.* University of Chicago Press.

Penner, F., Gambin, M., & Sharp, C. (2019). Childhood maltreatment and identity diffusion among inpatient adolescents: The role of reflective function. *Journal of Adolescence, 76,* 65–74.

Sharp, C. (2020). Adolescent personality pathology and the alternative model for personality disorders: Self development as nexus. *Psychopathology, 53*(3–4), 198–204.

Sharp, C., & Cervantes, B. R. (2023). Maladaptive self- and interpersonal functioning increments general psychiatric severity in the association with adolescent personality pathology. *Children (Basel), 10*(1), 120.

Sharp, C., Kerr, S., & Barkauskiene, R. (2022). The incremental utility of maladaptive self and identity functioning over general functioning for borderline personality disorder features in adolescents. *Personality Disorders, 13*(5), 474–481.

Sharp, C., Vanwoerden, S., Schmeck, K., Birkholzer, M., & Goth, K. (2021). An evaluation of age-group latent mean differences in maladaptive identity in adolescence. *Frontiers in Psychiatry, 12,* 730415.

Sharp, C., & Wall, K. (2021). DSM-5 level of personality functioning: Refocusing personality disorder on what it means to be human. *Annual Review of Clinical Psychology, 17,* 313–337.

Sharp, C., Wright, A. G. C., Fowler, J. C., Frueh, B. C., Allen, J. G., Oldham, J., & Clark, L. A. (2015). The structure of personality pathology: Both general ('g') and specific ('s') factors? *Journal of Abnormal Psychology, 124*(2), 387–398.

Tackett, J. L. (2006). Evaluating models of the personality–psychopathology relationship in children and adolescents. *Clinical Psychology Review, 26*(5), 584–599.

Vanwoerden, S., Franssens, R., Sharp, C., & De Clercq, B. (2022). The development of criterion A personality pathology: The relevance of childhood social functioning for young adult daily self-functioning. *Child Psychiatry and Human Development, 53*(6), 1148–1160.

CHAPTER 10

How does genetic research help us understand similarities and differences between personality and psychopathology?

Questions about the relative influences of nature and nurture have been central to discussions of personality and psychopathology since these topics have been discussed. The development of quantitative models that leverage known genetic relatedness of twins and other family members and, more recently, of sophisticated molecular approaches to examining the genome itself have begun to bring evidence to bear on these questions. In this chapter we asked experts to answer three questions about how genetic research can inform questions about the similarities and differences between personality and psychopathology:

Does genetic research support a personality-based conception of psychopathology?

What does genetic research say about how personality and psychopathology reflect the same phenomena?

How can genetic methods help distinguish personality from psychopathology?

Waszczuk generally takes the position that existing evidence supports similarities more than differences. She argues that psychopathology can be understood as extreme maladaptive traits, although she also emphasizes that more research needs to be done to determine whether this formulation holds across developmental stages and specific traits. Waszczuk emphasizes that this general conclusion is important because it means that evidence about personality traits in ongoing and future genetic studies can help inform the nature of psychopathology. Poore and Waldman describe and distinguish among several genetic methods that can be useful for answering these kinds of questions. They take a somewhat less optimistic view than Waszczuk, concluding that although there is multimethod evidence that genetic influences on personality and psychopathology overlap substantially, this overlap is not complete and there is also evidence that environmental influences on these domains differ.

PART I

Genetic evidence for personality in a hierarchical model of psychopathology

MONIKA A. WASZCZUK

Genetic research can inform psychiatric classification. Several recent literature reviews have discussed genetic evidence in support of dimensional and hierarchical conceptualizations of psychopathology (Smoller et al., 2019; Waszczuk et al., 2020), which are at the core of alternative classification approaches such as the hierarchical taxonomy of psychopathology (HiTOP) model (Kotov et al., 2017). The extant reviews have largely focused on psychiatric phenotypes. The current chapter extends this inquiry by reviewing genetic research on normal-range and maladaptive personality traits in the context of dimensional and hierarchical conceptualizations of psychopathology.

Genetic Liability Dimensions

The largest meta-analysis of taxometric research to date concluded that a vast majority of psychological variation is dimensional, including individual differences in all personality traits and almost all forms of psychopathology (Haslam et al., 2020). Thus, psychopathology constitutes the severe end of continuously distributed traits (Markon et al., 2011). The adaptive range of this continuum is thought to correspond to normal personality traits (Oltmanns et al., 2018). Indeed, broad patterns of alignment between personality traits and psychopathology have been explicated in empirical studies (Widiger et al., 2019).

There are multiple complementary explanations for the observed connections between personality and psychopathology, with shared underlying etiology playing a prominent role, in line with the spectrum model (South et al., 2010). The shared etiology is consistent with evidence that genetic liability to complex traits transcends boundaries between normality and psychopathology. Genetic influences on complex traits consist of hundreds of genetic variants, each with small effect, which in aggregate approximate a normal distribution (Plomin et al., 2009). As a result, genetic liability is continuously distributed on a dimension from heathy traits in the general population, which may encompass personality traits, to corresponding clinical diagnoses at the maladaptive end of the dimension.

Genetically informed studies can quantify the degree of shared genetic influences on personality traits and corresponding psychopathology dimensions. For example, across three twin samples, a heritable latent dimension was found to underlie neuroticism, depression symptoms, and major depressive disorder (MDD) diagnoses (Kendler et al., 2018). The latent dimension accounted for all genetic influences on depression symptoms and a significant proportion of genetic influences on neuroticism and MDD, with the latter two phenotypes also showing considerable unique genetic etiology. The substantial, but not complete, overlap on genetic liability dimensions of personality traits and corresponding psychopathology is consistent with the results of other twin studies (Hansell et al., 2012; Hettema et al., 2006).

Molecular genetic studies also support the argument that shared genetic liability underlies personality traits and corresponding psychopathology dimensions (Gupta et al., 2024; Linner et al., 2019). For example, a genome-wide association study (GWAS) of neuroticism identified 159 significant genetic loci, but GWAS conditional on (i.e., adjusted for) MDD showed that only 37 of these loci were unique to neuroticism, indicating a substantial genetic overlap (Gupta et al., 2024). Likewise, patterns of single-nucleotide-polymorphism (SNP)-based genetic correlations between personality and psychopathology demonstrate a degree of convergence that is consistent with phenotypic spectra. For example, neuroticism has the highest SNP-based genetic correlations with depression and anxiety, and general risk tolerance and (low) conscientiousness has the highest SNP-based genetic correlations with attention-deficit/hyperactivity disorder (ADHD). Structural equation modeling (SEM) methods can be applied to GWAS summary statistics to further inform genetic liability dimensions (Grotzinger et al., 2019). In one such genomic SEM (gSEM) study, neuroticism had the largest genetic correlation with internalizing factor, whereas conscientiousness had the largest negative genetic correlations with externalizing and neurodevelopmental factors (Waldman et al., 2020). Overall, molecular genetic data are consistent with data that indicate that the partial overlap on genetic liability dimensions underlies personality traits and corresponding psychopathology.

Although GWAS and twin models focus on common genetic variants, rare genetic variants can also inform genetic liability dimensions. Rare variants are observed more frequently in patients with severe psychopathology (Jacquemont et al., 2022), suggesting that there may be differences in genetic architecture at extremes of severity distributions. Therefore, rare variants are likely to contribute to the discontinuity in the genetic liability shared between normal personality traits and clinical levels of corresponding psychopathology, distinguishing personality from psychopathology.

The estimates of shared genetic liability between personality and psychopathology dimensions can be affected by a range of psychometric and methodological issues. The two domains are usually assessed using separate instruments; for example, psychiatric diagnoses that consider temporal features and impairment are often used to measure psychopathology, whereas personality traits tend to be self-reported, introducing method-specific variance that can lower estimates of genetic overlap (Waszczuk et al., 2023). Conversely, genetic liability dimensions can be overestimated because individuals with severe psychopathology are less likely to be included in genotyped biobanks and in typically powered community samples that constitute the majority of twin studies (Adams et al., 2020). Furthermore, SNP-based genetic correlations and gSEM analyses that rely on GWAS summary statistics are affected by the GWAS discovery sample sizes, phenotypes, and related methodological issues, which can alter estimates of genetic correlations (Waszczuk et al., 2023). Finally, the assessment of personality traits and psychopathology might not be at the same level as the phenotypic hierarchy. For example, if neuroticism corresponds to the internalizing factor, an investigation focusing only on the lower levels of internalizing factor, such as depressive symptoms, might identify a larger degree of dissociable genetic influences from neuroticism. The multivariate structural studies that are discussed in the next section can help explicate the alignment of genetic liability dimensions across the hierarchy.

Higher-Order Genetic Architecture

Patterns of genetic correlations observed across behavioral and molecular genetic studies of psychiatric phenotypes indicate a hierarchical architecture of genetic influences (Grotzinger et al., 2019; Waldman et al., 2020; Waszczuk et al., 2020). At the top of the hierarchy, a significant proportion of genetic influences is common to all psychiatric phenotypes, in line with a phenotypic general factor of psychopathology ("p-factor"). The remaining genetic risk is more specific and generally appears to parallel the phenotypic structure; that is, there are genetically coherent spectra of internalizing, externalizing, and thought disorder.

The parallel between phenotypic and genetic higher-order structure is observed in studies of normal personality traits (Gustavson et al., 2020; Turkheimer et al., 2014). Furthermore, genetic studies can inform whether higher-order genetic architectures of personality and psychopathology can be mapped onto each other, extending the spectrum model of the individual-differences continuum from normal traits (e.g., neuroticism) to corresponding psychopathology (e.g., depression) to a joint multivariate model. Indeed, personality traits demonstrate significant genetic correlations with higher-order factors of psychopathology. For example, several twin studies have identified a high genetic correlation between neuroticism and both general factor of psychopathology and internalizing factor (Hink et al., 2013; Poore et al., 2022).

A limited number of twin studies have comprehensively modeled the joint genetic architecture of personality and psychopathology using phenotypes spanning several higher-order spectra (Gjerde et al., 2023; Rosenström et al., 2019). In one study, the joint hierarchical genetic structure of 11 psychiatric disorders and 10 normal-range and maladaptive personality traits consisted of a highly heritable general factor of psychopathology influencing almost all phenotypes and two orthogonal moderately heritable internalizing and externalizing factors (Rosenström et al., 2019). The personality profile that best reflected the general factor was a high score on neuroticism and low scores on conscientiousness and agreeableness. However, in this study a statistically equivalent correlated factors model could also be fit to the data, and this model consisted of distinct but genetically correlated psychopathology and personality factors. The statistical equivalence of two structural genetic models highlights some of the challenges of comparing and interpreting complex multivariate architectures that combine personality and psychopathology.

The gSEM approach has also been used to test connections between genetic architectures of personality and psychopathology. A recent gSEM study derived a joint higher-order genetic structure using a range of personality trait and psychopathology phenotypes (Levey et al., 2021). Specifically, an internalizing genetic factor consisted of loadings from neuroticism alongside mood and anxiety disorder phenotypes. An externalizing genetic factor had major contributions from risk-taking behavior and cannabis use disorder phenotypes. A third genetic factor generally represented a neurocognitive domain, with no contribution from personality traits. Expanding the range of phenotypes, Gustavson et al. (2023) conducted gSEM that resulted in latent genetic factors of internalizing/neuroticism, externalizing (inclusive of risk-taking personality trait phenotypes), thought disorders, and compulsive disorders. Trait impulsivity demonstrated the largest positive genetic correlation with the externalizing factor, a moderate positive genetic correlation with the internalizing factor, a small positive genetic correlation with the thought disorders factor, and a small negative correlation with the compulsive disorders factor. Conversely, the residual trait urgency factor was specifically and strongly genetically correlated with the internalizing psychopathology factor.

Utility of Personality Traits in Psychiatric Genetics

Explaining shared genetic influences on personality and psychopathology across liability dimensions and hierarchical architecture has potential utility for advancing psychiatric genetic discovery. Personality traits that are markers of genetic vulnerability to psychopathology can serve as complimentary quantitative and transdiagnostic phenotypic targets in psychiatric GWAS (Waszczuk et al., 2023). For example, most of the genetic loci that were identified in the neuroticism GWAS are shared with MDD (Gupta et al., 2024). The advantage of personality phenotypes is that they are often more feasible to collect than psychiatric diagnoses or biomarkers are. This could help increase the GWAS sample size, which is one of the most important factors affecting gene discovery power. Moreover, dimensional personality instruments often demonstrate better psychometric properties than clinical measures, further improving GWAS performance. Finally, genetic datasets with personality phenotypes can be pooled with clinical datasets containing other genetically correlated traits to accelerate genetic discovery. For example, multivariate analyses of several risk-taking traits, ADHD, and substance use identified 579 significant loci associated with liability for externalizing, with over 100 loci constituting entirely novel discoveries (Linner et al., 2019).

Summary statistics from GWAS allow researchers to calculate polygenic scores (PGS), which are commonly used to translate molecular genetic discoveries to a wide range of research contexts (Lewis & Vassos, 2020). Personality PGS are useful in both predicting and understanding psychopathology (Hoy et al., 2023). Neuroticism PGS were found to be significantly associated with internalizing disorders such as depression, anxiety, and posttraumatic stress disorder (PTSD) in independent samples (Costantini et al., 2023; Docherty et al., 2018; Waszczuk et al., 2022). Personality PGS can also inform mechanistic studies. Risk-taking PGS were found to be significantly associated with altered neuroanatomy implicated in risky behaviors, which may ultimately advance models of the biological foundations of externalizing psychopathology

(Aydogan et al., 2021). Finally, pooling personality data in discovery GWAS can improve polygenic prediction. The aforementioned externalizing GWAS that combined data on risk-taking traits, ADHD, and substance use disorders resulted in an externalizing PGS that demonstrated some of the largest effect sizes observed for any PGS in psychiatric and behavioral genetics to date (Linner et al., 2019). The externalizing PGS significantly predicted a range of psychiatric outcomes in independent samples, most prominently substance use. Upcoming efforts to conduct considerably larger personality traits GWAS as well as future GWAS that combine genetically correlated personality traits and psychopathology promise to improve genetic prediction of mental health outcomes.

Conclusion

The current empirical evidence suggests that there is a considerable but not complete overlap in genetic liability dimensions of personality traits and corresponding psychopathology. Multivariate genetic research indicates that personality traits map onto hierarchical models of psychopathology. Attempts to fit a joint hierarchical genetic architecture of personality and psychopathology have resulted in meaningful higher-order factors that reflect phenotypic models, although there is yet no consensus on the joint genetic architecture. Genetic research is generally consistent with a personality-based conception of psychopathology, with implications for the utility of personality phenotypes for advancing molecular genetic research in psychiatry.

PART II

Exploring the shared genetic architecture between psychopathology and personality

HOLLY E. POORE and IRWIN D. WALDMAN

A large and long-standing body of literature has found substantial correlations between various forms of psychopathology and personality traits (John et al., 1994; Kotov et al., 2010; Watts et al., 2019). Consistent evidence of personality–psychopathology associations has led to the creation of several proposed models, which vary in their conceptualization of the causal or co-occurring nature of these relationships (Watson et al., 1994, 2008). Some models posit that personality and psychopathology are distinct constructs that causally influence each other via differing mechanisms (Durbin & Hicks, 2014; Watson et al., 1994, 2008). Other models characterize the associations between traits and disorders as stemming from shared liability and etiology. The spectrum model, which has arguably received the most attention of late, removes conceptual distinctions between traits and disorders and models them as indicators of the same continuum such that symptoms represent the extreme end of a continuous distribution.

Several of these models have received support (Durbin & Hicks, 2014; Watson et al., 2008; Watson et al., 1994), and current statistical tools are limited in their ability to favor one model over another. Genetically informed study designs represent one useful tool for understanding personality–psychopathology relationships. Quantitative genetic (e.g., twin) studies have long supported the hypothesis that psychopathology and personality share genetic and, to a lesser extent, environmental influences. Newer molecular and statistical genetic methods have also recently been used to address this question. In this chapter, we discuss methods used in twin, molecular, and statistical genetic studies that can be used to model the etiologic relationships between psychopathology and personality. When available, we review studies that have employed these methods to answer questions about the nature of the psychopathology and personality relationship.

Quantitative Genetic Studies

Quantitative genetic studies capitalize on the differences in trait correlations between identical (monozygotic) twins, who share 100% of their segregating DNA, and fraternal (dizygotic) twins, who share, on average, 50% of their segregating DNA, to estimate the genetic and environmental contributions to the trait (Neale & Cardon, 2013). These genetic influences can be further decomposed into additive effects, wherein genetic effects add up across chromosomal loci in a linear fashion, and nonadditive effects, wherein genetic influences result from the interaction of alleles within and across loci. Environmental influences can similarly be decomposed into two dimensions: (1) aspects of the trait-relevant environment that are shared between twins (shared environment) that make them similar for the trait and (2) aspects that differ between twins (nonshared environment) that make them similar for the trait. Twin studies assume that twins of both types have equivalent trait-relevant environments, an assumption that is generally supported in the literature (Felson, 2014; LoParo & Waldman, 2014). Thus, greater correlations between monozygotic relative to dizygotic twins imply genetic influences, whereas correlations between monozygotic twins less than one imply nonshared environmental influences.

Quantitative genetic methods can be used to parse the variance due to each type of genetic and environmental influence in a single trait as well as the degree to which common genetic and environmental influences contribute to cross-trait correlations. Several such multivariate models can be used to test alternative conceptualizations of the ways in which common and unique etiologic influence operate on related traits (Neale & Cardon, 2013). Cholesky decompositions partition the total variance in and covariance among multiple phenotypes into latent genetic and environmental components and can be used to simultaneously model shared and unique influences on the included phenotypes. In addition, they allow one to examine the proportion of the genetic component influencing the first trait that also influences, and thus may be causing, the second trait. Independent and common pathway models can also be used to model shared and unique influences. In independent pathway models, common latent and genetic environmental components influence related phenotypes directly, whereas in common pathway models the influence of these latent components on the related phenotypes are mediated through a higher-order factor (e.g., externalizing or internalizing) that represents the covariance shared among the phenotypes. In both models, phenotype-specific etiologic components are also estimated.

Multivariate quantitative genetic analyses have been used to explore shared etiologic influences on putatively distinct psychiatric disorders as well as between psychiatric disorders and other psychological traits, including personality. These analyses have shown shared genetic and, to a lesser extent, environmental influences between forms of psychopathology and a broad range of personality traits, including psychopathic traits, various forms of aggression, neuroticism, extraversion, agreeableness, conscientiousness, sensation seeking, impulsivity, and novelty seeking (Bienvenu et al., 2007; Blonigen et al., 2005; Kendler & Myers, 2014; Mann et al., 2017; Poore et al., 2022). In addition to bivariate genetic relationships between individual psychopathology and personality phenotypes, some studies suggest that shared etiologic influences exert influence on multiple phenotypes. In one such study, Kendler and colleagues (2014) demonstrated that genetic factors that influence externalizing disorders, including antisocial behavior and substance use disorders, also influence novelty seeking and extraversion. Similarly, genetic influences on internalizing disorders, such as depression and anxiety, also influence neuroticism and other personality traits (Kendler & Myers, 2014; Poore et al., 2022). Importantly, the degree of overlap in etiologic influences was higher among psychiatric disorders than between disorders and personality traits and personality traits retained a higher magnitude of unique genetic and environmental influences. Studies that model shared etiologic influences as operating through broad phenotypic factors (i.e., common pathway models) have shown similar overlap between psychiatric disorders and personality traits such that although most etiologic influences on each phenotype are captured by a higher-order factor, each phenotype retains unique genetic and environmental influences and the magnitude of unique influences tends to be higher for personality traits (Krueger et al., 2002; Young et al., 2000, 2009). Collectively, these findings from twin studies suggest that although there is consistent evidence of substantial overlap between the genetic influences on psychopathology and personality, both psychopathology and personality retain meaningfully unique variance.

Molecular Genetic Studies

In contrast to quantitative genetic studies, molecular-genetic studies identify specific genetic mechanisms that contribute to the development of a trait or the covariation between multiple traits. The most commonly used methodology in contemporary psychiatric and behavioral genetics is the genome-wide association study (GWAS), in which associations between a trait and millions of genetic markers across the genome are estimated. The move toward GWAS was partially driven by the poor replicability of candidate gene studies (Hewitt, 2012; Sullivan, 2007; Visscher et al., 2017) and mounting evidence that psychiatric disorders and related psychological traits are highly polygenic, meaning that they are influenced by many genetic variants of small effect. GWAS also generate summary statistics, regression coefficients, and their standard errors, reflecting the magnitude and significance of each SNP–trait association, which can be used in post-GWAS analyses to estimate the cumulative effects of genes and gene pathways (de Leeuw et al., 2015), interrogate the biological mechanism by which certain genes and gene pathways result in disease (e.g., bioannotation; Wang et al., 2020; Watanabe et al., 2017), model the shared genetic architecture among multiple traits (Bulik-Sullivan, Loh, et al., 2015; Frei et al., 2019), and test hypotheses about causal relationships between genetically correlated traits (O'Connor & Price, 2018; Sanderson et al., 2022).

The most commonly used method for estimating shared genetic influences from GWAS summary statistics is linkage disequilibrium score regression (LDSR; Bulik-Sullivan, Loh, et al., 2015). Linkage disequilibrium (LD) refers to any nonrandom association between genetic markers (e.g., single-nucleotide polymorphisms [SNPs]), which can be quantified using LD scores that represent an SNP's overall degree of correlation with other SNPs across the genome. In LDSR, each SNP's effect size is regressed on its LD score, with the assumption that if a trait is genetically influenced, variants that have a higher LD score will have higher effect sizes (Bulik-Sullivan, Loh, et al., 2015; Zheng et al., 2016). LDSR can be used to distinguish true polygenicity from noise and confounding factors, calculate SNP-based heritability of a trait, and calculate genetic correlations between two traits. For the latter function, the genetic covariance among two phenotypes, which is calculated by regressing the product of SNPs' effect sizes (i.e., *Z*-scores) from two GWAS on their LD scores, is normalized on SNP-based heritabilities to estimate the genetic correlation.

LDSR has been used to estimate genetic correlations among psychiatric disorders (Bulik-Sullivan, Finucane, et al., 2015) and between psychiatric disorders and cognitive (de la Fuente et al., 2021), sleep (Stein et al., 2018), physical health (Bahrami et al., 2020), and personality traits (Gupta et al., 2024). For example, recent GWASs have shown positive and moderate genetic correlations between cannabis use disorder and chronic pain (Levey et al., 2023), major depression and neuroticism

(Wray et al., 2018), and alcohol use disorder and risk taking (Zhou et al., 2023). Genetic correlations between broad spectra and personality traits have also been found for externalizing and internalizing, which were negatively correlated with agreeableness and positively correlated with neuroticism (Karlsson Linnér et al., 2021; Waldman et al., 2020). This finding of widespread pleiotropy across psychiatric disorders and related traits mirrors findings from the phenotypic structure of psychopathology literature (Kotov et al., 2017) as well as those from twin studies.

Although useful metrics, omnibus genetic correlations capture the average similarity between two traits across the whole genome, masking potentially discordant effects at different loci in the genome. For example, traits that are positively correlated at some loci and negatively correlated at other loci and are, therefore, substantially genetically related may appear to be uncorrelated. Therefore, additional methods to model the genetic overlap between two traits have been developed. Two such methods, bivariate causal mixture modeling (MiXeR; Frei et al., 2019) and local genetic correlations (e.g., local analysis of [co]variant association [LAVA]; Werme et al., 2022), can be used together to further model the polygenic overlap between traits. MiXeR quantifies polygenic overlap between pairs of traits by estimating the total number of genetic variants that influence both traits, influence one trait but not the other, and have no influence on either trait. Alternative models of the degree of polygenic overlap—partial, maximum, or minimum—between the two traits can also be tested and the best model selected using differences in the fit indices AIC (Akaike information criterion) and BIC (Bayesian information criterion). LAVA can be used to estimate the local genetic correlation between two traits at thousands of loci across the genome and can be extended to multivariate analyses, including partial correlations and multiple regressions.

The value of these methods in addition to traditional omnibus genetic correlations was recently illustrated in a study that examined the genetic relationships of schizophrenia, bipolar disorder, depression, and ADHD with neuroticism (Hindley et al., 2022). With the exception of depression, neuroticism was only moderately genetically correlated with the psychiatric disorders, suggesting modest genetic overlap. However, MiXeR analyses revealed that with the exception of depression, a model with complete overlap fit the relationships best. In particular, the causal genetic variants for the psychiatric disorders were subsumed in those for neuroticism, whereas neuroticism retained unique causal variants. The LAVA results also indicated more genetic overlap than would be expected given the omnibus genetic correlation, revealing a predominance of mixed-effect directions of local genetic correlations (60, 69, and 67% positive for schizophrenia, bipolar disorder, and ADHD, respectively).

Most of the evidence that psychiatric disorders and personality traits are genetically correlated come from GWAS focused on psychiatric disorders and, with the exception of neuroticism, genetic influences on personality traits are relatively poorly characterized in the current literature. The most recent neuroticism GWAS (Nagel et al., 2018), conducted in a sample of nearly 450,000 individuals, identified 136 genomic loci, implicating 599 genes influencing neuroticism. However, gene identification for other Big Five traits has lagged behind until recently. A new GWAS of all Big Five traits (Gupta et al., 2024) identified the first genome-wide significant loci for extraversion and agreeableness and identified novel loci for each other dimension. Mirroring phenotypic and twin studies, neuroticism and agreeableness were moderately genetically correlated, positively and negatively, respectively, with psychiatric traits including MDD, anxiety, manic behavior, and irritability. Conscientiousness was positively correlated with manic behavior and negatively with MDD, but these correlations were weak (r^Gs ~.15 and –.12, respectively). Extraversion was weakly and negatively correlated with anxiety, manic behavior, and MDD. Openness was positively correlated with anxiety, manic behavior, and MDD.

Given the strong genetic correlations of neuroticism with MDD and anxiety, the authors performed multitrait conditional and joint analysis (Zhu et al., 2018) to estimate genetic effects on neuroticism while conditioning on the genetic effects on MDD and anxiety, separately. After accounting for MDD, and to a lesser extent anxiety, the heritability and number of genome-wide significant loci for neuroticism were substantially attenuated, suggesting substantial genetic overlap. Finally, the authors applied Mendelian Randomization (MR; Sanderson et al., 2022), in which genetic variation is used to test models of the causal relationships between two variables, to test alternative models of the direction of causation between neuroticism, MDD, and anxiety. These results suggested a strong bidirectional relationship of neuroticism with MDD and anxiety.

Methods designed to model causality between genetically related traits can be useful for understanding the associations between psychopathology and personality. Mendelian Randomization is a widely used tool, results from which suggest causal relationships between many psychiatric disorders and related traits (Saccaro et al., 2022) including alcohol use disorder and depression (Grotzinger et al., 2022); tobacco use and schizophrenia (Wootton et al., 2020); and insomnia and ADHD, MDD, and PTSD (Sun et al., 2022). Despite its widespread use, findings about the presence and direction of causal relationships between similar traits are inconsistent in the literature (Saccaro et al., 2022). Furthermore, high polygenicity of and sample overlap between the traits of interest, which characterize the majority of studies in psychiatric genetics, limit the utility of MR analyses (O'Connor & Price, 2018). Latent Causal Variable (LCV) modeling is another approach to modeling causation (O'Connor & Price, 2018). In this approach, the degree to which a latent variable mediates the genetic correlation between two traits indicates the proportion of the genetic component for the first trait that is causal for the second trait. This approach is akin to the aforementioned Cholesky decomposition method, but it is applied in a molecular genetic context. LCV has yet to be used to disentangle the relationships between psychopathology and personality, although it has provided interesting insights in psychiatric genetics more broadly. For example, although cannabis use disorder is strongly genetically correlated with educational attainment, smoking initiation, and ADHD, LCV analyses did not demonstrate evidence of causal relationships between these traits (Johnson et al., 2020).

Additional recent advances in statistical genetics methods have facilitated investigation of genetic variants that exert influence on individual genetically correlated traits via broad latent factors that represent the variance shared among these phenotypes. One such tool is Genomic Structural Equation Modeling (gSEM; Grotzinger et al., 2019), which provides a flexible framework for applying SEM techniques to genetic covariance matrices that are derived from LDSR. Factors identified from SEM can then be used in subsequent gene-identification efforts, which can detect genetic associations that operate through broad factors.

This framework has several advantages for modeling the shared genetic architecture among related traits. First, when the goal is gene identification, the inclusion of genetically correlated traits with unique GWAS samples improves power to detect genetic associations beyond univariate analyses. Second, this framework enables one to model genetic variance that is shared among and unique to multiple phenotypes, potentially providing a more nuanced picture of shared genetic influences relative to simple genetic correlations. Third, the ability to identify broad latent factors facilitates exploration of the genetic correlations of broad spectra of psychopathology as well as residual factor indicators with the traits of interest. Finally, the number of Q_{SNPs}, SNPs that directly influence individual traits and are *not* mediated through the latent factor, can be used to adjudicate among alternative models, as increased Q_{SNPs} likely suggest poor fit of the model to the data (Clapp Sullivan et al., 2024). This distinction between genetic influences on disorders and traits arising from a latent factor versus those that directly influence the disorders and traits parallels the distinction between common versus independent pathway models described above.

A few notable applications of gSEM exemplify its utility and potential for further understanding psychopathology–personality relationships. In one study, the authors fit a five-factor model of impulsivity, analogous to the common phenotypic model, and estimated the genetic correlations between those impulsivity facets and a broad internalizing factor (Gustavson et al., 2020). They found differential genetic associations such that negative and positive urgency were more strongly related to internalizing than were other facets of impulsivity. In another study, an externalizing factor was identified with ADHD, substance use phenotypes, risk tolerance, and risky sexual behavior as indicators (Karlsson Linnér et al., 2021). Demonstrating the value of capitalizing on genetically correlated traits to boost power to detect genetic associations in a theory-driven model, this study identified far more significant genomic risk loci and produced a polygenic score more powerful than most GWAS of related traits to date.

Conclusions

Collectively, results from twin and molecular genetic studies consistently find genetic associations between psychiatric disorders and personality traits. The strongest relationships tend to be between neuroticism, MDD, and anxiety, as multiple studies and methods have demonstrated substantial overlap among these phenotypes. Agreeableness and conscientiousness are somewhat less strongly and negatively related to disorders across the externalizing and internalizing spectra. Finally, extraversion is weakly associated with certain externalizing and internalizing traits in the positive and negative direction, respectively, and openness is weakly or nonsignificantly associated with psychiatric disorders. However, even for pairs of traits with the strongest relationships, each psychopathology and personality dimension retains meaningful unique genetic variance, suggesting unique etiologic influences on the two domains. These patterns of associations broadly mirror findings from the phenotypic literature, potentially indicating that shared etiologic factors give rise to the oft-observed phenotypic relationships between psychopathology and personality. Last, although in their infancy, application of these statistical genetic approaches to data from future GWAS on larger samples can help to adjudicate among the pleiotropy, common pathway versus independent pathway, and causal directional models of personality–psychopathology described above.

PART I REFERENCES

Adams, M. J., Hill, W. D., Howard, D. M., Dashti, H. S., Davis, K. A., Campbell, A., . . . Porteous, D. (2020). Factors associated with sharing e-mail information and mental health survey participation in large population cohorts. *International Journal of Epidemiology, 49*(2), 410–421.

Aydogan, G., Daviet, R., Karlsson Linnér, R., Hare, T. A., Kable, J. W., Kranzler, H. R., . . . Nave, G. (2021). Genetic underpinnings of risky behaviour relate to altered neuroanatomy. *Nature Human Behaviour, 5*(6), 787–794.

Costantini, I., Sallis, H., Tilling, K., Major-Smith, D., Pearson, R. M., & Kounali, D. Z. (2023). Childhood trajectories of internalising and externalising problems associated with a polygenic risk score for neuroticism in a UK birth cohort study. *JCPP Advances, 3*(1), e12141.

Docherty, A. R., Moscati, A., Dick, D., Savage, J. E., Salvatore, J. E., Cooke, M., . . . Riley, B. P. (2018). Polygenic prediction of the phenome, across ancestry, in emerging adulthood. *Psychological Medicine, 48*(11), 1814.

Gjerde, L. C., Eilertsen, E. M., McAdams, T. A., Cheesman, R., Moffitt, T. E., Caspi, A., . . . Ystrom, E. (2023). The p factor of psychopathology and personality in middle childhood: genetic and gestational risk factors. *Psychological Medicine, 53*(9), 4275–4285.

Grotzinger, A. D., Rhemtulla, M., de Vlaming, R., Ritchie, S. J., Mallard, T. T., Hill, W. D., . . . Deary, I. J. (2019). Genomic structural equation modeling provides insights into the multivariate genetic architecture of complex traits. *Nature Human Behaviour, 3*(5), 513–525.

Gupta, P., Galimberti, M., Liu, Y., Beck, S., Wingo, A., Wingo, T., . . . Gelernter, J. (2024). A genome-wide investigation into the underlying genetic architecture of personality traits and overlap with psychopathology. *Nature Human Behavior, 8*(11), 2235–2249.

Gustavson, D. E., Friedman, N. P., Fontanillas, P., Elson, S. L., Team, a. R., Palmer, A. A., & Sanchez-Roige, S. (2020). The latent genetic structure of impulsivity and its relation to internalizing psychopathology. *Psychological Science, 31*(8), 1025–1035.

Gustavson, D. E., Morrison, C. L., Mallard, T. T., Jennings, M. V., Fontanillas, P., Elson, S. L., . . . Sanchez-Roige, S. (2023). Executive function and impulsivity predict distinct genetic variance in internalizing problems, externalizing problems, thought disorders, and compulsive disorders: A genomic structural equation modeling study. *Clinical Psychological Science, 12*(5), 865–881.

Hansell, N., Wright, M., Medland, S., Davenport, T., Wray, N., Martin, N., & Hickie, I. (2012). Genetic co-morbidity between neuroticism, anxiety/depression and somatic distress in a population sample of adolescent and young adult twins. *Psychological Medicine, 42*(6), 1249–1260.

Haslam, N., McGrath, M. J., Viechtbauer, W., & Kuppens, P. (2020). Dimensions over categories: A meta-analysis of taxometric research. *Psychological Medicine, 50*(9), 1418–1432.

Hettema, J. M., Neale, M. C., Myers, J. M., Prescott, C. A., & Kendler, K. S.

(2006). A population-based twin study of the relationship between neuroticism and internalizing disorders. *American Journal of Psychiatry, 163*(5), 857–864.

Hink, L. K., Rhee, S. H., Corley, R. P., Cosgrove, V. E., Hewitt, J. K., Schulz-Heik, R. J., . . . Waldman, I. D. (2013). Personality dimensions as common and broadband-specific features for internalizing and externalizing disorders. *Journal of Abnormal Child Psychology, 41,* 939–957.

Hoy, N., Lynch, S. J., Waszczuk, M. A., Reppermund, S., & Mewton, L. (2023). Transdiagnostic biomarkers of mental illness across the lifespan: A systematic review examining the genetic and neural correlates of latent transdiagnostic dimensions of psychopathology in the general population. *Neuroscience and Biobehavioral Reviews, 155*(2), 105431.

Jacquemont, S., Huguet, G., Klein, M., Chawner, S. J., Donald, K. A., van den Bree, M. B., . . . Earl, R. K. (2022). Genes to mental health (G2MH): A framework to map the combined effects of rare and common variants on dimensions of cognition and psychopathology. *American Journal of Psychiatry, 179*(3), 189–203.

Kendler, K. S., Gardner, C. O., Neale, M. C., Aggen, S., Heath, A., Colodro-Conde, L., . . . Gillespie, N. A. (2018). Shared and specific genetic risk factors for lifetime major depression, depressive symptoms and neuroticism in three population-based twin samples. *Psychological Medicine, 49*(16), 2745–2753.

Kotov, R., Krueger, R. F., Watson, D., Achenbach, T. M., Althoff, R. R., Bagby, M., . . . Zimmerman, M. (2017). The hierarchical taxonomy of psychopathology (HiTOP): A dimensional alternative to traditional nosologies. *Journal of Abnormal Psychology, 126*(4), 454.

Levey, D. F., Stein, M. B., Wendt, F. R., Pathak, G. A., Zhou, H., Aslan, M., . . . Overstreet, C. (2021). Bi-ancestral depression GWAS in the Million Veteran Program and meta-analysis in > 1.2 million individuals highlight new therapeutic directions. *Nature Neuroscience, 24*(7), 954–963.

Lewis, C. M., & Vassos, E. (2020). Polygenic risk scores: From research tools to clinical instruments. *Genome Medicine, 12*(1), 44.

Linner, K. R., Biroli, P., Kong, E., Meddens, S. F. W., Wedow, R., Fontana, M. A., . . . Beauchamp, J. P. (2019). Genome-wide association analyses of risk tolerance and risky behaviors in over 1 million individuals identify hundreds of loci and shared genetic influences. *Nature Genetics, 51*(2), 245–257.

Markon, K. E., Chmielewski, M., & Miller, C. J. (2011). The reliability and validity of discrete and continuous measures of psychopathology: a quantitative review. *Psychological Bulletin, 137*(5), 856.

Oltmanns, J. R., Smith, G. T., Oltmanns, T. F., & Widiger, T. A. (2018). General factors of psychopathology, personality, and personality disorder: Across domain comparisons. *Clinical Psychological Science, 6*(4), 581–589.

Plomin, R., Haworth, C. M., & Davis, O. S. (2009). Common disorders are quantitative traits. *Nature Reviews Genetics, 10*(12), 872–878.

Poore, H. E., Watts, A. L., Friedman, H. P., & Waldman, I. D. (2022). A broad internalizing dimension accounts for the genetic associations between personality and individual internalizing disorders. *Journal of Psychopathology and Clinical Science, 131*(8), 857.

Rosenström, T., Gjerde, L. C., Krueger, R. F., Aggen, S. H., Czajkowski, N. O., Gillespie, N. A., . . . Ystrom, E. (2019). Joint factorial structure of psychopathology and personality. *Psychological Medicine, 49*(13), 2158–2167.

Smoller, J. W., Andreassen, O. A., Edenberg, H. J., Faraone, S. V., Glatt, S. J., & Kendler, K. S. (2019). Psychiatric genetics and the structure of psychopathology. *Molecular Psychiatry, 24*(3), 409–420.

South, S. C., Eaton, N. R., & Krueger, R. F. (2010). The connections between personality and psychopathology. In T. Millon, R. F. Krueger, and E. Simonsen (Eds.), *Contemporary directions in psychopathology: Scientific foundations of the DSM-V and ICD-11* (pp. 242–262). Guilford Press.

Turkheimer, E., Pettersson, E., & Horn, E. E. (2014). A phenotypic null hypothesis for the genetics of personality. *Annual Review of Psychology, 65*, 515–540.

Waldman, I. D., Poore, H. E., Luningham, J. M., & Yang, J. (2020). Testing structural models of psychopathology at the genomic level. *World Psychiatry, 19*(3), 350–359.

Waszczuk, M. A., Docherty, A. R., Shabalin, A. A., Miao, J., Yang, X., Kuan, P.-F., . . . Luft, B. J. (2022). Polygenic prediction of PTSD trajectories in 9/11 responders. *Psychological Medicine, 52*(10), 1981–1989.

Waszczuk, M. A., Eaton, N. R., Krueger, R. F., Shackman, A. J., Waldman, I. D., Zald, D. H., . . . Ormel, J. (2020). Redefining phenotypes to advance psychiatric genetics: Implications from hierarchical taxonomy of psychopathology. *Journal of Abnormal Psychology, 129*(2), 143.

Waszczuk, M. A., Jonas, K. G., Bornovalova, M., Breen, G., Bulik, C. M., Docherty, A. R., . . . Krueger, R. F. (2023). Dimensional and transdiagnostic phenotypes in psychiatric genome-wide association studies. *Molecular Psychiatry, 28*(12), 4943–4953.

Widiger, T. A., Sellbom, M., Chmielewski, M., Clark, L. A., DeYoung, C. G., Kotov, R., . . . Mullins-Sweatt, S. (2019). Personality in a hierarchical model of psychopathology. *Clinical Psychological Science, 7*(1), 77–92.

PART II REFERENCES

Bahrami, S., Steen, N. E., Shadrin, A., O'Connell, K., Frei, O., Bettella, F., . . . Andreassen, O. A. (2020). Shared genetic loci between body mass index and major psychiatric disorders: A genome-wide association study. *JAMA Psychiatry, 77*(5), 503–512.

Bienvenu, O. J., Hettema, J. M., Neale, M. C., Prescott, C. A., & Kendler, K. S. (2007). Low extraversion and high neuroticism as indices of genetic and environmental risk for social phobia, agoraphobia, and animal phobia. *American Journal of Psychiatry, 164*(11), 1714–1721.

Blonigen, D. M., Hicks, B. M., Krueger, R. F., Patrick, C. J., & Iacono, W. G. (2005). Psychopathic personality traits: Heritability and genetic overlap with internalizing and externalizing psychopathology. *Psychological Medicine, 35*(5), 637–648.

Bulik-Sullivan, B. K., Finucane, H. K., Anttila, V., Gusev, A., Day, F. R., Loh, P. R., . . . Neale, B. M. (2015). An atlas of genetic correlations across human diseases and traits. *Nature Genetics, 47*(11), 1236–1241.

Bulik-Sullivan, B. K., Loh, P. R., Finucane, H. K., Ripke, S., Yang, J., Schizophrenia Working Group of the Psychiatric Genomics, Consortium, . . . Neale, B. M. (2015). LD Score regression distinguishes confounding from polygenicity in genome-wide association studies. *Nature Genetics, 47*(3), 291–295.

Clapp Sullivan, M. L., Schwaba, T., Harden, K. P., Grotzinger, A. D., Nivard, M. G., & Tucker-Drob, E. M. (2024). Beyond the factor indeterminacy problem using genome-wide association data. *Nature Human Behaviour, 8*(2), 205–218.

de la Fuente, J., Davies, G., Grotzinger, A. D., Tucker-Drob, E. M., & Deary, I. J. (2021). A general dimension of genetic sharing across diverse cognitive traits inferred from molecular data. *Nature Human Behavior, 5*(1), 49–58.

de Leeuw, C. A., Mooij, J. M., Heskes, T., & Posthuma, D. (2015). MAGMA: Generalized gene-set analysis of GWAS data. *PLOS Computational Biology, 11*(4), e1004219.

Durbin, C. E., & Hicks, B. M. (2014). Personality and psychopathology: A stagnant field in need of development. *European Journal of Personality, 28*(4), 362–386.

Felson, J. (2014). What can we learn from twin studies? A comprehensive evaluation of the equal environments assumption. *Social Science Research, 43*, 184–199.

Frei, O., Holland, D., Smeland, O. B., Shadrin, A. A., Fan, C. C., Maeland, S., . . . Dale, A. M. (2019). Bivariate causal mixture model quantifies polygenic overlap between complex traits beyond genetic correlation. *Nature Communications, 10*(1), 2417.

Grotzinger, A. D., Mallard, T. T., Akingbuwa, W. A., Ip, H. F., Adams, M. J., Lewis, C. M., . . . Schizophrenia Working Group of the Psychiatric Genetics Consortium. (2022). Genetic architecture of 11 major psychiatric disorders at biobehavioral, functional genomic and molecular genetic levels of analysis. *Nature Genetics, 54*(5), 548–559.

Grotzinger, A. D., Rhemtulla, M., de Vlaming, R., Ritchie, S. J., Mallard, T. T., Hill, W. D., . . . Tucker-Drob, E. M. (2019). Genomic structural equation modelling provides insights into the multivariate genetic architecture of complex traits. *Nature Human Behaviour, 3*(5), 513–525.

Gupta, P., Galimberti, M., Liu, Y., Beck, S., Wingo, A., Wingo, T., . . . Levey, D. F. (2024). A genome-wide investigation into the underlying genetic architecture of personality traits and overlap with psychopathology. *Nature Human Behaviour, 8*(11), 2235–2249.

Gustavson, D. E., Friedman, N. P., Fontanillas, P., Elson, S. L., Palmer, A. A., & Sanchez-Roige, S. (2020). The latent genetic structure of impulsivity and its relation to internalizing psychopathology. *Psychological Science, 31*(8), 1025–1035.

Hewitt, J. K. (2012). Editorial policy on candidate gene association and candidate gene-by-environment interaction studies of complex traits. *Behavior Genetics, 42,* 1–2.

Hindley, G., Frei, O., Shadrin, A. A., Cheng, W., O'Connell, K. S., Icick, R., . . . Roelfs, D. (2022). Charting the landscape of genetic overlap between mental disorders and related traits beyond genetic correlation. *American Journal of Psychiatry, 179*(11), 833–843.

John, O. P., Caspi, A., Robins, R. W., Moffitt, T. E., & Stouthamer-Loeber, M. (1994). The "Little Five": Exploring the nomological network of the five-factor model of personality in adolescent boys. *Child Development, 65*(1), 160–178.

Johnson, E. C., Demontis, D., Thorgeirsson, T. E., Walters, R. K., Polimanti, R., Hatoum, A. S., . . . Agrawal, A. (2020). A large-scale genome-wide association study meta-analysis of cannabis use disorder. *Lancet Psychiatry, 7*(12), 1032–1045.

Karlsson Linnér, R., Mallard, T. T., Barr, P. B., Sanchez-Roige, S., Madole, J. W., Driver, M. N., . . . Dick, D. M. (2021). Multivariate analysis of 1.5 million people identifies genetic associations with traits related to self-regulation and addiction. *Nature Neuroscience, 24*(10), 1367–1376.

Kendler, K. S., & Myers, J. (2014). The boundaries of the internalizing and externalizing genetic spectra in men and women. *Psychological Medicine, 44*(3), 647–655.

Kotov, R., Gamez, W., Schmidt, F., & Watson, D. (2010). Linking "Big" personality traits to anxiety, depressive, and substance use disorders: A meta-analysis. *Psycholological Bulletin, 136*(5), 768–821.

Kotov, R., Krueger, R. F., Watson, D., Achenbach, T. M., Althoff, R. R., Bagby, R. M., . . . Zimmerman, M. (2017). The hierarchical taxonomy of psychopathology (HiTOP): A dimensional alternative to traditional nosologies. *Journal of Abnormal Psychology, 126*(4), 454–477.

Krueger, R. F., Hicks, B. M., Patrick, C. J., Carlson, S. R., Iacono, W. G., & McGue, M. (2002). Etiological connections among substance dependence, antisocial behavior, and personality: Modeling the externalizing spectrum. *Journal of Abnormal Psychology, 111*(3), 411–424.

Levey, D. F., Galimberti, M., Deak, J. D., Wendt, F. R., Bhattacharya, A., Koller, D., . . . Gelernter, J. (2023). Multi-ancestry genome-wide association study of cannabis use disorder yields insight into disease biology and public health implications. *Nature Genetics, 55*(12), 2094–2103.

LoParo, D., & Waldman, I. (2014). Twins' rearing environment similarity and childhood externalizing disorders: A test of the equal environments assumption. *Behavior Genetics, 44*(6), 606–613.

Mann, F. D., Engelhardt, L., Briley, D. A., Grotzinger, A. D., Patterson, M. W., Tackett, J. L., . . . Harden, K. P. (2017). Sensation seeking and impulsive traits as personality endophenotypes for antisocial behavior: Evidence from two independent samples. *Personality and Individual Differences, 105,* 30–39.

Nagel, M., Jansen, P. R., Stringer, S., Watanabe, K., De Leeuw, C. A., Bryois, J., . . . Muñoz-Manchado, A. B. (2018). Meta-analysis of genome-wide association studies for neuroticism in 449,484 individuals identifies novel genetic loci and pathways. *Nature Genetics, 50*(7), 920–927.

Neale, M., & Cardon, L. R. (2013). *Methodology for genetic studies of twins and families* (Vol. 67). Springer Science & Business Media.

O'Connor, L. J., & Price, A. L. (2018). Distinguishing genetic correlation from causation across 52 diseases and complex traits. *Nature Genetics, 50*(12), 1728–1734.

Poore, H. E., Watts, A. L., Friedman, H. P., & Waldman, I. D. (2022). A broad internalizing dimension accounts for the genetic associations between personality and individual internalizing disorders. *Journal of Psychopathology and Clinical Science, 131*, 857–867.

Saccaro, L. F., Gasparini, S., & Rutigliano, G. (2022). Applications of Mendelian randomization in psychiatry: A comprehensive systematic review. *Psychiatric Genetics, 32*(6), 199–213.

Sanderson, E., Glymour, M. M., Holmes, M. V., Kang, H., Morrison, J., Munafò, M. R., . . . Davey Smith, G. (2022). Mendelian randomization. *Nature Reviews Methods Primers, 2*(1), 6.

Stein, M. B., McCarthy, M. J., Chen, C.-Y., Jain, S., Gelernter, J., He, F., . . . Ursano, R. J. (2018). Genome-wide analysis of insomnia disorder. *Molecular Psychiatry, 23*(11), 2238–2250.

Sullivan, P. F. (2007). Spurious genetic associations. *Biological Psychiatry, 61*(10), 1121–1126.

Sun, X., Liu, B., Liu, S., Wu, D. J. H., Wang, J., Qian, Y., Ye, D., & Mao, Y. (2022). Sleep disturbance and psychiatric disorders: A bidirectional Mendelian randomisation study. *Epidemiology and Psychiatric Sciences, 31*, e26.

Visscher, P. M., Wray, N. R., Zhang, Q., Sklar, P., McCarthy, M. I., Brown, M. A., & Yang, J. (2017). 10 Years of GWAS discovery: Biology, function, and translation. *American Journal of Human Genetics, 101*(1), 5–22.

Waldman, I. D., Poore, H. E., Luningham, J. M., & Yang, J. (2020). Testing structural models of psychopathology at the genomic level. *World Psychiatry, 19*(3), 350–359.

Wang, G., Sarkar, A., Carbonetto, P., & Stephens, M. (2020). A simple new approach to variable selection in regression, with application to genetic fine mapping. *Journal of the Royal Statistical Society Series B: Statistical Methodology, 82*(5), 1273–1300.

Watanabe, K., Taskesen, E., van Bochoven, A., & Posthuma, D. (2017). Functional mapping and annotation of genetic associations with FUMA. *Nature Communications, 8*(1), 1826.

Watson, D., Clark, L. A., & Chmielewski, M. (2008). Structures of personality and their relevance to psychopathology: II. Further articulation of a comprehensive unified trait structure. *Journal of Personality, 76*(6), 1545–1586.

Watson, D., Clark, L. A., & Harkness, A. R. (1994). Structures of personality and their relevance to psychopathology. *Journal of Abnormal Psychology, 103*(1), 18–31.

Watts, A. L., Poore, H. E., Lilienfeld, S. O., & Waldman, I. D. (2019). Clarifying the associations between Big Five personality domains and higher-order psychopathology dimensions in youth. *Journal of Research in Personality, 82,* 103844.

Werme, J., van der Sluis, S., Posthuma, D., & de Leeuw, C. A. (2022). An integrated framework for local genetic correlation analysis. *Nature Genetics, 54*(3), 274–282.

Wootton, R. E., Richmond, R. C., Stuijfzand, B. G., Lawn, R. B., Sallis, H. M., Taylor, G. M. J., . . . Munafò, M. R. (2020). Evidence for causal effects of lifetime smoking on risk for depression and schizophrenia: A Mendelian randomisation study. *Psychological Medicine, 50*(14), 2435–2443.

Wray, N. R., Ripke, S., Mattheisen, M., Trzaskowski, M., Byrne, E. M., Abdellaoui, A., . . . the Major Depressive Disorder Working Group of the Psychiatric Genomics Consortium. (2018). Genome-wide association analyses identify 44 risk variants and refine the genetic architecture of major depression. *Nature Genetics, 50*(5), 668–681.

Young, S. E., Friedman, N. P., Miyake, A., Willcutt, E. G., Corley, R. P., Haberstick, B. C., & Hewitt, J. K. (2009). Behavioral disinhibition: Liability for externalizing spectrum disorders and its genetic and environmental relation to response inhibition across adolescence. *Journal of Abnormal Psychology, 118*(1), 117–130.

Young, S. E., Stallings, M. C., Corley, R. P., Krauter, K. S., & Hewitt, J. K. (2000). Genetic and environmental influences on behavioral disinhibition. *American Journal of Medical Genetics, 96*(5), 684–695.

Zheng, J., Erzurumluoglu, A. M., Elsworth, B. L., Kemp, J. P., Howe, L., Haycock, P. C., . . . Neale, B. M. (2016). LD Hub: A centralized database and web interface to perform LD score regression that maximizes the potential of summary level GWAS data for SNP heritability and genetic correlation analysis. *Bioinformatics, 33*(2), 272–279.

Zhou, H., Kember, R. L., Deak, J. D., Xu, H., Toikumo, S., Yuan, K., . . . Gelernter, J. (2023). Multi-ancestry study of the genetics of problematic alcohol use in over 1 million individuals. *Nature Medicine, 29*(12), 3184–3192.

Zhu, Z., Zheng, Z., Zhang, F., Wu, Y., Trzaskowski, M., Maier, R., . . . Yang, J. (2018). Causal associations between risk factors and common diseases inferred from GWAS summary data. *Nature Communications, 9*(1), 224.

CHAPTER 11

How does dimensional diagnosis change how we should think about psychiatric epidemiology?

Epidemiology is concerned with the frequency of diseases in the population or certain groups. Calculating such a frequency is complicated enough when diseases are discrete, but how can this be done when diagnoses are dimensional? In this section, we asked experts to answer three questions regarding the implications of dimensional diagnosis for psychiatric epidemiology:

Dimensional diagnosis directly challenges the idea that some people have a disorder and some do not: How does this affect the way epidemiologists think about establishing prevalence rates?

What should serve as the basis for determining cut scores for mental health problems?

How do cultural and local issues interact with how epidemiologists conduct psychopathology research?

Stein and Hartford frame these questions philosophically and assert an integrative position between diagnosis as objective or subjective. They argue that diagnosis can be understood as either categorical or dimensional depending on the purpose. Lines between health and illness must be drawn for practical reasons, but they do not have to be taken too seriously and can vary across time and place to the extent that diagnostic constructs themselves are understood to be fuzzy; what matters is developing a better understanding of associations between exposures and outcomes. In this respect, they point out that epidemiology has and continues to also inform diagnosis, not just the other way around. Markon also acknowledges the fuzziness of psychiatric concepts and further emphasizes that constructs may vary in their continuousness depending on the definition of that term, their underlying nature, and contextual factors. He offers several interesting ways in which we might think differently about epidemiology. He suggests that if most mental health concepts are generally continuous, perhaps psychiatric epidemiology should focus on characterizing distributions rather than calculating frequencies. Alternatively, perhaps frequencies could be calculated for consequences or significant symptoms of mental health problems rather than ostensible diseases themselves.

PART I

Philosophy of psychiatric epidemiology

A conceptual framework

DAN J. STEIN and ANNA HARTFORD

The use of dimensional diagnosis in psychiatric epidemiology research immediately raises questions at the intersection of philosophy. It turns out that the literature on philosophy of epidemiology is relatively sparse (Broadbent, 2013) and that on the philosophy of psychiatric epidemiology even sparser (Stein, 2023). In this chapter we provide a conceptual framework for considering issues at the intersection of philosophy and psychiatric epidemiology. We draw on a previous published framework that contrasts classical, critical, and integrative positions (Stein, 1991, 2021) and employ it to consider dimensional diagnosis in psychiatric epidemiology.

Classical View

A classical view of science and language emphasizes the importance of objective observation and the possibility that our descriptions of the world can be verified (Table 11.1). This position has its origins in the work of Plato—who emphasized universal "forms"—as well as the early Wittgenstein—who proposed a representational view of language (Stein, 2021). However, the position outlined here is intended to be a useful heuristic rather than a reflection of the work of any particular philosopher.

A classical view has emphasized the importance of "natural kinds"—discrete categories with necessary and sufficient criteria, an important example of which is the periodic table of chemical elements (Kincaid & Sullivan, 2014). In this perspective, it is possible "to carve nature at her

TABLE 11.1. Classical, Critical, and Integrative Philosophical Positions

	Classical position	Critical position	Integrative position
Philosophy of science	Science entails objective description of the world	Science is merely one approach to constructing our reality	Science is a social activity that allows knowledge of the world
Philosophy of language	Language allows verification of reality	Language allows validation of our constructs	Metaphors and models may have explanatory power
Categories versus dimensions	Natural kinds are often discrete categories, but they may also fall on dimensions	Human kinds, whether categorical or dimensional, are social constructs	There are different kinds of kinds, both categories and dimensions may be useful
Concepts of mental disorder	Diseases can be operationalized in terms of necessary and sufficient features	Social constructs differ across time and place and influence the expression and experience of illness	Disorders are theory bound and value laden, and underlying mechanisms can be discovered
Epidemiological constructs	Epidemiology allows objective description and measurement of disease	Epidemiological constructs are culture bound, influencing expression and experience of illness	Epidemiology is theory laden and value bound and yields explanatory accounts of disorders
Epidemiological explanations	Epidemiology finds laws that cover the relationships between exposures and health outcomes	Epidemiology provides one way of understanding health outcomes	Epidemiology provides explanatory accounts of health outcomes
Epidemiological values	Epidemiology is concerned with facts not values	Epidemiology reflects human values	Epidemiology entails a range of epistemic virtues

joints" (a phrase that has its origins in the work of Plato). However, this position may also focus on dimensions. The laws of nature, for example, describe the relationships between observable entities and may focus on categories or continua; thus, categorical mass is conserved during a chemical reaction, whereas wavelengths lie on a dimension and equal wave train velocity divided by frequency.

Just as natural kinds are universal and found across time and place, so the laws of nature transcend history and geography. The focus of the classical view is on the facts of the matter; science itself is a value-free endeavor. Thus, the classical position often views physics as the queen of the sciences: It exemplifies the discovery of universal natural laws, which hold irrespective of human perspectives or sociocultural values.

When applied to disease, a classical position again emphasizes the importance of rigorous observation. This may focus on categories; for example, disorders may be carefully operationalized, with necessary and sufficient criteria outlined. Alternatively, however, this position may use statistical approaches to establish the latent dimensions of disease; the hierarchical taxonomy of psychopathology (HiTOP) collaboration, for example, has emphasized how mental disorders fall into externalizing and internalizing spectra, which are in turn divided into more specific dimensions (Kotov et al., 2017).

Whether assessing categorical or dimensional constructs, epidemiological measures allow law-like associations between particular exposures and pathological outcomes to be determined. In a classical position, epidemiology may be conceptualized as value laden only in the sense that it provides a foundation for public health.

Psychiatric epidemiology has appropriately striven to employ rigorous measures. At the time of World War II, when many veterans reported psychiatric symptoms, the U.S. military developed the Neuropsychiatric Screening Adjunct, a symptom questionnaire based on the assumption that mental illness fell on a dimension of severity (De Vries et al., 2023). Adaptations of this instrument were employed in several major community studies of mental illness in the 1950s. The 1970s saw the development of the Feighner research diagnostic criteria, which were based on the assumption that mental disorders were categorical entities (Kendler et al., 2010). The Feighner criteria formed the basis for the subsequent development of DSM-III led by Robert Spitzer as well as a range of diagnostic interviews used in epidemiological studies.

The work of Feighner and colleagues has been termed "neo-Kraepelinian." Just as Kraepelin believed in universal disease entities, so a new wave of psychiatrists, impressed by advances in psychopharmacology and neuroscience, emphasized that mental disorders were characterized by biological dysfunctions (Klerman, 1978). This position seems reductionistic; multiple factors contribute to the etiology of mental disorders, and they seem not to have pathognomonic underlying lesions. Although Spitzer's focus on atheoretical operationalization is consistent with a classical position, he emphasized his disagreements with the neo-Kraepelinians (Wakefield, 2022). Similarly, epidemiologists who employed diagnostic interviews based on the DSM system would not have conceptualized themselves as neo-Kraepelinian.

Critical View

A critical view of science and language emphasizes that science is just one approach to constructing the world and the possibility that our constructions can be validated in dialogue with others (Table 11.1). This position has its origins in the work of counter-Enlightenment philosophers such as Vico and Herder, who emphasized the limitations of Enlightenment science and the value of other interpretations of the world (Berlin, 2000). Again, the position outlined here is intended to be heuristic rather than a reflection of the work of any particular thinker.

The critical view has emphasized the importance of "human kinds"—our social constructions are used to understand the world, but they also have an influence on those whom we categorize (Hacking, 1995). Thus, for example, when we label some as "mentally ill," this contributes to social discrimination. A critical view might highlight how science is a social activity, with normative ends. Viewing psychiatry as similar to physics is merely an attempt to legitimize its narratives; instead, a hermeneutic approach is appropriate, as it would be for a range of texts.

Whether we use categorical or dimensional approaches to labeling is a narrative choice, saying less about the objects that scientists are studying or about the relevant laws of nature and more about societal values (Horwitz & Grob, 2011; March & Oppenheimer, 2014). Human kinds vary from time to time and place to place and can only be understood within a particular sociocultural context. The focus of the critical view is less on scientific facts and laws and more on what constructions and narratives reveal about societies and cultures.

When applied to disease, a critical position may emphasize the importance of sociocultural issues such as social deviance. Epidemiological research may be used to interrogate how we label deviance and how we respond to it. Attempts to formulate epidemiological laws about such deviance may well be inappropriate; instead, we need to understand the lived experience of being labeled and to acknowledge that such lived experience may differ considerably across cultures. Furthermore, epidemiological research is explicitly value laden; it has the potential to alter social labeling and to ameliorate responses to those who are marginalized.

Psychiatric epidemiology has appropriately striven to address issues of stigmatization and to improve public health. Thus, for example, attitudinal and structural barriers to treatment of mental disorders have been carefully investigated. Global mental health has paid particular attention to the spectrum of conditions that lie between wellness and illness, to the social determinants of such conditions, and to the importance of advocating for policies that address such determinants (Patel et al., 2018).

Some who take a critical position might argue, however, that such work simply reinforces social constructions and narratives by erroneously conceptualizing mental disorders as medical conditions that deserve appropriate treatment (Mills, 2014). The difficulty with this position is that it elides the possibility that scientific advances may lead to better explanations of mental disorders and so to the potential for targeting these in innovative ways, whether via medical or societal interventions.

Integrative View

An integrative position attempts to draw on the strengths of the classical and critical positions while avoiding their weaknesses (Table 11.1). This position may be traced back to Aristotle, who was one of the fathers of biology (Leroi, 2014), and Dewey, who presaged much contemporary work on embodied cognition (Brinkmann, 2017). Aristotle notably argued that one had to adopt one's method to fit the nature of one's subject matter; "it is the mark of an educated man to look for precision in each class of things just so far as the nature of the subject admits; it is evidently equally foolish to accept probable reasoning from a mathematician and to demand from a rhetorician demonstrative proofs" (Aristotle, 1949).

The integrative position acknowledges that science is a social activity but at the same time argues that science advances by providing better and better explanations of the structures, processes, and mechanisms that underlie the phenomena of the world (Bhaskar, 1973, 1979). Thus, for example, the categorical elements of the periodic table can be understood on the basis of underlying atomic numbers, which fall on dimensions. Reality is complex and layered, encompassing a range of different kinds of kinds (Haslam, 2002) as well as different sorts of dimensions (Hopwood et al., 2023). Therefore, science employs a range of models and metaphors.

Rather than espousing the "hard naturalism" and scientism of the classical position or the hermeneutic focus and skepticism of the critical view, an integrative view may adopt a "soft naturalism" that recognizes the complexity of constructs and their explanations (De Caro & Macarthur, 2022). Constructs such as species (in biology) and disorders (in medicine) are "soft natural kinds"; they cannot easily be operationalized using necessary and sufficient criteria; they instead have fuzzy and vague borders, but they involve constellations of underlying mechanisms that help explain their phenomenology (Stein, 2022). The content and boundaries of disorders are necessarily culture bound insofar as they are conceptualized at a particular time and place, but it is not the case that "anything goes": The relevant facts and values can be reasonably debated (Stein, 1993).

An integrative view is consistent with conceptual pluralism, explanatory pluralism, and value pluralism. Conceptual pluralism emphasizes that the structures of the world can be described in a range of different but valid ways, including both categorical and dimensional approaches. Explanatory pluralism emphasizes that different explanations may validly contribute to knowledge; human behavior, for example, can be described using biological, psychological, or sociocultural models and metaphors. Science is theory bound and value laden, but its findings and its various values can be articulated and reasonably debated.

When applied to psychiatry and epidemiology, an integrative position may emphasize analogous points concerning conceptual pluralism, explanatory pluralism, and value pluralism.

Behavioral phenomena, for example, are complex and can be described using a range of categories and dimensions. Categories can be made dimensional (e.g., the number of diagnostic criteria for depression can be added to make a dimensional score), and dimensions can be converted into categories (e.g., those who have particular scores on depression scales can be said to have depression); epidemiological studies may benefit from including both categories and dimensions (Kessler, 2002; Kraemer et al., 2004).

Explanations of behavioral phenomena may include those focused on neurobiological, psychological, and sociocultural structures, processes, and mechanisms (Ruphy, 2017). Accordingly, epidemiological research on mental disorders investigates biological markers, psychological traits, and social determinants. Although disorder categories and dimensions are culture bound and may vary across time and place, underlying mechanisms may be universal. Thus, a number of associations between a range of exposures and mental disorder outcomes have been found across the globe.

Epidemiological science, like all sciences, involves a range of epistemic virtues including transparency and fallibility, and these can be reasonably debated. Epidemiological research can also help adjudicate between polices that emphasize different values: Work on substance use, for example, may usefully address the effects of supply reduction, demand reduction, and harm reduction.

Although epidemiology is theory bound and value laden it can make scientific progress, providing more powerful explanatory models and metaphors. John Snow's landmark discovery that people got sick from drinking at a particular water pump was possible because the cholera bacterium causes illness, although this bacterium was only later identified. The discovery of a link between cancer and smoking was possible because of real biological mechanisms underlying this association, although these continue to be studied.

From Nosology to Epidemiology and Back Again

Psychiatric epidemiology has long relied on diagnostic constructs that are derived from standard classifications. More recently, however, data from epidemiological studies of mental disorders have been used to optimize the nosology of these conditions (Stein et al., 2017). Here we consider a few examples of such work and how they are consistent with an integrative position in philosophy of psychiatric epidemiology.

In DSM-IV, generalized anxiety disorder (GAD) is diagnosed based on symptoms lasting for 6 months or longer. However, data from a community survey in the United States found that respondents who met criteria for GAD for shorter periods experienced as much distress and impairment (Kessler et al., 2005). This finding held in both high-income and low-and-middle-income countries, providing reassurance that the underlying mechanisms are universal (Lee et al., 2009). Thus, the recommendation was made to shorten the duration criterion (Kessler et al., 2005; Lee et al., 2009). Indeed, in ICD-11 the diagnostic guidelines for mental disorders purposefully avoid pseudo-precision. This is consistent with an integrative position that emphasizes that disorders are soft natural kinds with vague and fuzzy borders.

DSM-IV criteria for GAD also emphasize that worries must be "excessive." However, epidemiological data indicated that individuals who meet all the criteria for GAD other than excessiveness have a somewhat milder presentation but are similar to excessive worriers in important ways (Ruscio et al., 2005). The singular determination that a particular set of symptoms is "excessive" may not necessarily provide a solution to the "line-drawing problem" (of where to draw the line between normality and pathology). Instead, determinations of pathology rely on a range of assessments of the degree of distress and impairment as well as inferences about dysregulation of underlying mechanisms (Stein, 2013; Stein et al., 2010).

A small minority of those exposed to a traumatic event develop posttraumatic stress disorder (PTSD), but subthreshold PTSD symptoms are common and may be clinically significant. In a World Mental Health Survey study, the 3% of individuals who met criteria for DSM-5 PTSD had higher distress and impairment. However, the additional 3.6% of individuals meeting only two or three of DSM-5 Criteria B–E also had elevated scores on such measures. This work allowed a rigorous proposal to define subthreshold PTSD for further research (McLaughlin et al., 2015).

Notably, thresholds for disorder may change over time, based on various considerations. Thus, for example, definitions of hypercholesterolemia have become broader over the years, as access to cholesterol-lowering drugs has become less expensive, allowing more cost-efficient treatment of even mild hypercholesteremia (Kessler et al., 2003). Making such decisions requires a careful weighing the relevant facts and values.

The World Mental Health Surveys comprise a particularly large and rigorous study that has shed light not only on how best to revise the nosology but also on multiple other psychiatric issues. It is noteworthy that the measures employed by this collaboration address both categories and dimensions and that particular variables (e.g., psychiatric disorders, childhood adversities) have been analyzed both as categories and dimensionally (Kessler et al., 2010; Scott et al., 2013).

Conclusion

This chapter has suggested that a conceptual framework for considering issues at the intersection of philosophy and epidemiology may be useful in addressing questions about the use of dimensional diagnosis in psychiatric epidemiology. From an integrative perspective, categorical and dimensional measures are both useful. Different cut points across studies contribute to inconsistent prevalence findings; more important are associations that hold across studies and that point to underlying universal causal mechanisms.

Statistical analyses of epidemiological data can usefully incorporate both categorical and dimensional constructs to investigate associations between exposures and outcomes. Advances in science occur when there is improved knowledge of how underlying structures, processes, and mechanisms account for phenomena. Thus, for example, work demonstrating that childhood adversities are associated with vulnerability to PTSD suggests that particular underlying mechanisms are at play, and deserve further investigation (Kessler et al., 2010).

Epidemiological research is not only theory bound but also value laden. Where we draw the line around a particular construct, for example, reflects considerations about a range of facts and values and is open to debate. Thus, for example, we may shift disease boundaries when more effective and cost-efficient treatments emerge (Kessler et al., 2003). Finally, although psychiatric epidemiology has relied on contemporary nosology, analyses of different sets of diagnostic criteria may contribute to optimization of the nosology (Stein et al., 2017).

PART II

Diagnoses as metrics in continuous approaches to psychopathology

KRISTIAN E. MARKON

Continuous diagnostic paradigms are not new but have now become ubiquitous and form the basis for a number of alternative nosological proposals in recent decades. With this renewed attention, it is important to consider potential challenges that might be faced with their even more widespread adoption, and approaches to fundamental issues in psychiatric and behavioral epidemiology might change as a result.

What, Exactly, Is Continuous in Continuous Models of Psychopathology?

To better understand potential issues in this area, it is important to first consider what, exactly, is continuous in continuous accounts of psychopathology. This certainly differs from model to model, but generally speaking, continuous models focus on a neuropsychological attribute, state, or process that is considered to be smoothly varying such that small changes in those attributes, states, or processes consistently occur with concomitantly small changes in frequency. These models contrast with discrete models, where changes in attributes, states, or processes are characterized by points or regions where values change differentially with relatively smaller or larger changes in frequency, as is the case when one moves from groups having a disease to those not having a disease. In continuous models, psychopathology is smooth in distribution with no obvious groupings; in discrete models, psychopathology is "lumpy" in distribution, with groups or classes of conditions.

Of course, a question immediately arises—"the distribution of what, exactly?" A measured psychological state? A neurobiological process? Some proposed etiologic factor? Functional impairments? The answers to these questions coincide with those about what the nature of psychopathology is, fundamentally, but nevertheless have practical consequences in terms of how to define its boundaries. A continuously varying mental state can be caused by discretely distributed etiologic factors, resulting in mixtures of mental states; similarly, mental states might be nonlinearly related to outcomes such that implied risk profiles are discrete even if the mental states are not.

This latter phenomenon points to a broader more abstract way of defining continuousness versus discreteness, which is homogeneity versus heterogeneity in differences within a psychopathology distribution. Continuous psychopathology is homogeneous throughout in the sense that a given change in level of the neuropsychological process or attribute is similar in how it manifests as another change in level of the process or attribute. A given change in less severe fear, for example, has changes in frequency and consequences that are similar to those of the same change in more severe fear. Severe fear will be less frequent and be associated with more impairment and greater levels of some neurobiological process, but *changes* in severe fear will have *changes* in impairments and neurobiology that are proportionally similar to *changes* in less severe fear.

It may be that continuousness as a concept has degrees itself (Hopwood et al., 2023) in the sense that there may be more or less continuous forms of psychopathology, each with implications for how to establish clinical thresholds for diagnosis, treatment, and prevalence. The extreme possibility—that there are solidly discrete categories of psychiatric illness—is probably not viable in general (Markon et al., 2011). However, there may be mixtures of continuous groups that only subtly differ from a purely continuous distribution, possibly due to known etiologic factors such as genetic syndromes; alternatively, some forms of psychopathology may be purely continuous in distribution but have nonlinear relationships with psychosocial or other functional outcomes (e.g., incarceration).

The Meaning of Diagnosis and Diagnostic Decision Thresholds

Moving to more continuous nosological paradigms will likely compel a shift in how psychiatric diagnoses are conceptualized, from the ascertainment of specific etiology to the ascertainment of either general etiology or intervention need. Syndromes of known discrete etiology, such as genetic disorders or localized neural lesions, will always be recognized, but the vast majority of psychopathologies of idiopathic or complex origin, continuous in distribution, will require conceptualization in terms of perceived intervention need and form. That is, what are the typical thresholds associated with intervention, either empirically in practice or as determined by protocol?

Body weight and temperature are good analogies in this respect. Obesity and fever are symptoms of known discrete diseases but also are sometimes diagnostically differentiated as conditions on their own because their causes are unknown or complex, otherwise require clinical attention, or both. Conventional thresholds used for defining a fever diagnosis (e.g., 38°C) arose from early studies of the distribution of body temperature and were largely arbitrarily defined based on observed distributions at that time (Mackowiak et al., 1992; Wunderlich & Seguin, 1871). As additional studies have been conducted, however, researchers have recognized that normative temperature varies by time of day, sex, era, and any number of other variables (Mackowiak et al., 1992; Wright & Auwaerter, 2020). As a result, different temperature thresholds for fever have been proposed for different settings based on thresholds' abilities to predict general criteria such as the presence of any confirmed infection, mortality, or other variables. Formal definitions of fever (Centers for Disease Control and Prevention, 2024) are in fact relatively subjective, allowing for reported feelings of fever and subjective clinician impressions of "warm." In this way, although body temperature per se is relatively objective, fever definition itself is a fuzzy concept, situationally dependent and in many ways reflecting an empirical characterization of what clinicians or clinics deem interventionally relevant or "noteworthy."

Common psychopathology dimensions, such as fear, dysphoria, and disinhibition, are similar to temperature in that their etiology is often unknown or complex and they often occur outside the context of a discernable discrete cause but still require clinical attention. They are closer to phenomenological conditions or types of "mental fever" in this respect than diseases or the underlying causes of fever per se. Like temperature thresholds for the diagnosis of fever, conventional diagnostic thresholds are ultimately empirically arbitrary but carry weight as established clinical constructs.

Diagnostic Thresholds as Metrics, and How to Characterize Psychopathology in Populations

How might questions about psychopathology in populations be approached if there are no clear ways to demarcate presence versus absence of mental disease

Certain psychopathology dimensions, such as dysphoria or positive emotion, have also never had conventional formal diagnostic thresholds, and such thresholds are arbitrary anyway, at least from the perspective of the dimensions' own distributions. Diagnoses ground questions about prevalence and similar issues in clinical significance; in the absence of diagnostic boundaries new groundings might be needed.

One approach is to treat psychopathology as continuous or quasi-continuous (for example, as is the case with symptom counts), without any attempt to attend to categorical diagnosis per se or thresholds associated with the latter. This approach would require abandoning concepts such as prevalence, focusing instead on the distribution of a given form of psychopathology and its characteristics, such as its mean, variance, and so forth. This avoids problems related to boundaries and potentially increases precision about what is being discussed. Characterizing modern normative distributions of body temperature, for instance, led to renewed discussion about what has been typical body temperature in different eras (Protsiv et al., 2020) and whether conventional fever thresholds might miss certain levels of illness (Smith & Clements, 2014). A similar focus in psychopathology might lead to greater precision about what is occurring and how it influences clinical decision making and societal resources.

There are admittedly problems with this approach. First and maybe most importantly, psychology and neurobehavioral science currently lack a good understanding of how the metrics of psychopathology measures translate into a metric of underlying illness. Thus, studying the distribution of a given operationalization in the form of a particular scale, test, or symptom count might be difficult to interpret vis-a-vis other operationalizations or of unclear meaning to society at large. What, for example, does zero on a given psychopathology measure mean? The absence of any illness? A certain level of illness? Even with continua, population scientific questions ideally are grounded in metrics that transcend particular measures and scales.

One might argue that questions about prevalence have as a core concern not necessarily diagnostic prevalence per se but concerns about the population rate at which levels of psychopathology reach a level associated with a significant criterion. This could be the prevalence of a discrete disease or syndrome state, but it could be any number of other things as well: the proportion of the population reaching some level of a continuum more often associated with clinical intervention than not, the proportion reaching some level of a continuum associated with identified etiologies, the proportion reaching a level associated with major psychosocial outcomes (for example, criminal conviction or incarceration), and so forth and so on.

Alternatively, it may be that certain indicators of different levels of a continuum, or their absence, themselves become meaningful in their own right. Severe markers might become a focus on their own, such as suicidality as markers of depression. In contrast, if a psychopathology continuum is often defined via counts of different behavioral and experiential markers, the absence of any of them could be a meaningful, if imperfect, criterion for lack of psychopathology and an appropriate target for prevalence studies.

It might be argued that this approach shifts the focus of inquiry into prevalence from psychopathology per se onto specific external criteria. However, it might just as reasonably be argued that this has always been the case, that formal diagnoses themselves reflect a particular institutional nosological decision about what constitutes "importance." The dominant prevalence of "not elsewhere classified" or "not otherwise specified" (NEC or NOS; Rajakannan et al., 2016) in health care settings points to existing formal diagnostic definitions not only being arbitrary but also possibly specific in a way that is not informative or useful in actual clinical settings, whatever the reasons might be. Shifting the focus more explicitly to consequentiality of continua in epidemiological studies from diagnosis per se to level of a specified criterion would arguably increase the precision with which population psychopathology is studied.

Variation in Diagnostic Processes

Being more explicit about the discrete criteria serving to grade different levels of psychopathology could also help better understand how those levels of psychopathology become instantiated in clinical decision making and care. Diagnostic judgments depend on characteristics of the clinician (Brechbiel & Keeley, 2019) as well as characteristics of the patient that are distinct from the psychopathology of interest (race; e.g., Hairston et al., 2019), and properties of psychopathology measures vary across different sociocultural groups and settings (e.g., Stevanovic et al., 2017). Separating psychopathology measures per se from defining criteria of interest (clinical care intervention, known causes, outcomes of interest) helps delineate the process by which expressed or experienced psychopathology is scaled in context.

Research on measurement invariance across cultures, for instance, has suggested that the same broad features of psychopathology are present across different sociocultural settings but that the specifics of how psychopathology is best assessed—and in particular, the thresholds for different indicators of psychopathology—vary (for example, He &

Li, 2021; Sorrel et al., 2021). This is broadly consistent with studies showing that diagnostic criteria sometimes differ in their utility across different cultures and that clinicians can have different thresholds for application of criteria depending on cultural context (e.g., drug seeking criteria are less useful in cultures where substances are less common or more societally stigmatized; Room et al., 1996). Even more broadly, continuous measures might relate to clinical status differently across cultures, depending on variables such as median level of education (as in the case of dementia; Prince et al., 2003).

By isolating the continuous level of psychopathology per se from discrete variables of interest that help scale the former—variables such as an expectation of clinical intervention, expectation of a known causal exposure, or likelihood of major sequelae, for example—it is possible to more precisely model the processes involved in arriving at clinical decisions. Doing so might improve the utility of assessments through recognition of how different measurement criteria or symptoms vary by context. Rather than assuming that a single fixed diagnostic definition applies equally across the population, research might help identify how important thresholds might be identified differently depending on sociodemographic, genetic, cultural, or other factors. Just as fever thresholds vary by factors such as age and sex, it might be appropriate to empirically identify thresholds that are optimally appropriate for one context as opposed to another or at least to quantify uncertainty in assessments due to variability in such factors.

Research on hierarchical dimensional models also points to ways in which different levels of specificity in measurement might apply to different individuals. In many ways, symptoms or indicators of a psychopathology continuum can often be thought of as very small subdimensions; to the extent that more specific symptoms or criteria (seeking more of a substance to avoid withdrawal, for example) vary in their validity across cultural and other scenarios, it may be that more prominent subdimensions (problems with a specific version of a substance) do also. Which level of specificity is appropriate might vary for different populations, which has important clinical and epidemiological implications.

Conclusions

Although they have a long presence in theory and research, continuous accounts of psychopathology have become prominent in formal nosological systems as well as scientific and clinical literature. Although the benefits of using continuous models have been well documented (Markon et al., 2011), questions might be raised about how to approach certain areas of inquiry about psychopathology in the population, such as those related to prevalence. Many of these questions can be addressed by refocusing inquiry on underlying issues, such as refocusing questions about prevalence onto questions about rates at which levels of psychopathology are severe enough to warrant clinical care, for example. Doing so has the advantage of clarifying questions at hand and potentially improving the accuracy of assessments across different scenarios.

PART I REFERENCES

Aristotle. (1949). The Nicomachean ethics of Aristotle. In *Everyman's library; no. 547.* Dent.

Berlin, I. (2000). *Three critics of the Enlightenment: Vico, Hamman, Herder.* Princeton University Press.

Bhaskar, R. (1973). *A realist theory of science.* Harvester Press.

Bhaskar, R. (1979). *The possibility of naturalism: A philosophical critique of the contemporary human sciences.* Routledge.

Brinkmann, S. (2017). *John Dewey: Science for a changing world.* Routledge.

Broadbent, A. (2013). *Philosophy of epidemiology.* Palgrave Macmillan.

De Caro, M., & Macarthur, D. (Eds.). (2022). *The Routledge handbook of liberal naturalism.* Routledge.

De Vries, Y. A., Bos, E. H., Roest, A. M., & De Jonge, P. (2023). Psychiatric epidemiology. In A. Tasman, M. B. Riba, R. D. Alarcón, C. A. Alfonso, S. Kanba, D. M. Ndetei, C. H. Ng, T. G. Schulze, & D. Lecic-Tosevski (Eds.), *Tasman's psychiatry* (pp. 1–41). Springer International.

Hacking, I. (1995). *Rewriting the soul: Multiple personality and the sciences of memory.* Princeton University Press.

Haslam, N. (2002). Kinds of kinds: A conceptual taxonomy of psychiatric categories. *Philosophy, Psychiatry, & Psychology, 9*(3), 203–217.

Hopwood, C. J., Morey, L. C., & Markon, K. E. (2023). What is a psychopathology dimension? *Clinical Psychology Review, 106,* 102356.

Horwitz, A. V., & Grob, G. N. (2011). The checkered history of American psychiatric epidemiology. *Milbank Quarterly, 89*(4), 628–657.

Kendler, K. S., Munoz, R. A., & Murphy, G. (2010). The development of the Feighner criteria: A historical perspective. *American Journal of Psychiatry, 167,* 134–142.

Kessler, R. C. (2002). The categorical versus dimensional assessment controversy in the sociology of mental illness. *Journal of Health and Social Behavior, 43,* 171–188.

Kessler, R. C., Brandenburg, N., Lane, M., Roy-Byrne, P., Stang, P. D., Stein, D. J., & Wittchen, H.-U. (2005). Rethinking the duration requirement for generalized anxiety disorder: Evidence from the National Comorbidity Survey Replication. *Psychological Medicine, 35*(7), 1073–1082.

Kessler, R. C., McLaughlin, K. A., Green, J. G., Gruber, M. J., Sampson, N. A., Zaslavsky, A. M., . . . Williams, D. R. (2010). Childhood adversities and adult psychopathology in the WHO World Mental Health Surveys. *British Journal of Psychiatry, 197*(5), 378–385.

Kessler, R. C., Merikangas, K. R., Berglund, P., Eaton, W. W., Koretz, D. S., & Walters, E. E. (2003). Mild disorders should not be eliminated from the DSM-V. *Archives of General Psychiatry, 60,* 1177–1122.

Kincaid, H., & Sullivan, J. (2014). *Classifying psychopathology: Mental kinds and natural kinds.* MIT Press.

Klerman, G. (1978). The evolution of a psychiatric nosology. In J. C. Shershow (Ed.), *Schizophrenia: Science and practice.* Harvard University Press.

Kotov, R., Krueger, R. F., Watson, D., Achenbach, T. M., Althoff, R. R., Bagby, R. M., . . . Zimmerman, M. (2017). The hierarchical taxonomy of psychopathology (HiTOP): A dimensional alternative to traditional nosologies. *Journal of Abnormal Psychology, 126*(4), 454–477.

Kraemer, H. C., Noda, A., & O'Hara, R. (2004). Categorical versus dimensional approaches to diagnosis: Methodological challenges. *Journal of Psychiatric Research, 38*(1), 17–25.

Lee, S., Tsang, A., Ruscio, A. M., Haro, J. M., Stein, D. J., Alonso, J., . . . Kessler, R. C. (2009). Implications of modifying the duration requirement of generalized anxiety disorder in developed and developing countries. *Psychological Medicine, 39*(7), 1163.

Leroi, A. M. (2014). *The lagoon: How Aristotle invented science* (S. MacPherson, Trans.). Viking Pengiun.

March, D., & Oppenheimer, G. M. (2014). Social disorder and diagnostic order: The US Mental Hygiene Movement, the Midtown Manhattan study and the development of psychiatric epidemiology in the 20th century. *International Journal of Epidemiology, 43*(Suppl. 1), i29–i42.

McLaughlin, K. A., Koenen, K. C., Friedman, M. J., Ruscio, A. M., Karam, E. G., Shahly, V., . . . Kessler, R. C. (2015). Subthreshold posttraumatic stress disorder in the World Health Organization World Mental Health Surveys. *Biological Psychiatry, 77*(4), 375–384.

Mills, C. (2014). *Decolonizing global mental health: The psychiatrization of the majority world.* Routledge, Taylor & Francis Group.

Patel, V., Saxena, S., Lund, C., Thornicroft, G., Baingana, F., Bolton, P., . . . UnÜtzer, J. (2018). The Lancet Commission on global mental health and sustainable development. *Lancet, 392,* 1553–1598.

Ruphy, S. (2017). *Scientific pluralism reconsidered: A new approach to the (dis) unity of science.* University of Pittsburgh Press.

Ruscio, A. M., Lane, M., Roy-Byrne, P., Stang, P. E., Stein, D. J., Wittchen, H.-U., & Kessler, R. C. (2005). Should excessive worry be required for a diagnosis of generalized anxiety disorder? Results from the US National Comorbidity Survey Replication. *Psychological Medicine, 35*(12), 1761–1772.

Scott, K. M., Alonso, J., De Jonge, P., Viana, M. C., Liu, Z., O'Neill, S., . . . Kessler, R. C. (2013). Associations between DSM-IV mental disorders and onset of self-reported peptic ulcer in the World Mental Health Surveys. *Journal of Psychosomatic Research, 75*(2), 121–127.

Stein, D. J. (1991). Philosophy and the DSM-III. *Comprehensive Psychiatry, 32*(5), 404–415.
Stein, D. J. (1993). Cross-cultural psychiatry and the DSM-IV. *Comprehensive Psychiatry, 34*(5), 322–329.
Stein, D. J. (2013). What is a mental disorder? A perspective from cognitive-affective science. *The Canadian Journal of Psychiatry, 58*(12), 656–662.
Stein, D. J. (2021). *Problems of living: Perspectives from philosophy, psychiatry, and cognitive-affective science.* Elsevier Academic Press.
Stein, D. J. (2022). Psychiatric disorders are soft natural kinds. *Philosophy, Psychiatry, & Psychology, 29*(3), 183–185.
Stein, D. J. (2023). Towards a philosophy of psychiatric epidemiology. *International Journal of Epidemiology, 52*(5), 1670–1672.
Stein, D. J., Phillips, K. A., Bolton, D., Fulford, K. W. M., Sadler, J. Z., & Kendler, K. S. (2010). What is a mental/psychiatric disorder? From DSM-IV to DSM-V. *Psychological Medicine, 40*(11), 1759–1765.
Stein, D. J., Scott, K. M., de Jonge, P., & Kessler, R. C. (2017). Epidemiology of anxiety disorders: From surveys to nosology and back. *Dialogues in Clinical Neuroscience, 19*(2), 127–136.
Wakefield, J. C. (2022). Klerman's "credo" reconsidered: Neo-Kraepelinianism, Spitzer's views, and what we can learn from the past. *World Psychiatry, 21*(1), 4–25.

PART II REFERENCES

Brechbiel, J. K., & Keeley, J. W. (2019). Pathways linking clinician demographics to mental health diagnostic accuracy: An international perspective. *Journal of Clinical Psychology, 75*(9), 1715–1729.
Centers for Disease Control and Prevention. (2024). Definitions of symptoms for reportable illnesses. Retrieved November 5, 2024, from *www.hhs.gov/guidance/document/cdc-defintion-symptoms-reportable-illnesses*
Hairston, D. R., Gibbs, T. A., Wong, S. S., & Jordan, A. (2019). Clinician bias in diagnosis and treatment. In M. Medlock, D. Shtasel, N. H. Trinh, & D. Williams (Eds.), *Racism and psychiatry* (pp. 105–137). Humana Press.
He, Q., & Li, J. J. (2021). Factorial invariance in hierarchical factor models of mental disorders in African American and European American youths. *Journal of Child Psychology and Psychiatry, 62*(3), 289–298.
Hopwood, C. J., Morey, L. C., & Markon, K. E. (2023). What is a psychopathology dimension? *Clinical Psychology Review, 106,* 102356.
Mackowiak, P., Wasserman, S., & Levine M. (1992). A critical appraisal of 98.6°F, the upper limit of the normal body temperature, and other legacies of Carl Reinhold August Wunderlich. *JAMA, 268,* 1578–1580.
Markon, K. E., Chmielewski, M., & Miller, C. J. (2011). The reliability and validity of discrete and continuous measures of psychopathology: A quantitative review. *Psychological Bulletin, 137*(5), 856–879.
Prince, M., Acosta, D., Chiu, H., Scazufca, M., & Varghese, M. (2003).

Dementia diagnosis in developing countries: A cross-cultural validation study. *The Lancet, 361*(9361), 909–917.

Protsiv, M., Ley, C., Lankester, J., Hastie, T., & Parsonnet, J. (2020) Decreasing human body temperature in the United States since the Industrial Revolution. *eLife, 9,* e49555.

Rajakannan, T., Safer, D. J., Burcu, M., & Zito, J. M. (2016). National trends in psychiatric not otherwise specified (NOS) diagnosis and medication use among adults in outpatient treatment. *Psychiatric Services, 67*(3), 289–295.

Room, R., Janca, A., Bennett, L. A., Schmidt, L., & Sartorius, N. (1996). WHO cross-cultural applicability research on diagnosis and assessment of substance use disorders: An overview of methods and selected results. *Addiction, 91*(2), 199–220.

Small E., & Clements, C. M. (2014). Defining fever: Likelihood of infection diagnosis as a function of body temperature in the emergency department. *Critical Care, 18,* 42.

Sorrel, M. A., García, L. F., Aluja, A., Rolland, J. P., Rossier, J., Roskam, I., & Abad, F. J. (2021). Cross-Cultural Measurement Invariance in the Personality Inventory for DSM-5. *Psychiatry Research, 304,* 114134.

Stevanovic, D., Jafari, P., Knez, R., Franic, T., Atilola, O., Davidovic, N., . . . Lakic, A. (2017). Can we really use available scales for child and adolescent psychopathology across cultures? A systematic review of cross-cultural measurement invariance data. *Transcultural Psychiatry, 54*(1), 125–152.

Wright, W. F., & Auwaerter, P. G. (2020). Fever and fever of unknown origin: Review, recent advances, and lingering dogma. *Open Forum Infectious Diseases,* 7(5), ofaa132.

Wunderlich C. A., & Seguin E. (1871). *Medical thermometry and human temperature.* William Wood.

CHAPTER 12

How does dimensional diagnosis change how we should think about psychotherapy research?

For several generations, the "gold-standard" approach to psychotherapy research was to sample people who meet criteria for a disorder and randomize them to different conditions to compare treatments. Because this model breaks down in a world in which disorders are not categories, the transition to dimensional approaches to diagnosis could have transformative effects on psychotherapy research. We asked experts three questions about this issue:

> *How should participants be sampled for psychotherapy research?*
>
> *How should treatments be organized in psychotherapy research?*
>
> *Will it make sense to focus treatment research on generating strategies that target major dimensions of psychopathology?*

Kerber et al. suggest that the transition to dimensional diagnosis encourages being more thoughtful and targeted about sampling, focusing on specific treatment mechanisms rather than therapy schools or packages, and considering both common and specific factors as they apply to both psychological treatments and dimensions of psychopathology. In essence, they argue that this transition is an opportunity to solve some of the oft-discussed issues in psychotherapy research. Stevens et al. take an even more progressive view, interpreting the transition to dimensional diagnosis as an opportunity to reconceptualize psychotherapy research from a complex systems perspective. This point of view is often idiographic and does not assume linear associations among variables and thus is a major departure from common research approaches. It would therefore require an entirely new way of thinking in research—but one with the virtue of aligning more closely with thinking in clinical practice.

PART I

How dimensional diagnosis transforms psychotherapy research

André Kerber, Thomas Munder,
and Johannes C. Ehrenthal

Three leading dimensional frameworks of psychopathology—the hierarchical taxonomy of psychopathology (HiTOP; Kotov et al., 2021), the DSM-5 alternative model of personality disorders (AMPD; American Psychiatric Association, 2013), and the ICD-11 classification of personality disorders (World Health Organization, 2022)—each reconceptualizes mental illness by integrating personality and clinical symptoms into hierarchies that embrace comorbidity rather than treating it as a nuisance. In all three systems, the overlap of syndromes and trait domains is considered as the very structure through which broad spectra of dysfunction are defined, whereas a clear conceptual distinction is drawn between a general severity dimension (the "p-factor" in HiTOP; impaired personality functioning in DSM-5 AMPD; and personality disorder severity in ICD-11) and the more fine-grained stylistic expression of psychopathology (maladaptive trait domains in DSM-5 and ICD-11; internalizing, externalizing, detachment, and thought-disorder spectra in HiTOP; Kerber et al., 2024). By moving decisively away from discrete diagnostic categories toward continuous trait-based dimensions, these models call for a shift in psychotherapy research toward transdiagnostic mechanisms—such as emotion regulation, cognitive flexibility, experiential exposure, and interpersonal learning—that cut across traditional disorders. Although this approach seemingly stands in stark contrast to the predominant disease models that stem from somatic medicine, in which pathogenic mechanisms cause a disorder that can be dichotomously assessed as either existing or absent, dimensional approaches offer distinct advantages for the future of psychotherapy research and practice. By reorienting around severity and style continua, psychotherapy research may produce more generalizable mechanism-based findings—ultimately providing more flexible efficient intervention frameworks that track and target the processes that underlie human suffering regardless of traditional diagnostic boundaries. Research based on dimensions could also provide new answers to the long-standing question of what is a more promising strategy for psychotherapy: a focus on similarities or differences between patients (e.g., Barlow, 2004; Wampold, 2007).

How Should Participants Be Sampled for Psychotherapy Research?

Theoretically, and speaking from a purely dimensional perspective of psychopathology, there is no such thing as a distinct mental disorder within an individual, which should make any sampling procedure challenging. If there is no such thing as anxiety disorder, who is in need of therapy? On a practical level, dimensional diagnoses require researchers to be more precise regarding what they consider central to their approach or study and how this relates to other relevant dimensions of psychopathology. For example, if researchers define high levels of problems in life as the main area of interest, they can allow other spectra, traits, or levels of personality function to vary or have to decide on why they want to keep some of these levels within a certain range. This of course, has implications for intervention planning as well as sample size calculation. Higher precision in conceptual thinking about sampling is therefore a key demand that can be delineated from dimensional approaches.

In a dimensional paradigm, sampling strategies for psychotherapy research must therefore extend beyond traditional diagnostic categories to embrace the richness of trait continua and the specific mechanisms under investigation. One approach is to assemble broadly representative cohorts—whether drawn from the general population or clinic settings—that span the full range of severity (from subclinical distress to profound impairment) and the principal spectra of dysfunction (internalizing, externalizing, thought disorder). Stratified sampling ensures that individuals with high internalizing traits, significant interpersonal dysfunction, or other targeted profiles are purposefully included, enhancing the study's generalizability and power to detect nuanced moderators of treatment response.

Alternatively, researchers may elect to leverage dimensional systems more selectively, recruiting participants who exemplify the particular trait domains or severity levels most relevant to their hypothesized mechanisms (e.g., focusing on elevated disinhibited externalizing when testing inhibitory-control interventions). It is also crucial to distinguish between population-representative samples, which offer broad external validity and insight into normative trait distributions, and clinical samples, which offer a deeper examination of severe presentations and treatment effects. Both designs carry trade-offs: population cohorts may underrepresent extreme scores, whereas clinical cohorts can overstate effect sizes or restrict the variability needed to identify cross-spectrum processes. By clarifying these choices upfront and aligning them with specific mechanistic questions, dimensional psychotherapy research can yield findings that are both scientifically rigorous and clinically meaningful. This is especially relevant, as many studies from the last few decades were optimized, also through sample selection, to produce large pre–post effects but did not result in similarly impressive long-term gains (Cuijpers et al., 2021).

All these sampling strategies are intended to obtain samples with large variance, which then serve as a starting point for correlational investigations of the links between dimensions (and their interactions) and psychotherapy processes and outcomes. In the sampling strategies of categorical research, these types of investigations are at least more challenging due to the difficulties of obtaining sufficient cell counts and the lower statistical power in categorical analyses. Thus, dimensional diagnoses provide an important foundation for testing models and hypotheses, in not just RCTs but also complex longitudinal designs (Philips & Falkenström, 2021).

How Should Treatments Be Organized and Assessed in Psychotherapy Research?

In traditional clinical thinking that views different mental disorders as distinct categories, it is natural to focus psychotherapeutic interventions on specific disorders. As is well known, this has led to lists of evidence-based psychotherapies, which are organized by types of mental disorders and for which only studies conducted on individuals with the disorder in question are accepted as evidence (see Division 12, American Psychological Association). Although this trend has weakened recently with the emergence of transdiagnostic approaches (Schaeuffele et al., 2021) or network models (Roefs et al., 2022), it is still dominant beyond the area of so-called emotional disorders (i.e., anxiety and depression).

For clinical thinking that sees mental disorders as expressions of different continua, a discussion about differential effectiveness is as important as in research on diagnostic groups. Initially, dimensional thinking does not result in clear subgroups for which specific psychotherapeutic approaches should be developed. It is therefore still unclear, for example, which subgroups formed by, say, the poles of a continuum are better treated by different interventions. To exaggerate somewhat, one could say that initially, the null hypothesis that generic psychotherapy, (i.e., without specialization) is valid, applies. Of course, there are robust findings on necessary specializations of psychotherapy for at least some diagnostic spectrums—for example, psychotic disorders (Lutgens et al., 2017), complex posttraumatic disorders (Karatzias et al., 2019), and borderline personality disorder (Cristea et al., 2017). Nevertheless, psychotherapy research focused on dimensional diagnosis might yield empirically and clinically more satisfying answers to questions of treatment specialization and adaptation.

Dimensional diagnosis necessitates organizing treatments around core psychopathological processes and transdiagnostic mechanisms rather than traditional diagnostic categories. Demonstrating the general effectiveness of a particular treatment does not provide evidence about how that treatment works (Cuijpers et al., 2019; Kazdin, 2007). Indeed, as Cronbach (1975) hypothesized, the effectiveness of any given treatment may depend on interactions between individual patient characteristics (aptitudes) and the treatment itself such that a treatment's effectiveness can vary substantially across different individuals. A better understanding of the underlying individual mechanisms of change could therefore inform the optimization of treatment options. One possible way to approach this is to analyze the association between the use of specific treatment techniques or methods and changes in specific psychopathological categories or spectra (Hill & Norcross, 2023). This approach typically assumes that symptom change is due to specific factors realized by a specific therapeutic technique (e.g., cognitive restructuring; Lemmens et al., 2016). Current evidence suggests that in psychotherapy, the effects are predominantly achieved through common factors (Norcross & Lambert, 2018) such as the therapeutic alliance, goal consensus, or collaboration (Wampold, 2015). For example, a meta-analysis of 295 studies encompassing over 30,000 patients found an overall association between alliance and outcome of $r = .28$, suggesting a positive relationship with symptom reduction that is independent of treatment type (Flückiger et al., 2018).

However, there is also emerging evidence on the relation of specific techniques to psychotherapy outcome (Grevenhaus et al., 2024). By organizing psychopathology based on empirical evidence into general severity and specific spectra rather than into categories with overlapping symptoms, a dimensional model such as the AMPD or HiTOP presumably enhances the precision with which treatment effects can be detected, as the error involved in categorical classification is reduced. Conventional diagnostic categories often conflate disparate symptom profiles (for example, two individuals meeting criteria for major depressive disorder may exhibit minimal symptom overlap), thereby obscuring the specific contributions of individual interventions. Consequently, Mullins-Sweatt and colleagues (2020) argue that each spectrum (e.g., internalizing, thought disorder, detachment, disinhibited or antagonistic externalizing) comes with a well-defined cluster of traits, symptoms, and mechanisms that can be targeted by particular techniques. When outcomes are evaluated along continuous trait dimensions—such as reductions in negative affectivity within the internalizing spectrum, enhancements in inhibitory control within disinhibition, or enhancement of mentalizing ability within the general severity domain—researchers can employ sophisticated mediation and moderation analyses to disentangle or test possible unique effects of techniques like cognitive restructuring, behavioral activation, or transference interpretations. This dimensional approach minimizes measurement error and increases statistical power by treating psychopathology as graded constructs rather than discrete entities. Moreover, by developing treatment taxonomies that map particular methods onto general severity and specific spectra, investigators can formulate and empirically test precise hypotheses regarding mechanism-specific change. As Mullins-Sweatt et al. (2020) conclude, only through such alignment of interventions with validated trait continua can psychotherapy research attain the granularity necessary to identify and optimize the active ingredients responsible for therapeutic benefit. At a minimum, dimensional approaches should allow for more rigorous tests of the long-standing controversy around the relative merits of the common factors of psychotherapy and of specific techniques.

To date, there remains limited insight into the interaction between specific techniques and common factors in the process of symptom change (Cuijpers et al., 2019; Tschacher et al., 2014). Furthermore, instruments used to measure common factors are often limited to the aspect of the therapeutic alliance, even though meta-analytic results also indicate the effectiveness of other common factors such as empathy, rupture repair, and emotional expression (Norcross & Lambert, 2018). Within a dimensional framework, common factors—such as empathic attunement, alliance formation, congruence/genuineness, real relationship, emotional expression, cultivating positive expectations, managing countertransference, and repairing alliance ruptures—primarily may mitigate broad impairments in self- and interpersonal functioning (Criterion A), thereby reducing overall severity (Kerber et al., 2024). In contrast, specific techniques may exert more circumscribed effects on specific traits or spectra. For instance, what is called "cognitive restructuring" in cognitive-behavioral therapy might preferentially decrease negative affectivity; what is called "transference analysis" in dynamic psychotherapies could selectively alter antagonistic traits; inhibition training could enhance impulse control within the disinhibited externalizing spectrum (Hopwood, 2018). In addition, this approach can help to communicate and build bridges between different therapy traditions, as it stimulates finding a common phenomenon-oriented language. This may foster finding similarities but also possible relevant differences between different traditions.

However, alternative perspectives remain tenable. It is possible that technique-specific interventions achieve broader gains by engaging common factors or that the distinction between general and specific processes is less clearly defined in practice. Consequently, psychotherapy research would benefit from designs that concurrently assess both common factors and discrete techniques, employ longitudinal analyses to test competing models, and explore whether common and specific factors of clinical psychological interventions yield differential effects across severity and style dimensions (Heim et al., 2025). Rather than adhering to fixed protocols for discrete disorders, a truly dimensional approach requires that treatments be conceptualized and evaluated along two orthogonal axes—severity/common factors versus style/specific techniques—and that empirical studies explicitly model how therapist–patient processes rooted in Criterion A traits/general severity interact with technique-specific effects on Criterion B traits/spectra.

Consequently, parallel to the assessment of general severity and specific style of (changes of) the individual psychopathology, assessments of treatments should be organized around common factors (alliance, empathy, etc.) and specific (psychodynamic, behavioral, humanistic, systemic) approaches and techniques. Disentangling common and specific variance in both assessments of psychopathology and treatments could finally leverage the potential of dimensional approaches and enhance precision in identifying which therapeutic elements drive symptom improvement across various disorders and dimensions of psychopathology. However, it must be noted that psychotherapy research is not independent from general research funding or which psychotherapy schools are represented in the grant committees, leading to relatively inflexible views on what is considered evidence based: Especially in times of reduced funding, it is virtually impossible to conduct RCTs to bring new approaches or existing ones with less controlled studies into guidelines (e.g., Leichsenring et al., 2024), ultimately hindering innovation and limiting patients' choice. Dimensional approaches to psychopathology and clinical psychological treatment may help build bridges across schools and paradigms, thereby advancing solutions to these challenges.

Will It Make Sense to Focus Treatment Research on Generating Strategies That Target Major Dimensions of Psychopathology?

Investigating treatment strategies with respect to major psychopathology dimensions offers a promising, dual-pronged approach that aligns with contemporary dimensional nosologies. On one hand, Hopwood and colleagues (2020) demonstrate how the HiTOP model can be used to integrate three broad clusters of therapeutic techniques—common factors, cognitive-behavioral methods, and relational interventions—by mapping them onto distinct hierarchical levels: common factors (e.g., alliance, empathy, rupture repair) correspond to the general severity axis; cognitive restructuring, exposure, skills training and motivational interviewing align with mid-level spectra such as internalizing, externalizing, and thought disorder; and relational analyses of transference and mentalizing or related constructs (Ehrenthal & Benecke, 2019) enrich our understanding of interpersonal dynamics within and across spectra.

On the other hand, Hopwood (2018) emphasizes that parsing out general severity (Criterion A in the AMPD, analogous to the HiTOP p-factor) from more stylistic trait-based expressions (Criterion B) can bring much-needed coherence to heterogeneous clinical presentations. Drawing on principles distilled from borderline personality treatment research—such as maintaining a structured therapeutic frame, fostering patient agency, and systematically connecting inner experiences to behavior—provides a blueprint for stabilizing broad personality dysfunction before targeting specific trait continua or spectra.

Consequently, both tailoring interventions to spectrum-specific mechanisms and disentangling severity from style warrant simultaneous attention. In practice, this means adopting hierarchical assessment protocols that first screen for general severity and then drill down into narrow traits, using standardized tools and ongoing process–outcome monitoring to guide case formulation and treatment adjustments. In research, it entails moving beyond category-based RCTs to designs that compare interventions across hierarchical levels, employing multidimensional outcome batteries (covering general distress, spectrum-level dysfunction, and trait-specific change), and developing an empirically derived taxonomy of technique–spectrum linkages within different dimensional perspectives, for example the HiTOP space. Such a comprehensive "both/and" strategy promises to clarify not only what works for whom but also how and why, thereby advancing more precise, mechanism-driven, and relational psychotherapy.

PART II

The application of complexity science and methods to psychotherapy research on dimensional diagnoses

TREVOR SANCHEZ STEVENS, ADELE M. HAYES, MERLIJN OLTHOF, and ANNA LICHTWARCK-ASCHOFF

The hierarchical taxonomy of psychopathology (HiTOP) model suggests that at the population level, symptoms are continuously distributed without clear cutoff points for pathology and that they tend to co-occur in a hierarchical and dimensional factor structure that crosses traditional diagnostic boundaries (Ruggero et al., 2019). This group-level structure, however, does not necessarily generalize to the individual level (Borsboom & Haslbeck, 2024; Molenaar, 2004). There is increasing interest in understanding how personality and psychopathology develop and are expressed within a person dynamically over time and across contexts (Hopwood et al., 2022; Wright et al., 2023, 2025; Zimmermann et al., 2019). Rather than having a static "true score" on these HiTOP dimensions, an individual and dynamic perspective recognizes that the patterns of thoughts, emotions, and behaviors that constitute personality and psychopathology wax and wane in intensity, arise from complex interactions between biopsychosocial processes that unfold across diverse timescales, and are expressed contextually as someone navigates the affordances and demands of their environment (DeYoung, 2015; Harkness et al., 2014; Hopwood et al., 2022; Wright et al., 2023; Zimmermann et al., 2019). A focus on contextualized within-person dynamics more closely matches the goals of modern clinical science and practice by guiding researchers to ask questions about when, where, why, and how patterns of functioning develop and move over time (Hayes & Andrews, 2020; S. Hayes et al., 2022; Morris et al., 2022). Embracing this complexity motivates the need for methods that can incorporate the rich data and theory needed to inform intervention (Olthof, Hasselman, Oude Maatman, et al., 2023; Wright & Hopwood, 2022).

A Complex Adaptive Systems Framework

Complexity science offers theory and methods that embrace the challenge of understanding and intervening in evolving complex systems and can be applied to psychological science (Hasselman, 2022). The science of complex adaptive systems (CAS) seeks to discover and apply general principles of how systems behave and change over time (Mitchell, 2009). A complex system is composed of many interdependent parts that interact such that whole-system behavior is not well understood when individual components or subsystems are studied in isolation. Larger, more complex systems often have nested subsystems as elements themselves. Complex systems are driven by reciprocal, nonlinear interactions between components, such as feedback loops that can amplify or inhibit system dynamics. Over time, these interactions can result in new higher-order patterns of system behavior (i.e., emergence; Olthof, Hasselman, Oude Maatman, et al., 2023).

Some complex systems are adaptive; their behavior patterns reorganize and adapt to their environment and shifting internal dynamics (Mitchell, 2009). Such systems develop over time through a process of variation, selection by context, and retention of adaptive patterns of behavior—retaining information about previous system states and contexts (S. Hayes et al., 2022; Mitchell, 2009). CAS can settle into stable patterns called attractors, a set of preferred states to which the system repeatedly returns across time and contexts—a characteristic style of behaving. This stability gives coherence to the system and provides a pattern of behavior that has adequately survived past contexts. Although attractor states are essential to the integrity of a system, a system must also retain enough variability to adapt flexibly to changing contexts (Olthof, Hasselman, Oude Maatman, et al., 2023). Attractor states can become tightly integrated with repeated activation across time and contexts, locking down system dynamics through mutual overregulation (Lenton et al., 2021). Systems with strong attractors can become entrenched and resistant to change, insensitive to new information and shifting conditions. When perturbations occur, strong connections between components tend to pull the system back into the attractor. Lasting change in these systems may require destabilization of the existing attractor (increasing system variability and allowing it to explore new states) and the formation and environmental support of alternative attractors (changing the environment or relationships between parts to foster a new pattern; Olthof, Hasselman, Oude Maatman, et al., 2023).

Application of CAS Perspective to Clinical Phenomena

From a complexity science lens, personality and psychopathology can be considered multimodal (biopsychosocial) sets of attractors in a complex adaptive system of interdependent thoughts, feelings, and behaviors that interact with the environment over time (Fried, 2022; Hayes & Andrews, 2020; Schiepek et al., 2016). Researchers have formulated theories of personality (Cramer et al., 2012; DeYoung, 2015; Sosnowska et al., 2020) and psychopathology (Granic et al., 2018; Olthof, Hasselman, Oude Maatman, et al., 2023) to account for the pathological patterns that keep a system stuck in distress and dysfunction and guide intervention efforts. For instance, negative thoughts (self-criticism and hopelessness) can trigger emotional reactions (sadness and guilt), leading to behavioral withdrawal and inactivity, which in turn can exacerbate feelings of loneliness and reinforce negative thoughts, thereby perpetuating a depressive cycle. This feedback loop can be supported or disrupted by the context of the behaviors and the resources and demands of the environment. Entrenched feedback loops and unsupportive contexts can lock down the system so that disconfirming new information that could tip the system into more functional patterns is instead avoided, deflected, or assimilated (Hayes & Andrews, 2020).

Issues in Psychotherapy Research

From a CAS perspective, psychotherapy research is focused on developing a scientific understanding of how to identify and disrupt unhealthy stuck patterns and facilitate the emergence of new, more functional patterns. High levels of interdependence in psychopathological processes call for intervention studies to target and measure multiple dimensions of functioning at multiple levels of analysis and to consider their interrelations over time (Olthof, Hasselman, Oude Maatman, et al., 2023; Wright & Hopwood, 2022). Furthermore, causation in psychological change is multiply determined, idiosyncratic, contextual, and complex—responses to interventions tend to be probabilistic not deterministic. Given this complexity, how should psychotherapy research identify treatment targets, sample participants, and organize intervention delivery and what methods and measures can be used to capture the dynamics of change in this context?

What Are the Treatment Targets?

From a CAS perspective, psychotherapy is designed to shift a person from entrenched dysfunctional attractors toward more flexible and functional attractors that allow clients to meet the demands of their changing environments over time and support more valued behaviors (Hayes & Andrews, 2020; S. Hayes et al., 2022). Rather than treating individual symptoms (e.g., feelings of worthlessness, avoidance) or broader pathological dimensions (e.g., internalizing behaviors) or disorders (e.g., depression), treatments would target the processes and environmental influences that connect symptoms, prevent new learning, and maintain psychopathological patterns (Tschacher & Haken, 2019). Clinicians can focus on identifying and disrupting the within-person dynamics of maladaptive patterns and feedback loops between thoughts, feelings, and behaviors (e.g., introducing mindfulness to disrupt avoidance patterns). They can also facilitate shifts out of maladaptive attractors by helping clients change or create environments that support more valued and functional behaviors (e.g., involving family in changing one's home environment). Psychotherapy has traditionally focused on disrupting maladaptive patterns (e.g., exposure therapy, behavioral activation, cognitive restructuring); a CAS perspective also emphasizes the importance of creating and stabilizing new patterns to support better functioning after treatment (Hayes & Andrews, 2020).

How Should We Sample Study Participants?

Psychotherapy research should be concerned with understanding the processes and outcomes of clinical interventions in the full range of individuals who could benefit from treatment (Morris et al., 2022). In a categorical system, this population is identified by diagnostic cutoffs and labels. A systems-related approach would focus more on levels of functional impairment, distress, and degree of entrenchment or "stuckness" (chronicity and recurrence)—which can be considered indicators of system health, apart from the content of personality and psychopathology (Ruggero et al., 2019; see Wright et al., 2025, for an approximation of this approach). In CAS terms, functional impairment reflects a mismatch between system behavior and the environment such that adaptive goals are not being met. Distress reflects the internal dynamics of the system straining to meet environmental demands. Stuckness refers to the level of pattern entrenchment reflected by the system's history, chronicity, recurrence, or pull to return to old patterns. These properties can help define when a client has a problem that may benefit from clinical intervention.

From a CAS perspective, dynamic patterns of thoughts, feelings, behaviors, and the environment are the treatment targets and, thus, can inform sampling and should be tracked over time (Olthof, Hasselman, Aas, et al., 2023). These patterns can be characterized by their dynamics (how the parts of the pattern interact, such as an avoidance feedback loop) and their content (thoughts, behaviors, and feelings that form the pattern, such avoiding social rejection). One-time assessments are merely snapshots of a dynamic process. Rather than collecting a sample of participants with "major depressive disorder" based on a one-time intake appointment, a CAS approach might instead collect data over time during a baseline period and select participants based on important characteristics of pathological patterns such as feedback loops or cycles, attractor strength, and sensitivity to context. Dense sampling over time can reveal trajectories and profiles of change throughout treatment, facilitating the study of nonlinear processes such as sudden gains and losses, periods of destabilization and sensitivity, or levels of system resilience (Hayes & Andrews, 2020; Olthof, Hasselman, Aas, et al., 2023; Olthof, Hasselman, Oude Maatman, et al., 2023; Schiepek et al., 2016). Because change processes in dynamic systems unfold over multiple interacting timescales, measurement frequency should be determined by the timescale of the processes of interest (Hopwood et al., 2022). Careful consideration should be given to how context affects the expression of psychopathology and how to account for this in sampling and measurement strategies. For example, in daily assessments, participants might note their current location, whether they are alone or with others, activities they are engaged in, situational perceptions, and other contextual features. Samples based on clinically relevant system dynamics (e.g., dysfunction, distress, stuckness of patterns) rather than static diagnostic categories allow for analyses of more personalized intervention targets and the use of higher resolution methods for tracking moving patterns.

How Should Treatments Be Organized?

CAS-informed therapeutic approaches are often structured in three phases: mapping system behavior, disrupting maladaptive attractors, and developing more functional attractors. Specific intervention strategies are then selected based on the case conceptualization and the change processes to mobilize. For example, exposure-based cognitive therapy for depression (EBCT; A. Hayes et al., 2022), integrative psychotherapy (Schiepek et al., 2016), and process-based therapy (Ong et al., 2024) follow this organization. The first phase of treatment in these approaches focuses on defining and mapping system components and their interconnections, which is achieved through clinical interviewing and possibly intensive longitudinal monitoring. Clinicians and clients collaboratively identify dynamic patterns that maintain dysfunction as targets for intervention and valued and functional system states as treatment goals (Ong et al., 2024; Schiepek et al., 2016). After identifying and mapping maladaptive attractors, clinicians can conceptualize which set of therapeutic operations and environmental changes might most effectively disrupt stuck patterns and facilitate a transition to more adaptive behavior (Hayes & Andrews, 2020). The final phase of treatment focuses on building new attractors to maintain treatment gains and to compete with or inhibit the pull to previous pathological patterns (Hayes & Andrews, 2020). Building more functional attractors can involve sparking positive emotions, increasing social engagement, and strengthening more positive views of the self.

What Methods Can Be Used for CAS-Informed Psychotherapy Research?

Randomized controlled trials have been invaluable in evaluating the efficacy of psychotherapy; however, they do not capture the complexity of *how* psychological change occurs (Hayes & Andrews, 2020). Traditional psychotherapy research designs focus on changes in aggregated disorder-based symptoms that are assessed before and after treatment. Aggregating symptoms into sum scores overlooks their differential clinical importance and client-specific variability in change processes (Fried, 2022). In addition, sparse assessment during treatment leaves researchers with little data to study how clinical change unfolds, especially nonlinear change (e.g., sudden gains or symptom spikes; Hayes & Andrews, 2020).

The interdisciplinary nature of complex systems research has yielded many approaches for organizing and analyzing dynamic and multimodal data. In addition to traditional population-based studies, a CAS perspective centers on and values deep analyses of individual systems and their evolution over time. In the case of psychotherapy research, this view revives the relevance of in-depth case studies. Following the principle of "first analyze, then aggregate" (Rose, 2016), CAS research can study within-person dynamics and then look for patterns or differences in these dynamics at the group level (Olthof, Hassellman, Aas, et al., 2023). The breadth of complexity science prohibits a full review of available methods, but we highlight several tools and examples that could be relevant to psychotherapy research.

Intensive Longitudinal Data

Modeling dynamic systems requires densely sampling system behaviors at the appropriate timescales. For instance, psychotherapy researchers can collect multivariate intensive longitudinal data (ILD) using smartphone-based surveys and remote sensors to monitor system behavior in its natural context throughout the day (Bringmann et al., 2022). It is important to note that there are theoretical and methodological issues to consider when collecting ILD (Hopwood et al., 2022; Kaurin et al., 2023).

Dynamic Statistical Network Models

Dynamic statistical network models use multivariate time series data to idiographically model a client as a system of variables that are connected over time (Borsboom et al., 2021; Bringmann et al., 2022). Changes in the network structure and dynamics have been investigated as early warning signs for transitions in psychological functioning (Haslbeck et al., 2020; Scheffer et al., 2009; Wichers et al., 2019). These models are extensions of the general linear model and provide person-level network estimates of average correlations at one or few timescales, including hypothesis tests and confidence intervals. Although the apparent interpretability of these methods is a strength, they struggle to comprehensively model the behavior of nonlinear nonstationary systems that can develop on multiple timescales (Hasselman & Bosman, 2020).

Recurrence-Based Methods

Recurrence-based methods offer another approach to studying nonlinear nonstationary complex system behavior in a relatively assumption-free framework. These methods examine how a system returns to similar states over time (Hasselman & Bosman, 2020). A system's state is based on the particular values of a set of relevant system variables $[X, Y, Z]$ at a given time, forming a coordinate in an N-dimensional state space. Studying how these systems travel in the state space and recur can reveal patterns and insights into system dynamics. For example, a person might initially be stuck in a rigid pattern with recurring sadness, rumination, and inactivity and later transition to a more flexible regime with a higher diversity of states. Recurrence analysis offers methods to quantify and visualize these patterns (Hasselman, 2022; Heino, 2021). Examples of recurrence methods used in psychotherapy research include work on destabilizing patterns in parent–child interactions (Lichtwarck-Aschoff et al., 2012) and examining changes in text structure in an expressive writing intervention for women with breast cancer (Lyby et al., 2019).

State Space Grids

State space grids (SSGs) provide another method that tracks a system's movement through state space (Hollenstein, 2013). SSGs map a time series of system states onto a grid, showing occurrences and transitions between states. These grids offer a low-dimensional depiction of both system topology and dynamics, helping to identify attractors or transition points. Quantitative measures can be extracted from these plots for analysis of system behavior. In psychotherapy research, SSGs have been used to study system variability and treatment outcomes in cognitive therapy for personality disorders (Hayes & Yasinski, 2015) and in cognitive behavioral therapy for youth with anxiety (Carper et al., 2022).

Machine-Learning Methods

Machine-learning methods can provide psychotherapy researchers with versatile tools for extracting and analyzing information from noisy high-dimensional data sets generated by CAS (Krakauer, 2023; Lalk et al., 2024; Tang et al., 2020). Machine-learning methods can help facilitate information decomposition of complex systems (e.g., identify which subcomponents drive system-level behavior), reconstruct causal networks (via complexity-based measures of causality and random forests), and extract features from unstructured data such as text, video, or images (Lalk et al., 2024; Tang et al., 2020).

"Qualitative methods" capture rich contextual information about processes of psychological change and can be used in mixed-methods designs to complement and cross-validate quantitative findings from time-series analyses. For example, Olthof et al. (2024) used qualitative information gathered from participants to further characterize transition and resilience processes in quantitative time-series data. Hulsmans et al. (2024) used intensive qualitative analysis of patient records to study mechanisms of change for clinically relevant transitions. De Smet et al. (2024) used qualitative data to contextualize items from experience-sampling methods and study the validity of dynamic network models for capturing clients' reported experiences.

Conclusion

A CAS approach to psychological science situates the emerging development of a more dynamic and individualized approach to personality and psychopathology within a broader interdisciplinary framework. A CAS perspective can help shape theory and methods in psychotherapy research for analyzing the formation and change of dynamic patterns that develop into personality and pathology within a person across time and contexts. A CAS lens for studying the treatment of maladaptive patterns moves beyond a categorical perspective on psychopathology and has implications for the research and development of psychotherapeutic interventions. Methods from CAS can be used to model system changes and understand the dynamics of when, where, how, and why change occurs within a person throughout therapy. Embracing the dynamic complexity of psychopathology may paradoxically help to simplify psychotherapy research and practice by identifying general principles of psychological system change that can be applied transdiagnostically.

PART I REFERENCES

American Psychiatric Association. (2013). *Diagnostic and statistical manual of mental disorders* (5th ed.). Author.

Barlow, D. H. (2004). Psychological treatments. *American Psychologist, 59*(9), 869–878.

Cristea, I. A., Gentili, C., Cotet, C. D., Palomba, D., Barbui, C., & Cuijpers, P. (2017). Efficacy of psychotherapies for borderline personality disorder: A systematic review and meta-analysis. *JAMA Psychiatry, 74*(4), 319.

Cronbach, L. J. (1975). Beyond the two disciplines of scientific psychology. *American Psychologist, 30*(2), 116–127.

Cuijpers, P., Karyotaki, E., Ciharova, M., Miguel, C., Noma, H., & Furukawa, T. A. (2021). The effects of psychotherapies for depression on response, remission, reliable change, and deterioration: A meta-analysis. *Acta Psychiatrica Scandinavica, 144*(3), 288–299.

Cuijpers, P., Reijnders, M., & Huibers, M. J. H. (2019). The role of common factors in psychotherapy outcomes. *Annual Review of Clinical Psychology, 15*, 207–231.

Ehrenthal, J. C., & Benecke, C. (2019). Tailored treatment planning for individuals with personality disorders. In U. Kramer (Ed.), *Case formulation for personality disorders* (pp. 291–314). Elsevier.

Flückiger, C., Del Re, A. C., Wampold, B. E., & Horvath, A. O. (2018). The alliance in adult psychotherapy: A meta-analytic synthesis. *Psychotherapy, 55*(4), 316–340.

Grevenhaus, C. J., Flückiger, C., Theimer, L., & Benecke, C. (2024). Does technique matter? A multilevel meta-analysis on the association between psychotherapeutic techniques and outcome. *Research in Psychotherapy: Psychopathology, Process, and Outcome, 27*(2), 803.

Heim, P., Brose, A., Böttche, M., Peters, E. M., Ehrenthal, J. C., Knaevelsrud, C., & Kerber, A. (2025). Mechanisms of change in naturalistic mental health care settings: Study protocol for a longitudinal multimethod study. *BMJ Open, 15*(10), e106741.

Hill, C. E., & Norcross, J. C. (2023). Skills and methods that work in psychotherapy: Observations and conclusions from the special issue. *Psychotherapy, 60*(3), 407–416.

Hopwood, C. J. (2018). A framework for treating DSM-5 alternative model for personality disorder features. *Personality and Mental Health, 12*(2), 107–125.

Hopwood, C. J., Bagby, R. M., Gralnick, T., Ro, E., Ruggero, C., Mullins-Sweatt, S., . . . Zimmermann, J. (2020). Integrating psychotherapy with the hierarchical taxonomy of psychopathology (HiTOP). *Journal of Psychotherapy Integration, 30*(4), 477–497.

Karatzias, T., Murphy, P., Cloitre, M., Bisson, J., Roberts, N., Shevlin, M., . . . Hutton, P. (2019). Psychological interventions for ICD-11 complex PTSD symptoms: Systematic review and meta-analysis. *Psychological Medicine, 49*(11), 1761–1775.

Kazdin, A. E. (2007). Mediators and mechanisms of change in psychotherapy research. *Annual Review of Clinical Psychology, 3,* 1–27.

Kerber, A., Ehrenthal, J. C., Zimmermann, J., Remmers, C., Nolte, T., Wendt, L. P., . . . Knaevelsrud, C. (2024). Examining the role of personality functioning in a hierarchical taxonomy of psychopathology using two years of ambulatory assessed data. *Translational Psychiatry, 14*(1), 340.

Kotov, R., Krueger, R. F., Watson, D., Cicero, D. C., Conway, C. C., DeYoung, C. G., . . . Wright, A. G. C. (2021). The hierarchical taxonomy of psychopathology (HiTOP): A quantitative nosology based on consensus of evidence. *Annual Review of Clinical Psychology, 17,* 83–108.

Leichsenring, F., Abbass, A., Fonagy, P., Levy, K. N., Lilliengren, P., Luyten, P., . . . Steinert, C. (2024). WHO treatment guideline for mental disorders. *The Lancet Psychiatry, 11*(9), 676–677.

Lemmens, L. H. J. M., Müller, V. N. L. S., Arntz, A., & Huibers, M. J. H. (2016). Mechanisms of change in psychotherapy for depression: An empirical update and evaluation of research aimed at identifying psychological mediators. *Clinical Psychology Review, 50,* 95–107.

Lutgens, D., Gariepy, G., & Malla, A. (2017). Psychological and psychosocial interventions for negative symptoms in psychosis: Systematic review and meta-analysis. *British Journal of Psychiatry, 210*(5), 324–332.

Mullins-Sweatt, S. N., Hopwood, C. J., Chmielewski, M., Meyer, N. A., Min, J., Helle, A. C., & Walgren, M. D. (2020). Treatment of personality pathology through the lens of the hierarchical taxonomy of psychopathology: Developing a research agenda. *Personality and Mental Health, 14*(1), 123–141.

Norcross, J. C., & Lambert, M. J. (2018). Psychotherapy relationships that work III. *Psychotherapy, 55*(4), 303–315.

Philips, B., & Falkenström, F. (2021). What research evidence is valid for psychotherapy research? *Frontiers in Psychiatry, 11,* 625380.

Roefs, A., Fried, E. I., Kindt, M., Martijn, C., Elzinga, B., Evers, A. W. M., . . . Jansen, A. (2022). A new science of mental disorders: Using personalised, transdiagnostic, dynamical systems to understand, model, diagnose and treat psychopathology. *Behaviour Research and Therapy, 153,* 104096.

Schaeuffele, C., Schulz, A., Knaevelsrud, C., Renneberg, B., & Boettcher, J.

(2021). CBT at the crossroads: The rise of transdiagnostic treatments. *International Journal of Cognitive Therapy, 14*(1), 86–113.

Tschacher, W., Junghan, U. M., & Pfammatter, M. (2014). Towards a taxonomy of common factors in psychotherapy-results of an expert survey: Taxonomy of common factors in psychotherapy. *Clinical Psychology & Psychotherapy, 21*(1), 82–96.

Wampold, B. E. (2007). Psychotherapy: The humanistic (and effective) treatment. *American Psychologist, 62*(8), 857–873.

Wampold, B. E. (2015). How important are the common factors in psychotherapy? An update. *World Psychiatry, 14*(3), 270–277.

World Health Organization. (2022). *ICD-11: International classification of diseases* (11th rev.). Author.

PART II REFERENCES

Borsboom, D., Deserno, M., Rhemtulla, M., Epskamp, S., Fried, E. I., McNally, R., . . . Waldorp, L. (2021). Network analysis of multivariate data in psychological science. *Nature Reviews Methods Primers, 1*(1), 58.

Borsboom, D., & Haslbeck, J. (2024). Integrating intra-and interindividual phenomena in psychological theories. *Multivariate Behavioral Research,* 1–20.

Bringmann, L. F., Albers, C., Bockting, C., Borsboom, D., Ceulemans, E., Cramer, A., . . . Wichers, M. (2022). Psychopathological networks: Theory, methods and practice. *Behaviour Research and Therapy, 149,* 104011.

Carper, M. M., Silk, J. S., Ladouceur, C. D., Forbes, E. E., McMakin, D., Ryan, N., & Kendall, P. C. (2022). Changes in affective network variability among youth treated for anxiety disorders. *Child Psychiatry & Human Development, 53,* 526–537.

Cramer, A. O., Van der Sluis, S., Noordhof, A., Wichers, M., Geschwind, N., Aggen, S. H., . . . Borsboom, D. (2012). Dimensions of normal personality as networks in search of equilibrium: You can't like parties if you don't like people. *European Journal of Personality, 26*(4), 414–431.

De Smet, M., Imaani Quintens, L., Debeer, D., Van Nieuwenhove, K., Jongerling, J., & Meganck, R. (2024). A mixed methods idiographic network approach for adolescent-specific assessment and care: A proof of concept. *Qualitative Psychology.* Advanced online publication.

DeYoung, C. G. (2015). Cybernetic Big Five theory. *Journal of Research in Personality, 56,* 33–58.

Fried, E. I. (2022). Studying mental health problems as systems, not syndromes. *Current Directions in Psychological Science, 31*(6), 500–508.

Granic, I., Lewis, M. D., & Lichwarck-Aschoff, A. (2018). Complex pathways to psychopathology. *Psychological Inquiry, 29*(3), 145–150.

Harkness, A. R., Reynolds, S. M., & Lilienfeld, S. O. (2014). A review of systems for psychology and psychiatry: Adaptive systems, Personality Psychopathology Five (PSY-5), and the DSM-5. *Journal of Personality Assessment, 96*(2), 121–139.

Haslbeck, J. M. B., Bringmann, L. F., & Waldorp, L. J. (2020). A tutorial on estimating time-varying vector autoregressive models. *Multivariate Behavioral Research, 56*(1), 120–149.

Hasselman, F. (2022). The complex systems approach to behavioural science. Available at *https://complexity-methods.github.io/book*

Hasselman, F., & Bosman, A. M. (2020). Studying complex adaptive systems with internal states: A recurrence network approach to the analysis of multivariate time-series data representing self-reports of human experience. *Frontiers in Applied Mathematics and Statistics, 6,* 9.

Hayes, A. M., & Andrews, L. A. (2020). A complex systems approach to the study of change in psychotherapy. *BMC Medicine,*

Hayes, A. M., & Yasinski, C. (2015). Pattern destabilization and emotional processing in cognitive therapy for personality disorders. *Frontiers in Psychology, 6,* 107.

Hayes, A. M., Yasinski, C., & Alpert, E. (2022). The application of exposure principles to the treatment of depression. In J. A. J. Smits, J. Jacquart, J. Abramowitz, J. Arch, & J. Margraf (Eds.), *Clinical guide to exposure therapy: Beyond phobias* (pp. 317–345). Springer International.

Hayes, S. C., Ciarrochi, J., Hofmann, S. G., Chin, F., & Sahdra, B. (2022). Evolving an idionomic approach to processes of change: Towards a unified personalized science of human improvement. *Behaviour Research and Therapy, 156,* 104155.

Heino, M. T., Knittle, K., Noone, C., Hasselman, F., & Hankonen, N. (2021). Studying behaviour change mechanisms under complexity. *Behavioral Sciences, 11*(5), 77.

Hollenstein, T. (2013). *State space grids.* Springer.

Hopwood, C. J., Bleidorn, W., & Wright, A. G. (2022). Connecting theory to methods in longitudinal research. *Perspectives on Psychological Science, 17*(3), 884–894.

Hulsmans, D., Otten, R., Poelen, E., van Vonderen, A., Daalmans, S., Hasselman, F., . . . Lichtwarck-Aschoff, A. (2024). A complex systems perspective on chronic aggression and self-injury: Case study of a woman with mild intellectual disability and borderline personality disorder. *BMC Psychiatry, 24*(1), 378.

Kaurin, A., King, K. M., & Wright, A. G. (2023). Studying personality pathology with ecological momentary assessment: Harmonizing theory and method. *Personality Disorders: Theory, Research, and Treatment, 14*(1), 62.

Krakauer, D. C. (2023). Unifying complexity science and machine learning. *Frontiers in Complex Systems, 1,* 1235202.

Lalk, C., Steinbrenner, T., Kania, W., Popko, A., Wester, R., Schaffrath, J., . . . Rubel, J. (2024). Measuring alliance and symptom severity in psychotherapy transcripts using BERT topic modeling. *Administration and Policy in Mental Health and Mental Health Services Research, 51*(4), 509–524.

Lichtwarck-Aschoff, A., Hasselman, F., Cox, R., Pepler, D., & Granic, I. (2012). A characteristic destabilization profile in parent-child interactions associated with treatment efficacy for aggressive children. *Nonlinear Dynamics-Psychology and Life Sciences, 16*(3), 353.

Lenton, T. M., Kohler, T. A., Marquet, P., Boyle, R. A., Crucifix, M., Wilkinson, D. M., & Scheffer, M. (2021). Survival of the systems. *Trends in Ecology & Evolution, 36*(4), 333–344.

Lyby, M. S., Mehlsen, M., Jensen, A. B., Bovbjerg, D. H., Philipsen, J. S., & Wallot, S. (2019). Use of recurrence quantification analysis to examine associations between changes in text structure across an expressive writing intervention and reductions in distress symptoms in women with breast cancer. *Frontiers in Applied Mathematics and Statistics, 5,* 37.

Mitchell, M. (2009). *Complexity: A guided tour.* Oxford University Press.

Molenaar, P. C. (2004). A manifesto on psychology as idiographic science: Bringing the person back into scientific psychology, this time forever. *Measurement, 2*(4), 201–218.

Morris, S. E., Sanislow, C. A., Pacheco, J., Vaidyanathan, U., Gordon, J. A., & Cuthbert, B. N. (2022). Revisiting the seven pillars of RDoC. *BMC Medicine, 20*(1), 220.

Muris, P., Meesters, C., Van Melick, M., & Zwambag, L. (2001). Self-reported attachment style, attachment quality, and symptoms of anxiety and depression in young adolescents. *Personality and Individual Differences, 30*(5), 809–818.18.1–13.

Olthof, M., Bunge, A., Maciejewski, D., Hasselman, F., & Lichtwarck-Aschoff, A. (2024). Transitions and resilience in ecological momentary assessment: A multiple single-case study. *Journal for Person Oriented Research, 10*(2), 89–99.

Olthof, M., Hasselman, F., Aas, B., Lamoth, D., Scholz, S., Daniels-Wredenhagen, N., . . . Lichtwarck-Aschoff, A. (2023). The best of both worlds? General principles of psychopathology in personalized assessment. *Journal of Psychopathology and Clinical Science, 132*(7), 808–819.

Olthof, M., Hasselman, F., Oude Maatman, F., Bosman, A. M., & Lichtwarck-Aschoff, A. (2023). Complexity theory of psychopathology. *Journal of Psychopathology and Clinical Science, 132*(3), 314.

Ong, C. W., Ciarrochi, J., Hofmann, S. G., Karekla, M., & Hayes, S. C. (2024). Through the extended evolutionary meta-model, and what ACT found there: ACT as a process-based therapy. *Journal of Contextual Behavioral Science, 32,* 100734.

Rose, T. (2016). *The end of average: How to succeed in a world that values sameness.* Penguin UK.

Ruggero, C. J., Kotov, R., Hopwood, C. J., First, M., Clark, L. A., Skodol, A. E., . . . Zimmermann, J. (2019). Integrating the hierarchical taxonomy of psychopathology (HiTOP) into clinical practice. *Journal of Consulting and Clinical Psychology, 87*(12), 1069–1084.

Scheffer, M., Bascompte, J., Brock, W. A., Brovkin, V., Carpenter, S. R., Dakos, V., Held, H., van Nes, E., Rietkerk, M., & Sugihara, G. (2009). Early-warning signals for critical transitions. *Nature, 461*(7260), 53–59.

Schiepek, G., Eckert, H., Aas, B., Wallot, S., & Wallot, A. (2016). *Integrative psychotherapy: A feedback-driven dynamic systems approach.* Hogrefe.

Sosnowska, J., Kuppens, P., De Fruyt, F., & Hofmans, J. (2020). New directions in the conceptualization and assessment of personality: A dynamic systems approach. *European Journal of Personality, 34,* 988–998.

Tang, Y., Kurths, J., Lin, W., Ott, E., & Kocarev, L. (2020). When machine learning meets complex systems: Networks, chaos, and nonlinear dynamics. *Chaos: An Interdisciplinary Journal of Nonlinear Science, 30*(6), 063151.

Tschacher, W., & Haken, H. (2019). *The process of psychotherapy.* Springer International.

Wichers, M., Schreuder, M. J., Goekoop, R., & Groen, R. N. (2019). Can we predict the direction of sudden shifts in symptoms? Transdiagnostic implications from a complex systems perspective on psychopathology. *Psychological Medicine, 49*(3), 380–387.

Wright, A. G., & Hopwood, C. J. (2022). Integrating and distinguishing personality and psychopathology. *Journal of Personality, 90*(1), 5–19.

Wright, A. G., Pincus, A. L., & Hopwood, C. J. (2023). Contemporary integrative interpersonal theory: Integrating structure, dynamics, temporal scale, and levels of analysis. *Journal of Psychopathology and Clinical Science, 132*(3), 263.

Wright, A. G. C., Ringwald, W. R., & Zimmermann, J. (2025). Measuring psychopathology in daily life. *Clinical Psychological Science, 13*(3), 649–663.

Zimmermann, J., Woods, W., Ritter, S., Happel, M., Masuhr, O., Jaeger, U., . . . Wright, A. (2019). Integrating structure and dynamics in personality assessment: First steps toward the development and validation of a personality dynamics diary. *Psychological Assessment, 31*(4), 516–531.

CHAPTER 13

What is the difference between personality traits and psychopathology symptoms/functioning?

In the medical model, personality is conceptualized in terms of personality disorders, which are distinguished from other kinds of disorders. However, dimensional models that are organized around personality traits cast doubt on this distinction and raise new questions about how personality traits can be distinguished from the specific symptoms or dysfunctions that people present with. In this section, we asked the authors to answer three questions related to how personality and symptoms/functioning could be distinguished.

> *If personality structure organizes individual differences in psychopathology, what is the difference between symptoms and traits?*
>
> *How can this difference be measured?*
>
> *What kinds of research designs will be needed to separate personality traits from symptoms and functioning?*

The authors present very different perspectives on this issue, in part because their scope differs. DeYoung and Krueger concentrate on psychopathology writ large, whereas Herpertz focuses on personality disorders in particular. They also use different theoretical models: DeYoung and Krueger Big Five Cybernetic Theory and Herpertz the alternative model of personality disorders (AMPD). These differences influence their respective definitions of dysfunction. DeYoung and Krueger define dysfunction in terms of the frustration of both general and specific goals and Herpertz as the broad and global Levels of Personality Functioning Scale (LPFS) dimension from the AMPD. The AMPD and DSM more generally distinguish specific dysfunctions from the LPFS dimension, leaving room for the kinds of dysfunctions articulated by DeYoung and Krueger to coexist with the LPFS. However, whereas DeYoung and Krueger assert that the constructs measured by the LPFS should be conceptualized as traits cast doubt on the AMPD criterion A/B distinction and thus the validity of personality disorder as a unique class of psychopathology, Herpertz tries to find a way to remain within the boundaries of the medical model and asserts that the distinction between personality and other psychopathology has clinical utility. She calls for further multimethod research to distinguish the kinds of dysfunction captured by the LPFS from both traits and dysfunction associated with other kinds of disorder.

PART I

Psychopathology, personality, and cybernetics

Dimensional diagnosis should prioritize dysfunction over symptoms

COLIN G. DEYOUNG and ROBERT F. KRUEGER

The discovery that mental disorders are dimensional rather than categorical has posed a challenge for conceptualization and diagnosis of psychopathology (Haslam et al., 2020; Kotov et al., 2017). The challenge is further deepened by the discovery that variation in features of psychopathology is hard to differentiate from normal personality variation. Quantitative investigations of the covariance of features of psychopathology have indicated that their major patterns of covariation—that is, their major dimensions—are largely the same as the major dimensions of normal variation in personality (Stepp et al., 2012; Suzuki et al., 2015; Widiger et al., 2019). Four of the major dimensions of psychopathology (internalizing, antagonism, disinhibition, and detachment) are clearly and empirically identifiable as four of the so-called Big Five personality traits (Neuroticism, low Agreeableness, low Conscientiousness, and low Extraversion, respectively). The fifth of the Big Five, Openness/Intellect, is a bit more complicated to harmonize with psychopathology, but psychoticism or thought disorder seems to be a variant of openness to experience (Widiger et al., 2019; DeYoung & Krueger, 2018a). The close correspondence between personality and psychopathology raises the question of how having an unusual or extreme personality is distinct from being mentally ill. In this chapter, we attempt to answer this question with reference to our theory of psychopathology as cybernetic dysfunction (DeYoung & Krueger, 2018a, 2018b, 2023)—cybernetics being the study of goal-directed systems that self-regulate via feedback.

Defining Our Terms

To provide a coherent answer, several concepts need to be defined, including personality, psychopathology, symptoms, and dysfunction. We accept the common usage of "personality" in psychology as referring to *all persistent between-person variation in emotion, motivation, cognition, and behavior* (e.g., Baumert et al., 2017). From this perspective, any persistent feature of psychopathology is already clearly encompassed within personality, and we accept this implication. However, we also embrace a distinction between two different categories of elements of personality: personality traits and characteristic adaptations (DeYoung, 2015). We define personality traits as *probabilistic descriptions of relatively stable patterns of emotion, motivation, cognition, and behavior in response to classes of stimuli that have been present in human environments over evolutionary time,* and we argue that they result from variation in parameters of evolved mechanisms that are present in every intact human brain (such as reward and punishment systems). In contrast, characteristic adaptations are *relatively stable goals, interpretations, and strategies, specified in relation to a person's particular life circumstances and learned during the person's lifetime.* Liking to talk a lot is a personality trait, as one could meaningfully differentiate people in any culture throughout human history in terms of their talkativeness, but habitually hanging out in sports bars is a characteristic adaptation, as many cultures have not had sports bars so the description has meaning only in specific contexts. Our understanding of psychopathology hinges on this distinction.

We define psychopathology as *persistent failure to move toward one's goals due to failure to generate effective new goals, interpretations, or strategies when existing ones prove unsuccessful* (and we take this to be synonymous with "cybernetic dysfunction"). Goals are understood broadly to encompass any desired state of the world including not just explicit and specific representations of the desired future but also broad, vague, and even potentially unconscious desires, values, and basic needs. Goals can involve both desired subjective states and desired objective conditions of the world. Although it can be hard for both individuals and clinicians observing them to know exactly what are all of an individual's goals or to understand how they are prioritized, there is a fact of the matter, so psychopathology is not merely a value judgment. Our definition entails that psychopathology requires the failure of characteristic adaptations. People develop psychopathology when their learned goals, interpretations, and strategies cease being effective in moving them toward their important goals and they are also unable to adapt by developing new goals, interpretations, and/or strategies that would allow them to get their goal pursuit back on track (DeYoung & Krueger, 2018a, 2018b, 2023).

Our approach to psychopathology entails something that may at first seem surprising but on closer inspection is consistent with common approaches to mental illness: Symptoms of psychopathology (including observable signs as well as subjective experiences) are not necessarily indicative of psychopathology. A symptom is a clue, an indicator of risk, not an infallible indicator of the presence of illness. People with severe symptoms are more likely to be mentally ill, but they are not necessarily mentally ill. (A dramatic illustration of this point is a study showing that a group of healthy, self-professed psychics who experience daily auditory hallucinations were indistinguishable from a group of psychotic patients on standard clinical measures of hallucinations; Powers et al., 2017.) In DSM-5, most disorders require for their diagnosis not only the presence of certain symptoms but also the presence of "distress or impairment in social, occupational, or other important areas of functioning." DSM-5 explains this by noting that "it has not been possible to completely separate normal and pathological symptom expressions contained in diagnostic criteria" (American Psychiatric Association, 2013, p. 21). From our perspective, this lack of separation is not a failure of medical science but rather an inescapable fact about symptoms.

Most symptoms of psychopathology are simply personality traits if they are persistent. For example, people differ in their levels of anxiety and in their tendency to hear voices (Linscott & van Os, 2013). In our theory, there is no level of anxiety or degree of voice-hearing that inherently indicates mental illness. Instead, what must be identified separately from the presence of any particular symptom is cybernetic dysfunction, the failure of characteristic adaptations. It is only when someone's anxiety or auditory hallucinations (or any other symptoms) cause them to be unable to pursue their important goals effectively that they become mentally ill.

There are several different definitions of "dysfunction" (Wouters, 2003), and we think that our cybernetic definition of dysfunction as failure of goal pursuit and adaptation is more relevant to both lay and medical understandings of mental illness than is the evolutionary definition of dysfunction that is embraced by Wakefield (1992) in his definition of mental illness as "harmful dysfunction" (DeYoung & Krueger, 2018a). From the evolutionary perspective, dysfunction is operation in a manner contrary to that which was selected by evolution, but this makes determining whether patterns of behavior are dysfunctional extremely difficult (Bolton, 2008). Although we prefer a different definition of dysfunction, what our theory shares with Wakefield's is the idea that there is an objective component to identifying psychopathology that rests on identifying dysfunction rather than being tethered primarily to the presence of symptoms.

Rethinking Diagnosis

Given the cybernetic dysfunction perspective, how should dimensional systems be used to carry out diagnosis? The most prominent dimensional system for describing psychopathology is the Hierarchical Taxonomy of Psychopathology (HiTOP), which organizes features of psychopathology according to their patterns of covariation (Kotov et al., 2017, 2021). A remaining task of the HiTOP consortium is to extend HiTOP from a descriptive system for research and case characterization to a system for diagnosis of mental disorder. Merely quantifying the severity of many symptoms is not enough for treatment decisions. To allow diagnosis, two additional determinations are being considered by the consortium: (1) deciding on a threshold for every HiTOP dimension above which mental disorder is deemed to be present, and (2) identifying when dysfunction is present alongside symptoms.

From our perspective, thresholds on symptom dimensions should not be used for diagnosing mental disorder. One might establish practical thresholds of risk on each dimension (these would be semiarbitrary but based on research to establish risk associated with a given level), and sometimes risk might warrant intervention for prevention. Nonetheless, extremity of symptoms is neither necessary nor sufficient for diagnosis. Although HiTOP is a classification of features of psychopathology, it is possible to have a so-called "feature of psychopathology" without having psychopathology, for the reasons discussed above in relation to defining "symptoms." The constructs that are organized by HiTOP are reasonably considered features of psychopathology because they are common risks for or consequences of cybernetic dysfunction. Therefore, someone diagnosed with mental illness will most likely have elevated symptoms on at least one dimension, but this is not a necessary condition, and it is possible for someone to have cybernetic dysfunction even without extremity on any symptom dimension (DeYoung & Krueger, 2018a, 2023).

In relation to the determination of dysfunction, one must first define it. Rather than using common medical definitions of dysfunction related to disability, occupational impairment, social problems, or subjective distress, we recommend a more individualized conception of cybernetic dysfunction, which requires assessment of people's goals and their progress in pursuing them and adapting in the face of challenges to that pursuit. (Here we do not mean just people's perceptions of their progress in goal pursuit, which are important but may be biased in various ways, but also their actual progress, which requires assessment of their life circumstances to evaluate.) Naturally, goals related to occupation, relationships, and subjective emotional experiences are likely to be important for many people, but we should not rely on a one-size-fits-all approach that assumes everyone has the same major goals and needs.

For similar reasons, we do not consider the concept of "self and interpersonal dysfunction," found in the new DSM and ICD dimensional models of personality disorder, to be a viable alternative to cybernetic dysfunction. These DSM and ICD models assume that a lack of empathy or capacity for intimacy is necessarily dysfunctional. Although these qualities may often cause cybernetic dysfunction, they do not always do so (for people who are satisfied without intimate social relationships or who manage to achieve them despite difficulty; cf. DeYoung & Tiberius, 2023). We view these interpersonal features as personality traits, involved in psychopathology only when they are accompanied by cybernetic dysfunction (DeYoung & Krueger, 2023). Note that we are not arguing against the importance of self and interpersonal difficulties like those described by the new DSM and ICD models. Indeed, we think they are important symptom dimensions in their own right and not simply redundant with other maladaptive traits (DeYoung & Krueger, 2025; Sharp & Wall, 2021). Furthermore, one of the self-related constructs in the DSM and ICD models (lack of self-direction) bears a fairly close resemblance to cybernetic dysfunction, so we can imagine assessments related to that construct that could be compatible with our theory (DeYoung & Krueger, 2018a). In general, although it makes sense in the process of diagnosis to investigate categories of goals in which dysfunction often occurs, we emphasize the need to tie determination of dysfunction to the person's particular goals.

Allowing individuals' particular goals to determine the criteria for dysfunction makes our theory more flexible in cross-cultural applications than many other approaches to diagnosis. Different cultures will shape individuals' goals in different ways, and our approach considers any valued goal to be relevant for diagnosis. Additionally, when considering mental illness in different cultures, our theory allows one to be sensitive to the fact that different cultures have different values while nonetheless acknowledging that cultural forces can contribute to mental illness. For example, in a culture that demonizes homosexuality, our theory prevents that culture from declaring homosexuality to be a mental illness (because cybernetic dysfunction is the only necessary and sufficient criterion for diagnosis and homosexual people are just as capable, in principle, of pursuing their personal goals as anyone else), but it does allow one to describe how the culture conflicts with homosexual people's goals in a way that may lead to higher incidence of mental illness (e.g., dysfunctional depression or anxiety) in that population.

Once cybernetic dysfunction is identified as present, then the full symptom profile is useful to understand potential contributing causes of dysfunction and to guide treatment. The duration of symptoms is also likely to be informative. Here, we should note that although most widely recognized persistent symptoms of psychopathology are personality traits, a few, like harmful drug use or phobias of certain types of stimuli, are technically characteristic adaptations. However, this is not particularly relevant to our argument here, and the only meaningful difference between "symptoms" and "personality," as concepts, is that features of personality must be persistent by definition, whereas symptoms can be of any duration (DeYoung et al., 2022). If a symptom (or any other psychological state) persists sufficiently long, it is a trait or at least a characteristic adaptation and in either case is part of personality.

Our perspective implies that there are no such things as personality disorders distinct from other mental disorders (DeYoung & Krueger, 2025). (Note that this does not mean we view the new DSM and ICD models for personality disorder as misguided—self and interpersonal problems need to be recognized and treated—but we object to labeling them as "personality disorder.") Having unusual or extreme personality traits is never necessary or sufficient to identify psychopathology, and all mental disorders involve personality in the sense that they entail a failure of characteristic adaptations. Although diagnosis using the term "personality disorder" is never appropriate, the question of whether symptoms are persistent or confined to a single episode may nonetheless provide useful information for treatment decisions. It is also important to remember that traits are not perfectly stable. Someone with a persistently high trait level of a given symptom dimension, but without psychopathology, is at risk for shifting, at some point, to an even higher level that is then more likely to cause dysfunction (DeYoung et al., 2022). Such cases are much more common than cases in which someone with a low level of a given symptom dimension starts experiencing symptoms that are much more severe than their typical trait levels. But of course, the latter kind of cases do occur. Psychopathology can be brief, whereas personality is by definition persistent. Nonetheless, whether a brief episode or a persistent problem, mental illness should be diagnosed based on the presence of cybernetic dysfunction.

A Research Agenda

Although symptoms can be traits when persistent, it is reasonable in measurement to refer to features of psychopathology as "traits" when they are measured with a general time frame (asking what people are like typically or in general) and as "symptoms" when they are measured with a specific time frame (e.g., over the last 2 weeks or month; DeYoung et al., 2022). Researchers should systematically identify the time frame (also called a "recall period") at which symptoms are empirically indistinguishable from traits in questionnaire measurement, and symptoms should not be assessed with a recall period longer than whatever that turns out to be. For this research, it is crucial that the trait and symptom framings are assessed for the same constructs, preferably with the same or only minimally modified items.

After establishing an effective operational distinction between trait and symptom measures, researchers will be better able to study the difference between passing episodes of psychopathology and more persistent problems. Assessment of symptom dimensions (assessed with either symptom or trait framing) will continue to be important for research on the causes of psychopathology and on individual differences in treatment effectiveness. However, high-quality research on psychopathology will also require separate assessments of dysfunction. One important priority is to ensure that assessments of symptoms and traits do not explicitly confound these constructs with cybernetic dysfunction. Hopwood et al. (2022) make a similar prescription, but their understanding of dysfunction is looser and includes behaviors that are not necessarily cybernetically dysfunctional, such as lying, feeling ashamed, or engaging in criminal behavior. These are risk factors rather than inherent failures of goal pursuit, and they become dysfunctional only when they cause people to be unable to meet their goals and needs.

Another top priority is to develop good measures of cybernetic dysfunction. We believe the most effective format for such measures will be semistructured interviews, which will aid in the idiographic assessment of people's goal hierarchies, their life circumstances, and their attempts at adaptation (DeYoung & Krueger, 2018a, 2023). Standardized questionnaire measures of cybernetic dysfunction may also be useful, but efforts should be made to ensure that respondents are thinking in terms of their specific goals, needs, and values when they respond to items. Such questionnaire measures are likely to covary most strongly with internalizing symptoms (Clark & Ro, 2014), in part because they will be contaminated with the evaluative bias (sometimes called "demoralization") that is most reflected in internalizing symptoms (Pettersson et al., 2014; Tellegen et al., 2006) and in part because subjective distress (which is central to internalizing) is the most typical consequence of most instances of psychopathology.

If cybernetic dysfunction is empirically classifiable as a component of the internalizing spectrum within HiTOP, this does not invalidate its designation as the criterion for psychopathology. Cybernetic dysfunction also qualifies as a trait, under our definition, if it is pervasive and persistent, but that too does not invalidate it (and when we contrast "traits" with "dysfunction" in this chapter, we mean "traits other than general severity of cybernetic dysfunction"). Some questions in science are definitional rather than empirical. To address a question empirically, one must decide what to measure, and deciding what to measure depends on one's definition of the construct under study. In other words, regardless of its relations to various symptom dimensions, cybernetic dysfunction should be the criterion one is attempting to predict in research on psychopathology rather than being treated as just one predictor among many. The presence of a traditional diagnosis is not a good alternative criterion because both the development of HiTOP and our theoretical endeavor have been driven by the inadequacy of the current diagnostic system.

In summary, we need to measure cybernetic dysfunction separately from symptoms and traits. (Even people who prefer a definition of dysfunction that is different from our cybernetic definition would be wise to attempt to separate dysfunction from symptoms and traits in measurement given that symptoms are indicators of risk rather than illness per se.) This approach will allow understanding of the conditions under which symptoms and traits are associated with dysfunction. Longitudinal designs may be helpful for differentiating cases in which symptoms contribute causally to cybernetic dysfunction versus cases in which symptoms result from cybernetic dysfunction. In any case, however, it is always the dysfunction that indicates psychopathology, not the symptoms. Combining the theoretical clarity that we have tried to achieve in this chapter with novel empirical inquiry to formalize cybernetic dysfunction could improve dimensional diagnosis and provide a framework for more effective intervention.

PART II

What is the difference between personality traits and personality disorder symptoms/functioning?

Sabine C. Herpertz

In answering the questions posed by the editors, I will focus on the alternative model of personality disorders (AMPD) of DSM-5 Section III because it explicitly attempts to distinguish personality functioning (Criterion A) from personality traits (Criterion B). Thereby, dysfunction is regarded as a holistic unidimensional construct common to all personality disorders (Morey et al., 2014). It is related to the capability to reflect on one's characteristic ways of thinking, feeling, and behaving; to be aware of one's agency; to have knowledge of the goals and motives that drive one's behavior and social interaction with others; and to be able to see oneself from the perspective of others. Pathological traits stylistically describe "tendencies of feeling, thinking, and behaving in relatively consistent ways across time and across situations" (American Psychiatric Association, 2013, p. 772) that significantly contribute to functional impairments and symptoms as their clinical manifestations.

Meanwhile there is a lively discussion concerning whether both criteria are necessary for personality disorder diagnosis and whether the assessment of maladaptive traits and thus Criterion B may be sufficient in subsequent models of personality disorder classification. Arguments group around issues of incremental validity, suggesting a substantial relationship between Criteria A and B (Sleep et al., 2019) that questions two separate criteria on the basis of the pattern of empirical covariation (Zimmermann et al., 2022). In the following chapter I will choose a basically conceptual approach with a focus on the clinical relevance of both criteria, which compiles five arguments in favor of keeping a two-step diagnosis as forwarded in the DSM-5 AMPD and quite analogously in ICD-11.

Dysfunction Best Captures the Conceptual Framework of Illness

From early on to today's conceptualizations, personality disorder is a "pattern of inner experience and behavior that leads to distress or impairment" (American Psychiatric Association, 2013, p. 645). Consequently, this definition incorporates suffering (the traditional term) or dysfunction (the actual term) as the entry criterion for personality disorder. A classification of severity of dysfunction, as reflected in the level of personality functioning (LPF), seeks to operationalize the overall degree of dysfunction that is needed to define illness and to capture the clinically relevant difference between dysfunction that is related to personality disorder and dysfunction that is not related to personality disorder. It relates to individuals' ability to solve life tasks involving the development of integrated representations of self and others (Livesley et al., 1994), to live in a social community, and to take on and maintain roles in society. The assessment of severity is required to make decisions about the need for treatment including its level and dosage to safeguard transitions to mental health services. Dysfunction manifests as symptoms that reflect maladaptive patterns of cognition, emotional experience, emotional expression, and behaviors. Thereby, the conceptualization of dysfunction (instead of impairment) has to be related to the overall organization of the personality (Wakefield, 2008), meaning that personality-related dysfunction is a specific construct that has to be differentiated from dysfunction linked to other psychopathologies to the extent possible. Notably, dysfunctions in individuals with personality disorder may be similar to those in other mental disorders on a purely descriptive level (e.g., low cognitive empathy in individuals with schizophrenia or chronic depression).

Personality traits, even when they are extreme, are not necessarily pathological (Livesley et al., 1994; Clark & Ro, 2014) and are not sufficient to define illness, although high scores on maladaptive trait measures are likely to be accompanied by dysfunction (Morey et al., 2022) and can be regarded as disposition or risk for symptoms. In conclusion, the assessment of severity of dysfunction should be separated from the description of traits, an argument shared by HiTOP and DeYoung (DeYoung et al., 2022).

Dysfunction Reflects Fundamental Psychological and Biological Systems at the Core of Personality Disorder

Functional impairments reflect basic processes that are closely linked to the fundamental psychological and biological mechanisms that underlie mental health and illness and can be effectively related to abnormalities in brain circuits that are involved in processes related to the self and others (Herpertz et al., 2018). More specifically, high intralimbic functional connectivity indicating disruptions in core brain networks that mediate mentalization and affective processing were found to underlie self and interpersonal personality impairments in personality disorder (Traynor et al., 2023). Analogous to the high covariation of self and interpersonal dysfunction (Zimmermann et al., 2015), their reciprocity in the development of brain circuits related to the self and others highly overlap, supporting the notion that self and interpersonal dysfunction are inseparable constructs.

Interestingly, Criterion A can be recognized in the National Institute of Mental Health's Research Domain Criteria (RDoC), the domain of systems for social processing, in particular, which subsumes perception and understanding of the self and of others in addition to social communication. Because the RDoC seeks to define the biological, physiological, and behavioral mechanisms through which mental health risk and protective factors operate, Criterion A allows one to go beyond a solely behavioral phenotype and deepens the understanding of the nature of personality disorder in terms of varying degrees of dysfunctions in fundamental psychological and biological systems.

There is also an increasing number of studies that seek to identify the neurobiological basis of traits. As traits are defined as fairly enduring, one would expect a relatively high temporal stability in the relationship between personality traits and network aspects of the brain (Markett et al., 2018). However, a recent meta-analysis on structural neuroimaging data came to the conclusion that no replicable deviations from the norm could be found in relation to any personality trait (Chen & Canli, 2022). Most functional neuroimaging studies on traits focus on neuroticism, with a recent meta-analysis reporting significant positive correlations between neuroticism and resting-state brain activity (Lin et al., 2023). Although increased activity in the middle temporal gyrus, the striatum, and the hippocampus might reflect negative affectivity, enhanced fear learning, and reward processing, negative correlations in the superior temporal gyrus and the supramarginal gyrus might suggest maladaptive social cognitive processes.

(Dys)function Captures Dynamic Aspects of Personality Disorder Best

Personality and personality disorder are less stable than the traditional concept has suggested for decades. There are both stable and dynamic aspects to personality. Personality disorder symptoms may be most sensitive to actual situational factors, but impairments in personality functioning may capture more persistent core vulnerability characteristics of personality pathology, whereas traits may be most stable (Weekers et al., 2024). Thereby, more general and more specific factors can be differentiated in the longitudinal course of personality disorder. Although the general factor, which is related to symptoms and dysfunctions, showed high fluctuations between assessment points in this study, indicating low stability, decrement over time, and relatedness to broad indicators of psychosocial functioning, specific features, such as traits, were found to show higher mean stability of individual stylistic differences. Furthermore, measurements of functional impairments presented with high stress-related fluctuations (Sinnaeve et al., 2021). The assumption of slow and gradual changes of traits were concluded from a number of observational longitudinal studies that show modest changes occurring over relatively long periods (Roberts, 2006), with test–retest correlations of traits ranging between .74 and .78 (Hopwood et al., 2011). One reason for stability is that traits as basic tendencies are highly genetically based (Livesley et al., 1998), whereas dysfunction and symptoms strongly interact with environmental challenges that can be more or less met with adaptive capacities (Morey & Hopwood, 2013).

Traits, compared to functional impairments and personality disorder symptoms, are a poorer reflection of the dynamic processes that underlie and contextualize personality disorder. Clinicians learn in the encounter with their patients that the personality dynamics they observe over short or long terms across treatment cannot be adequately captured in traits that are preferably assessed in cross-sectional self-report data. The trait concept does not reflect a model that can explain how personality manifests in and changes across various situations, how personality is influenced by social relationships, how the person feels on the inside, and how the person appears on the outside. Traits show stability at more or less brief intervals despite age-normative changes across longer intervals, particularly in the transition from adolescence to adulthood (Roberts et al., 2006). No doubt, traits have also be shown to change along psychotherapy, probably not globally but in particular facets of trait domains (Roberts et al., 2017).

The Diagnosis of Personality Disorder Implicates the Evaluation of Metacognitive Processes in the Sense of a Reflexive Self

The diagnosis of personality disorder implicates the evaluation of metacognitive processes—namely, a reflexive self. The capability to critically reflect on one's thoughts, emotions, and behaviors and to place one's own mental processes in a biographical continuum of basic needs, motives, and goals determines the level of self-functioning. Therefore, it is not surprising that self-dysfunction is likely to be the best predictor of the level of global functioning and even of psychosocial functioning (Buer Christensen et al., 2020). Consequently, self-functioning as compared to interpersonal functioning may be the prominent description level that reflects a disorganization of personality or a "general adaptive failure of a subjective intrapsychic system needed to fulfill adult life tasks" (Sharp & Wall, 2021, p. 19). At the same time, self-functioning cannot be separated from interpersonal functioning because its basis is acquired in the context of a person's early social relationships and results in the capacity to mentalize and thus to understand mental states in self and others (Fonagy & Target, 1997).

Psychotherapy Needs to Target Self-Functioning in Close Interaction with Interpersonal Processes

Criterion A is suggested to have high predictive validity for treatment outcome and helps to consider the intensity and style of treatment needed as well as the risk of treatment drop-out (Busmann et al., 2019). Compared to pathological traits, dysfunction is closer to mental distress and the problems that patients experience (Bach & Tracy, 2022) and thus can be more easily integrated in therapist–patient communication and motivation to change.

Because psychotherapy is developing toward setting a focus on psychological functions of cognition, emotion, behavior, etc. rather than their contents, thus targeting the relationship of a patient to his/her own experience (Hayes & Hofmann, 2021), self-functioning appears to play a major role in processes of change. Particularly when initiating processes of change, mentalizing capacity, which has become the target of mentalization-based therapy (MBT; Bateman & Fonagy, 2016), allows clients to reflect on what one is and would like to be. The understanding of processes that underlie the origin, development, and maintenance of dysfunction has become an integral part also of the third wave of cognitive-behavioral therapy (CBT)—for example, using mindfulness and acceptance techniques to focus on the awareness of and the relationship to one's thoughts (Segal et al., 2004). Another example is schema therapy, wherein the focus lies in the inner models of self and others and the level of personality functioning is conceptualized as healthy adult functioning that is able to detect and regulate emotions, understand reality, to be self-directed, and to maintain a coherent and positive self-concept (Bach & Bernstein, 2019).

Interestingly, interventions that have been shown to modulate traits also refer to self-functioning when addressing an individual's awareness of beliefs, expectations, and motives—namely, the awareness of the discrepancy between the desired and actual self (Stieger et al., 2021). Many techniques of dialectical behavior therapy (DBT) refer to the trait negative affectivity, but DBT goes beyond when educating mindfulness and validating the patient's experiences, thereby strengthening the self.

During psychotherapy, the level of self-functioning is expected to develop in exchange with autobiographic narratives, rules, and ethical orientations that have been learned in the relationship with significant others and have led to characteristic wishes, motives, and beliefs that underlie adult relationships. Thereby, the episodes of one's own life story are conceptually linked, integrating the remembered past, present, and possible future into an overarching, no longer merely momentary continuity of the self. One's own life becomes narratable and thus an essential part of one's own identity. This gives rise to the self-concept, which generates meaning out of one's traits (Sharp & Wall, 2021). Importantly psychotherapy also targets interpersonal functioning, not only when focusing on patients' problems in interpersonal relationships but already on a more global level when working with the therapeutic alliance, as the most important common effect of psychotherapy.

In conclusion, Criterion A provides the fabric of psychotherapy targets (Hutsebaut, 2023). Because the psychotherapy process always captures a metacognitive level by improving self-direction, mentalizing capacity, and emotion regulation, the mechanisms of change involved in most evidence-based psychotherapies directly refer to changes in self-functioning. Consequently, successfully targeting self-functioning appears to be a prerequisite to mitigating maladaptive traits. Psychotherapy could be further developed in the way to individualize the allocation to treatment modules that target specific mechanisms of impaired functioning related to the self and to the interpersonal realm and their psychobiological signatures, also considering their severity levels (Schramm et al., 2024).

How Can the Differences between Traits, Functional Impairments, and Symptoms Be Measured?

Dimensional measures of personality pathology should continue measuring Criteria A and B separately. Trait domains and facets should be coded truly dimensionally considering the bipolarity of maladaptive traits, and due to reports of high convergent validity between self-report and interview (Nuzum et al., 2019), assessment can be carried out without a structured interview to take clinicians' restricted time into consideration. The measurement of functional impairments requires an interview that in the best case is enriched by informants' reports. Tools have to be designed that assess the dynamic nature and context dependence of personality pathology, functional impairments in particular, and thus to also better capture change.

Further Research Designs Needed

The last decade has seen remarkably intensive research into the dimensional classification of personality disorder. At the same time, this research is still in its infancy. One area in which more research is needed is further specifying the differentiation between personality-related dysfunctioning/symptoms and traits and providing a conceptual and methodological framework for treatment development and an evidence base on which to make differentiated recommendations on what works for whom (Kramer et al., 2022).

To specify and discriminate personality dysfunction from general inability that may also occur from specific forms of psychopathology (depression, anxiety, conduct disorder, etc.), longitudinal studies are required. Large sample sizes along the continuum of the severity levels of impairment and recruited such that they reflect diversity in clinical symptoms are needed. Longitudinal data of children and of adolescents along trajectories are necessary to pursue questions on the stability of functional impairments and traits over the life cycle or on the early precursors and developmental modulators of latent vulnerability to personality disorder.

Performance-based experimental as well as real-time measures should be used to reflect the bidirectionality of interpersonal and environmental influences, how the social environment affects an individual's behavior, and how the individual's behavior in turn affects the behaviors of others toward the individual. To capture interpersonal dysfunction that hinders well-being in everyday life, performance measurements in tasks should go beyond single-person designs and include groups of participants who are assessed repeatedly while they interact.

To come to a mechanistic understanding of the development of dysfunctions and traits and their interaction and to provide knowledge about the causality between symptoms, functions, and traits, these constructs require a joint assessment by multiple methods (Zimmermann et al., 2022). Such designs would allow research to contribute information concerning whether pathological traits are behaviorally anchored expressions of underlying impairments in basic domains of the self and the communication with others (Sharp & Wall, 2021) or whether functional impairments are instead negative consequences of maladaptive traits.

Psychological assessments should be combined with (neuro)biological measurements. Computational models based on machine-learning approaches can deal with different levels of analysis and advance the understanding of personality disorder by integrating large datasets from diverse modalities into unifying mechanistic frameworks. These frameworks are expected to describe specific configurations of neural circuit activities that underlie Criteria A and B with respect to functioning in everyday life and clinical problems. Thereby, the trait model has to be extended that has been traditionally conceptualized as "pragmatic abstractions with no special biological value" (Yarkoni, 2015).

To more deeply understand the dynamics of symptoms, functional impairments, and traits in personality disorder, complex designs with parallel assessments are needed to distinguish between- and within-person processes, the latter including a granular examination of the intraindividual dynamics in exchange with the environment with a focus on timelines and moment-to-moment assessments. Experience-sampling designs that collect data in various time frames and contexts allow researchers to capture when and how change occurs and whether changes in the course of therapy predict consequential outcomes, such as remission or later relapse (Roberts et al., 2017). For example, machine-learning approaches that use recurrent neural networks (RNNs) as a main analytical and theoretical tool for time-series data can provide the tools for tracking and understanding the temporal fluctuations in dysfunctions in personality disorder (Haines & Beauchaine, 2020). Comprehensive datasets from large-scale samples are needed to arrive at a data-driven approach to personality pathology to be able to draw inferences on causal architectures and to identify personality indices that have predictive value for their effects on long-term personality functioning and real-life outcomes, thus yielding forward predictions or forecasting the implications of interventions.

Conclusion

Focusing on the clinical utility of the two-step-diagnosis currently forwarded by the AMPD appears to be a suitable approach to diagnosing personality disorder. Notably, the severity of functional impairments tracks dynamically with patients' suffering, clinical functioning, and symptoms as well as with short-term intraindividual variability, changing context, long-term developmental trajectories, and finally most important, with change under treatment. The differentiation between the self and the interpersonal level of dysfunction, although artificial, is close to topics that psychotherapy works with but may need to be merged in a unidimensional factor structure in a next step to reflect their mutual interaction. Trait specifiers are, nevertheless, needed to describe the stylistic features that are typical of the individual concerned and should include both extreme poles of the trait domains that may interact with functioning.

PART I REFERENCES

American Psychiatric Association. (2013). *Diagnostic and statistical manual of mental disorders* (5th ed.). Author.

Baumert, A., Schmitt, M., Perugini, M., Johnson, W., Blum, G., Borkenau, P., . . . Wrzus, C. (2017). Integrating personality structure, personality process, and personality development. *European Journal of Personality, 31*(5), 503–528.

Bolton, D. (2008). *What is mental disorder? An essay in philosophy, science, and values.* Oxford University Press.

Clark, L. A., & Ro, E. (2014). Three-pronged assessment and diagnosis of personality disorder and its consequences: Personality functioning, pathological traits, and psychosocial disability. *Personality Disorders: Theory, Research, and Treatment, 5*(1), 55–69.

DeYoung, C. G. (2015). Cybernetic Big Five theory. *Journal of Research in Personality, 56,* 33–58.

DeYoung, C. G., Chmielewski, M., Clark, L. A., Condon, D. M., Kotov, R., Krueger, R. F., . . . HiTOP Normal Personality Workgroup. (2022). The distinction between symptoms and traits in the hierarchical taxonomy of psychopathology (HiTOP). *Journal of Personality, 90,* 20–33.

DeYoung, C. G., & Krueger, R. F. (2018a). A cybernetic theory of psychopathology. *Psychological Inquiry, 29,* 117–138.

DeYoung, C. G., & Krueger, R. F. (2018b). Understanding psychopathology: Cybernetics and psychology on the boundary between order and chaos. *Psychological Inquiry, 29,* 165–174.

DeYoung, C. G., & Krueger, R. F. (2023). A cybernetic perspective on the nature of psychopathology: Transcending conceptions of mental illness as statistical deviance and brain disease. *Journal of Psychopathology and Clinical Science, 132*(3), 228–237.

DeYoung, C. G., & Krueger, R. F. (2025). What does personality have to do with mental disorder? A cybernetic perspective. In K. Banicki & P. Zachar (Eds.), *Conceptualizing personality disorder: Perspectives from philosophy, psychological science, and psychiatry I* (pp. 181–195). Cambridge University Press.

DeYoung, C. G., & Tiberius, V. (2023). Value fulfillment from a cybernetic perspective: A new psychological theory of well-being. *Personality and Social Psychology Review, 27,* 3–27.

Haslam, N., McGrath, M. J., Viechtbauer, W., & Kuppens, P. (2020). Dimensions over categories: A meta-analysis of taxometric research. *Psychological Medicine, 50*(9), 1418–1432.

Hopwood, C. J., Wright, A. G., & Bleidorn, W. (2022). Person–environment transactions differentiate personality and psychopathology. *Nature Reviews Psychology, 1*(1), 55–63.

Kotov, R., Krueger, R. F., Watson, D., Achenbach, T. M., Althoff, R. R., Bagby, R. M., . . . Zimmerman, M. (2017). The hierarchical taxonomy of psychopathology (HiTOP): A dimensional alternative to traditional nosologies. *Journal of Abnormal Psychology, 126*(4), 454–478.

Kotov, R., Krueger, R. F., Watson, D., Cicero, D. C., Conway, C. C., DeYoung, C. G., . . . Wright, A. G. (2021). The hierarchical taxonomy of psychopathology (HiTOP): A quantitative nosology based on consensus of evidence. *Annual Review of Clinical Psychology, 17,* 83–108.

Linscott, R. J., & van Os, J. (2013). An updated and conservative systematic review and meta-analysis of epidemiological evidence on psychotic experiences in children and adults: On the pathway from proneness to persistence to dimensional expression across mental disorders. *Psychological Medicine, 43*(6), 1133–1149.

Pettersson, E., Mendle, J., Turkheimer, E., Horn, E. E., Ford, D. C., Simms, L. J., & Clark, L. A. (2014). Do maladaptive behaviors exist at one or both ends of personality traits? *Psychological Assessment, 26*(2), 433–446.

Powers, A. R., Kelley, M. S., & Corlett, P. R. (2017). Varieties of voice-hearing: Psychics and the psychosis continuum. *Schizophrenia Bulletin, 43,* 84–98.

Sharp, C., & Wall, K. (2021). DSM-5 level of personality functioning: Refocusing personality disorder on what it means to be human. *Annual Review of Clinical Psychology, 17,* 313–337.

Stepp, S. D., Yu, L., Miller, J. D., Hallquist, M. N., Trull, T. J., & Pilkonis, P. A. (2012). Integrating competing dimensional models of personality. *Personality Disorders: Theory, Research, and Treatment, 3,* 107–126.

Suzuki, T., Samuel, D. B., Pahlen, S., & Krueger, R. F. (2015). DSM-5 alternative personality disorder model traits as maladaptive extreme variants of the five-factor model: An item-response theory analysis. *Journal of Abnormal Psychology, 124,* 343–354.

Tellegen, A., Ben-Porath, Y. S., Sellbom, M., Arbisi, P. A., McNulty, J. L., & Graham, J. R. (2006). Further evidence on the validity of the MMPI-2 Restructured Clinical (RC) scales: Addressing questions raised by Rogers, Sewell, Harrison, and Jordan and Nichols. *Journal of Personality Assessment, 87,* 148–171.

Wakefield, J. C. (1992). Disorder as harmful dysfunction: A conceptual critique of *DSM-III-R's* definition of mental disorder. *Psychological Review, 99,* 232–247.

Widiger, T. A., Sellbom, M., Chmielewski, M., Clark, L. A., DeYoung, C. G., Kotov, R., . . . Wright, A. G. C. (2019). Personality in a hierarchical model of psychopathology. *Clinical Psychological Science, 7,* 77–92.

Wouters, A. G. (2003). Four notions of biological function. *Studies in history and philosophy of science part C: Studies in history and philosophy of biological and biomedical sciences, 34,* 633–668.

PART II REFERENCES

Bach, B., & Bernstein, D. P. (2019). Schema therapy conceptualization of personality functioning and traits in ICD-11 and DSM-5. *Current Opinion in Psychiatry, 32*(1), 38–49.

Bach, B., & Tracy, M. (2022). Clinical utility of the alternative model of personality disorders: A 10th year anniversary review. *Personality Disorders: Theory, Research, and Treatment, 13*(4), 369.

Bateman, A., & Fonagy, P. (2016). *Mentalization based treatment for personality disorders: A practical guide.* Oxford University Press.

Buer Christensen, T., Eikenaes, I., Hummelen, B., Pedersen, G., Nysæter, T.-E., Bender, D. S., . . . Selvik, S. G. (2020). Level of personality functioning as a predictor of psychosocial functioning—Concurrent validity of Criterion A. *Personality Disorders: Theory, Research, and Treatment, 11*(2), 79.

Busmann, M., Wrege, J., Meyer, A. H., Ritzler, F., Schmidlin, M., Lang, U. E., . . . Euler, S. (2019). Alternative model of personality disorders (DSM-5) predicts dropout in inpatient psychotherapy for patients with personality disorder. *Frontiers in Psychology, 10*, 952.

Chen, Y.-W., & Canli, T. (2022). "Nothing to see here": No structural brain differences as a function of the Big Five personality traits from a systematic review and meta-analysis. *Personality Neuroscience, 5*, e8.

Clark, L. A., & Ro, E. (2014). Three-pronged assessment and diagnosis of personality disorder and its consequences: Personality functioning, pathological traits, and psychosocial disability. *Personality Disorders: Theory, Research, and Treatment, 5*(1), 55.

DeYoung, C. G., Chmielewski, M., Clark, L. A., Condon, D. M., Kotov, R., Krueger, R. F., . . . Mullins-Sweatt, S. N. (2022). The distinction between symptoms and traits in the hierarchical taxonomy of psychopathology (HiTOP). *Journal of Personality, 90*(1), 20–33.

Fonagy, P., & Target, M. (1997). Attachment and reflective function: Their role in self-organization. *Development and Psychopathology, 9*(4), 679–700.

Haines, N., & Beauchaine, T. P. (2020). Moving beyond ordinary factor analysis in studies of personality and personality disorder: A computational modeling perspective. *Psychopathology, 53*(3–4), 157–167.

Hayes, S. C., & Hofmann, S. G. (2021). "Third-wave" cognitive and behavioral therapies and the emergence of a process-ased approach to intervention in psychiatry. *World Psychiatry, 20*(3), 363–375.

Herpertz, S. C., Bertsch, K., & Jeung, H. (2018). Neurobiology of Criterion A: Self and interpersonal personality functioning. *Current Opinion in Psychology, 21*, 23–27.

Hopwood, C. J., Donnellan, M. B., Blonigen, D. M., Krueger, R. F., McGue, M., Iacono, W. G., & Burt, S. A. (2011). Genetic and environmental influences on personality trait stability and growth during the transition to adulthood: A three-wave longitudinal study. *Journal of Personality and Social Psychology, 100*(3), 545.

Hutsebaut, J. (2023). Isn't Criterion A rather than B the language of psychotherapy? Comment on Sauer-Zavala et al.(2022). *Personality Disorders: Theory, Research, and Treatment, 14*(4), 385–387.

Kramer, U., Eubanks, C. F., Bertsch, K., Herpertz, S. C., McMain, S., Mehlum, L., . . . Zimmermann, J. (2022). Future challenges in psychotherapy research for personality disorders. *Current Psychiatry Reports, 24*(11), 613–622.

Lin, J., Li, L., Pan, N., Liu, X., Zhang, X., Suo, X., . . . Gong, Q. (2023). Neural correlates of neuroticism: A coordinate-based meta-analysis of resting-state functional brain imaging studies. *Neuroscience & Biobehavioral reviews, 146,* 105055.

Livesley, W. J., Jang, K. L., & Vernon, P. A. (1998). Phenotypic and genetic structure of traits delineating personality disorder. *Archives of General Psychiatry, 55*(10), 941–948.

Livesley, W. J., Schroeder, M. L., Jackson, D. N., & Jang, K. L. (1994). Categorical distinctions in the study of personality disorder: Implications for classification. *Journal of Abnormal Psychology, 103*(1), 6.

Markett, S., Montag, C., & Reuter, M. (2018). Network neuroscience and personality. *Personality Neuroscience, 1,* e14.

Morey, L. C., Berghuis, H., Bender, D. S., Verheul, R., Krueger, R. F., & Skodol, A. E. (2014). Toward a model for assessing level of personality functioning in DSM-5, part II: Empirical articulation of a core dimension of personality pathology. In S. K. Huprich & C. J. Hopwood (Eds.), *Personality assessment in the DSM-5* (pp. 50–56). Routledge.

Morey, L. C., Good, E. W., & Hopwood, C. J. (2022). Global personality dysfunction and the relationship of pathological and normal trait domains in the DSM-5 alternative model for personality disorders. *Journal of Personality, 90*(1), 34–46.

Morey, L. C., & Hopwood, C. J. (2013). Stability and change in personality disorders. *Annual Review of Clinical Psychology, 9,* 499–528.

Nuzum, H., Ready, R. E., & Clark, L. A. (2019). Comparability of self-and other-rated personality structure. *Psychological Assesessment, 31*(6), 741.

Roberts, B. W. (2006). Personality development and organizational behavior. *Research in Organizational Behavior, 27,* 1–40.

Roberts, B. W., Luo, J., Briley, D. A., Chow, P. I., Su, R., & Hill, P. L. (2017). A systematic review of personality trait change through intervention. *Psychological Bulletin, 143*(2), 117.

Roberts, B. W., Walton, K. E., & Viechtbauer, W. (2006). Patterns of mean-level change in personality traits across the life course: A meta-analysis of longitudinal studies. *Psychological Bulletin, 132*(1), 1.

Schramm, E., Elsaesser, M., Jenker, C., Hautzinger, M., & Herpertz, S. C. (2024). Algorithm-based modular psychotherapy vs. cognitive-behavioral therapy for patients with depression, psychiatric comorbidities and early trauma: A proof-of-concept randomized controlled trial. *World Psychiatry, 23*(2), 257–266.

Segal, Z. V., Teasdale, J. D., & Williams, J. M. G. (2004). Mindfulness-based cognitive therapy: Theoretical rationale and empirical status. In S. C. Hayes, V. M. Follette, & M. M. Linehan (Eds.), *Mindfulness and acceptance: Expanding the cognitive-behavioral tradition* (pp. 45–65). Guilford Press.

Sharp, C., & Wall, K. (2021). DSM-5 level of personality functioning:

Refocusing personality disorder on what it means to be human. *Annual Review of Clinical Psychology, 17,* 313–337.

Sinnaeve, R., Vaessen, T., van Diest, I., Myin-Germeys, I., van den Bosch, L. M., Vrieze, E., . . . Claes, S. (2021). Investigating the stress-related fluctuations of level of personality functioning: A critical review and agenda for future research. *Clinical Psychology & Psychotherapy, 28*(5), 1181–1193.

Sleep, C. E., Lynam, D. R., Widiger, T. A., Crowe, M. L., & Miller, J. D. (2019). An evaluation of DSM–5 Section III personality disorder Criterion A (impairment) in accounting for psychopathology. *Psychological Assessment, 31*(10), 1181.

Stieger, M., Flückiger, C., Rüegger, D., Kowatsch, T., Roberts, B. W., & Allemand, M. (2021). Changing personality traits with the help of a digital personality change intervention. *Proceedings of the National Academy of Sciences, 118*(8), e2017548118.

Traynor, J. M., Wrege, J. S., Walter, M., & Ruocco, A. C. (2023). Dimensional personality impairment is associated with disruptions in intrinsic intralimbic functional connectivity. *Psychological Medicine, 53*(4), 1323–1333.

Wakefield, J. C. (2008). The perils of dimensionalization: Challenges in distinguishing negative traits from personality disorders. *Psychiatric Clinics of North America, 31*(3), 379–393.

Weekers, L. C., Hutsebaut, J., Rovers, J., & Kamphuis, J. H. (2024). Head-to-head comparison of the alternative model for personality disorders and Section II personality disorder model in terms of predicting patient outcomes 1 year later. *Personality Disorders: Theory, Research, and Treatment, 15*(2), 101–109.

Yarkoni, T. (2015). Neurobiological substrates of personality: A critical overview. In M. Mikulincer, P. R. Shaver, M. L. Cooper, & R. J. Larsen (Eds.), *APA handbook of personality and social psychology: Vol. 4. Personality processes and individual differences* (pp. 61–83). American Psychological Association.

Zimmermann, J., Böhnke, J. R., Eschstruth, R., Mathews, A., Wenzel, K., & Leising, D. (2015). The latent structure of personality functioning: Investigating Criterion A from the alternative model for personality disorders in DSM-5. *Journal of Abnormal Psychology, 124*(3), 532.

Zimmermann, J., Hopwood, C. J., & Krueger, R. F. (2022). The DSM-5 Level of Personality Functioning Scale. In R. F. Krueger & P. H. Blaney (Eds.), *Oxford textbook of psychopathology* (4th ed., pp. 579–603). Oxford University Press.

CHAPTER 14

If psychopathology is dimensional, what are personality disorders?

There is increasing momentum toward reorganizing psychopathology diagnosis around dimensions that closely resemble personality traits. Given the long-standing assumption that personality was most relevant for personality disorders, such a reorganization leaves important questions about what constitutes personality disorders unanswered. We asked experts to answer three questions about the nature of personality disorders:

If personality and psychopathology share a common individual differences structure, what is specific about personality disorders?

Is there a role for personality disorder in an integrative model of personality and psychopathology?

If so, how can the distinct features of personality disorders be conceptualized and measured?

Miller and colleagues take a relatively traditional approach by defining personality disorders as precocious, pervasive, and persistent and criticize contemporary models that focus on self and interpersonal dysfunction. In contrast, Wright and Mostajabi argue that self and interpersonal dysfunction are the distinguishing features of personality disorders. The approach both sets of authors take to answering these questions does not represent the full spectrum of views on these questions but offers two perspectives on how best to conceptualize personality and personality pathology.

PART I

Personality disorders are distinguished by precociousness, pervasiveness, and persistence, but distinctions are blurry and fraught

JOSHUA D. MILLER, NATHANIEL L. PHILLIPS, THOMAS A. WIDIGER, and DONALD R. LYNAM

Scholars (e.g., Costa & Widiger, 1994) have long argued that personality disorders can be conceptualized and assessed using a general model of personality—the five-factor model (FFM). That is, personality disorders represent long-standing difficulties negotiating life's challenges as they relate to specific personality domains (e.g., pervasive negative emotionality represented by neuroticism; pervasive difficulties getting along with others in work/school, friendships, and romance represented by disagreeableness). Research has shown that personality disorders have relatively unique trait profiles across the 30 facets of the FFM (Lynam & Widiger, 2001). Moreover, FFM facets can be used to assess personality disorders (Miller et al., 2004) in a manner that retains their nomological nets (even borderline personality disorder; Trull et al., 2003) and an FFM-driven conceptualization can explain the patterns of comorbidity and sex differences in the personality disorders (Lynam & Widiger, 2001, 2008). In fact, a very similar model was proposed by the DSM-5 Personality Disorder Workgroup to replace the traditional personality disorders categories in DSM-5, albeit with an emphasis on maladaptive personality traits and functioning. It has been only within the last 7 years (HiTOP; Kotov et al., 2017) that it has been suggested that all forms of psychopathology might be understood via a slightly expanded version of this model. When modeled together, personality disorders and other forms of psychopathology are integrated into five or six dimensions (Kotov et al., 2017) termed internalizing, antagonistic externalizing, disinhibited externalizing, detachment, thought disorder, and somatoform.

The separation between personality disorders and other forms of psychopathology was emphasized in DSM-III, where they were primarily delineated for the pragmatic purpose of getting clinicians to pay more attention to personality pathology. Following this separation, various rationales for the division were offered. First, personality disorders were described as enduring patterns of acting, thinking, and feeling. Unlike other forms of psychopathology that might have episodic or fluctuating symptoms, personality disorders were assumed to be stable over time and situations. Second, they were assumed to negatively affect multiple domains of functioning—relationships, work, and other social interactions. Third, it was believed that personality disorders almost always arose by late childhood/early adulthood; in fact, several personality disorders had recognizable child/adolescent counterparts (e.g., conduct disorder and antisocial personality disorder).[1] We summarize these differences as the three P's—"pervasiveness" (in terms of breadth of the traits and their influence), "persistence" (both cross-situationally and temporally),[2] and "precociousness" (in terms of their early emergence). We believe this is a fairly good starting point for deciding how and whether personality disorders should be separated from other forms of psychopathology. It is true that these criteria do not differentiate personality disorders from other disorders as well as initially believed. However, this is not primarily because they do not characterize personality disorders but because these criteria are true of many disorders (e.g., Oldehinkel & Ormel, 2023; Powers & Casey, 2015).

One approach to differentiating personality disorders from other psychiatric disorders that we believe is problematic is the one offered by Wright et al. (2022), who have argued that what separates personality disorders from other psychiatric disorders (e.g., major depression; eating

---

[1]Another common but seemingly inaccurate notion is that personality disorders are more ego-syntonic than other psychiatric disorders. However, several studies have shown that individuals with personality disorder symptoms can self-report on these symptoms with the same relative accuracy with respect to self–other convergence (Oltmanns & Oltmanns, 2020), generally dislike these traits, would like to reduce them, and acknowledge the impairment associated with them (e.g., Sleep et al., 2019, 2022).

[2]Wright et al. (2022) suggest that personality disorders are not as stable as initially thought, but this is partially driven by the more behaviorally focused symptoms (e.g., nonsuicidal self-injury) rather than trait-based symptoms. In addition, personality disorder stability estimates are difficult to interpret given other methodological features including regression to the mean and ascertaining and assessing psychiatric patients when particularly clinically distressed (Clark, 2005; d'Huart et al., 2023).

disorders) is the former's interpersonal nature, which they explicate via contemporary integrative interpersonal theory (CIIT).[3] We believe there are several issues with this model. First, it is unnecessary. The interpersonal traits that Wright et al. describe, dominance and warmth, already exist in the FFM and, by extension, the HiTOP model. Second, the Wright et al. model is insufficient to characterize the breadth of personality pathology in general and, more specifically, the traditional personality disorders included in psychiatric nosologies. The personality disorders require non-interpersonal traits for their full descriptions. What is antisocial personality disorder without deficient impulse control (i.e., high disinhibition)? What is borderline personality disorder without high negative affect? What is obsessive–compulsive personality disorder without compulsivity (i.e., maladaptive conscientiousness)? A description of personality disorders as interpersonal only is bereft of important content. Adoption of CIIT as the model for all personality disorders would narrow coverage of the traditional personality disorders and expand coverage to include many other disorders that have not been traditionally defined as personality disorders. In their proposal, Wright et al. (2022) acknowledge that the boundary between personality-based "interpersonal disorders" and other Axis I disorders may be blurry but expend remarkably little effort addressing this issue, despite that it is a critical tenet of their model.

Third, we do not believe this model can discriminate personality disorders from other forms of psychopathology. CIIT is based on deficits in self and interpersonal functioning; Wright et al. (2022) write, "maladaptive self-processes include distorted construals, affective dysregulation, and motivational or self-dysregulation" (p. 1094). The authors go on to give examples of these in relation to personality disorders, such as "extreme desires to be close to others as in the traditional dependent category, to stay away from others as in the traditional avoidant category, or to vacillate between these extremes as in the traditional borderline category are examples of motivational dysregulation" (p. 1094) But these same distorted construals of self and others and attachment difficulties play primary roles in any number of psychiatric disorders including eating disorders (e.g., inaccurate appraisal of weight/body shape and implications for self/other love; attachment difficulties, Jewell et al., 2023), major depressive disorder (e.g., attributional errors related to self and others; attachment problems; Muris et al., 2001), social anxiety disorder (e.g., attributional errors related to interpersonal perceptions; attachment problems; Eng et al., 2001), substance use disorder (e.g., attachment

[3]Wright et al. also assert that "interpersonal disorders" will be seen as a less stigmatizing term than personality disorders. However, this is an empirical question and the initial data are not supportive (Stanton et al., 2025).

difficulties, Gidhagen et al., 2018), schizophrenia (e.g., social cognition; Green et al., 2015), and so on. Interpersonal/self difficulties as well as negative interpersonal consequences are nearly ubiquitous across disorders and certainly not in the "trivial" manner suggested by Wright and Mostajabi. Although CIIT may be well-situated to describe the interpersonal processes that contribute to, maintain, and moderate outcomes in psychiatric disorders, interpersonal dysfunction is itself ill-suited to separating personality disorders from other psychiatric disorders.

Fourth, not only does the model not work in theory to distinguish personality disorders, it doesn't work in practice. Criterion A of the alternative model of personality disorders (AMPD) is meant to reference the sorts of problems in self and other functioning that are fundamental to CIIT. But the current instantiation of that criterion, the Levels of Personality Functioning Scale (LPFS), does not distinguish personality disorders from other forms of psychopathology. To date, several studies have examined the ability of the Criterion A to distinguish between personality disorders and other forms of psychopathology. In a clinical community sample, Few et al. (2013) found the median correlation between the subscales of the LPFS with symptoms of anxiety and depression to be higher than the median correlation with the symptoms of the 10 DSM-5 personality disorders (i.e., median r's = .46 and .36). Using an online community sample enriched for mental health treatment-seeking, Sleep, Lynam, et al. (2019) found that the median correlation between the LPFS total score and a variety of "Axis I" symptoms was practically equivalent to the median correlation between the LPFS total and personality disorder symptoms (i.e., .61 vs. .58). In fact, Kerber et al. (2024) found that personality functioning scales are almost "pure markers" of a generalized psychopathology factor in a very large ($N > 27{,}000$) ambulatory study that took place over 2 years. Specifically, using a bifactor approach, they found that personality functioning "scales had the highest loadings on the general factor and lowest loadings on specific factors" (p. 8). The notion that self and other deficits will be specific to personality pathology is demonstrably false. Deficits in self and other functioning are not capable of distinguishing personality disorders from other forms of psychopathology.[4]

Fifth, many to most of the LPFS components are explicitly traits, such as "deceit and coercion" (American Psychiatric Association, 2013, p. 754) for antisocial and "rigidity and stubbornness" (American

[4]Wright et al. (2022) also suggest that CIIT recognizes dynamics that are not present within the trait model, but dynamics are readily incorporated within a run-of-the-mill trait model like the FFM or the HiTOP model. Only a "straw man" version of a trait model would argue it that it doesn't allow for responsivity to situations, contexts, or relationships (Widiger, 2022).

Psychiatric Association, 2013, p. 768) for obsessive–compulsive characteristics. Others are explicit representations of DSM-IV diagnostic criteria, such as "failure to conform to lawful or culturally normative ethical behavior" for antisocial (American Psychiatric Association, 2013, p. 754) and "intense, unstable, and conflicted close relationships" (American Psychiatric Association, 2013, p. 756) for borderline. Even when the impairment concerns an intrapsychic disturbance in the sense of self, it is still a trait. To the extent that an impaired sense of self reflects a characteristic or consistent expression of the self, it can be readily understood as a personality trait (Widiger & Hines, 2022). "Personality traits are enduring patterns of perceiving, relating to, and thinking about the environment and oneself" (American Psychiatric Association, 2013, p. 647). A characteristically inaccurate or distorted sense of self is an example of an enduring pattern of perceiving and thinking about oneself. Indeed, some of the DSM-5 Criterion A impairments and Criterion B traits are virtually identical. For example, there is no meaningful distinction between a "lack of concern for feelings, needs, or suffering of others; lack of remorse after hurting or mistreating another" (American Psychiatric Association, 2013, p. 764) and a "lack of concern for feelings or problems of others; lack of guilt or remorse about the negative or harmful effects of one's actions on others" (American Psychiatric Association, 2013, p. 764). The former is a Criterion A self-impairment and the latter is a Criterion B trait.

Sixth, we are concerned that the model is overreliant on theory that, as Wright and Mostajabi write in their chapter, may not be "amenable to scientific inquiry." The current overarching movement toward a dimensional reorganization of psychopathology is based on decades of robust empirical evidence, showing that this conceptualization better captures the nature and overlap of general psychopathology and personality disorders. Reorganizing personality disorders as interpersonal disorders based on theory without sufficient evidence, in our opinion, contradicts the principles of this important advancement. We question how, in the absence of "high-quality" empirical evidence, the reorganization of the majority personality disorders as interpersonal can be viewed as necessary and/or beneficial.

Ultimately, we question whether any attempted distinction between "Axis I and II" disorders can be entirely successful and harken back to Lilienfeld and Marino's (1995) discussion of Roschian concepts vis-à-vis mental disorders. They note that Roschian concepts "which are mental constructions that are typically used to categorize entities in the natural environment (e.g., bird, fruit, mountain), are characterized by unclear boundaries and an absence of defining (i.e., criterial) features" (p. 416). Pervasiveness, precociousness, and persistence are criteria that (reasonably) have been used to describe differences between personality disorders and other psychiatric disorders, but these distinctions often fail due to aptness of the "three P's" with respect to many forms of psychopathology.

We believe that there is likely no singular criterion or criteria that can regularly distinguish between the two and that such comparisons are fraught by nature. Trait models of personality describe basic tendencies to deal with various evolutionary challenges (Nettle, 2006; attention to threat—neuroticism). Precocious, persistent, and pervasive dysfunction in any of the domains featured in trait models (e.g., being under or oversensitive to threat; being too deliberate vs. too spontaneous; being too focused on group harmony and cooperation vs. being too focused on agentic competition-oriented relations) can represent personality disorders; however, only some configurations of personality pathology are specifically interpersonal in nature (e.g., Widiger et al., 2023). In our opinion, proponents of the reframing of personality disorders as "interpersonal disorders" fail to acknowledge that personality disorders, broadly speaking, are related to dysfunction across all major domains of personality including the non-interpersonal domains of neuroticism—emotional stability, conscientiousness–disinhibition, and openness–closedness. Wright and colleagues (2022) elide this distinction, writing "also within the interpersonal domain are behaviors, such as the rigidity associated with the traditional obsessive–compulsive category, impulsivity characteristic of the traditional antisocial category, and of the push–pull attachment sequences characteristic of the traditional borderline category" (pp. 1092–1093). But notably, the authors provide little empirical data to support these contentions.[5] Of course, these disorders, like all psychiatric disorders, have interpersonal *consequences* but there is little evidence to suggest that the core of all personality disorders is interpersonal in nature.

Is There a Role for Personality Disorder in an Integrative Model of Personality and Psychopathology?

There is clear and compelling evidence that a comprehensive model of psychopathology must include personality disorders if it is to provide sufficient coverage of psychological problems. The personality disorders are prevalent in the general community (Winsper et al., 2020) and

---

[5]In fact, obsessive–compulsive personality disorder is largely unrelated—empirically (Samuel & Widiger, 2008) and theoretically (Lynam & Widiger, 2001)—to interpersonal domains of personality.

treatment-seeking populations (Beckwith et al., 2014), are related to substantial distress and impairment (e.g., Pompili et al., 2005; Whisman et al., 2007), and have meaningful societal implications (e.g., Bode et al., 2017; Gatner et al., 2023). More importantly, the inclusion of personality disorder symptoms helps bolster the formation of major domains of psychopathology (e.g., negative affectivity: borderline personality disorder; thought disorder; schizotypal and schizoid personality disorders) or form the foundation of others (e.g., antagonistic externalizing: borderline and narcissistic personality disorders; detachment: avoidant and schizoid personality disorders). A failure to include personality disorders would lead to an impoverished description of psychopathology in not only the interpersonal realm but also the realm of emotional dysregulation and under/over regulation of impulses.

If So, How Can the Distinct Features of Personality Disorders Be Conceptualized and Measured?

We suggest conceptualizing personality disorders as configurations of extreme and/or maladaptive variants of basic personality traits paired with concrete evidence of impairment. This may be done by focusing on the three P's during basic personality assessment by identifying whether the extreme and/or maladaptive trait(s) are relatively long-standing (e.g., Rose et al., 2024), early arising (Chanen & Thompson, 2019), and associated with meaningful dysfunction in critical life domains (i.e., work, relationships, physical health, psychological well-being; Mullins-Sweatt & Widiger, 2010). It may be the case that this conceptualization captures other forms of psychopathology (e.g., early arising and persistent depression and anxiety; the hyperactivity–oppositional defiant disorder–conduct disorder cluster). This is understandable given the reconceptualization of other forms of psychopathology using higher-order spectra that are very similar to basic models of personality in most of their features, including the three Ps. This approach has the added benefits of being parsimonious, relatively easy to implement, and requiring little inference on the part of patients or care providers about internal dynamics that are emphasized in the models favored by Wright and colleagues (2022). We believe such models are unnecessary and that there were good reasons that models such as this were abandoned in DSM III in favor of a more descriptive approach.

PART II

The personality disorders as disorders of self and social functioning

AIDAN G. C. WRIGHT and JANAN MOSTAJABI

During the run-up to the *Diagnostic and Statistical Manual of Mental Disorders, Fifth Edition* (DSM-5; American Psychiatric Association, 2013), the personality disorder field was abuzz with hope and excitement about the possibility of significant changes to the how personality pathology would be represented in the manual, most notably a shift away from problematic categories toward a dimensional model. However, the enthusiasm and optimism gave way to acrimonious infighting during the process. This was perhaps unavoidable because answering the seemingly straightforward question of "How should we dimensionalize personality disorders?" forced the DSM Personality and Personality Disorders Workgroup to engage with the much more difficult question of "What are personality disorders?" This process put a spotlight on this more fundamental question, and it has captured much of the field's attention since. Answering the questions that organize this chapter continue this fieldwide discourse.

Nearly everyone agrees that the 10 personality disorder diagnoses in Section II of DSM-5 are a problematic way to organize the classification of this important form of psychopathology and therefore they need to be replaced.[6] The point of disagreement that lingers and that we address here is whether, moving forward, personality disorders should be defined primarily as interpersonal disorders (here interpersonal includes both self and social functioning; Wright & Nielsen, 2025)

[6]It is difficult to take as intellectually serious those who argue in favor of retaining the current discrete categorical model of 10 diagnoses on conceptual grounds, so we will not address this perspective here.

or whether they should be defined using just maladaptive "traits" that include content beyond interpersonal functioning. It is clear to us that much of the debate is a philosophical one, not one that is amenable to direct scientific inquiry, although data are often conscripted to reinforce one's viewpoint. Differences of opinion about what should be considered personality disorder as opposed to another form of psychopathology may just be a matter of taste.

Nevertheless, we make the argument that diagnostic systems are currently primarily organized around domains of dysfunction and that within these domains the personality disorders is where most of the primary interpersonal dysfunction is located; therefore, they are first and foremost interpersonal disorders, even if across the current 10 diagnoses there are features that tap into additional content domains that are not explicitly interpersonal on their surface (e.g., dysregulated emotions, impulsive behavior, disordered thought). ICD-11 now officially reflects this view, requiring only self and social impairments for a diagnosis, and in the provisional DSM-5 Section III alternative model of personality disorders (AMPD; American Psychiatric Association, 2013) self and social impairments are required for a diagnosis (Criterion A) but one must also include additional specification of the type of dysfunction through a set of maladaptive personality traits (Criterion B). In either of these systems, self and social impairments are recognized to be dimensional, ranging from modest to severe. These systems also each include a set of dimensional "traits" that have emerged from the psychometric tradition in clinical and personality psychology. The DSM-5 trait domains include antagonism, detachment, disinhibition, negative affectivity, and psychoticism, whereas in ICD-11 psychoticism is excluded and anankastia is added. As noted, rating these traits is a requirement if using the DSM-5 diagnostic system, but they are optional in the ICD-11 system. Thus, the perspective that interpersonal dysfunction is the core of personality disorder is now reflected in the most updated diagnostic systems.

However, detractors from this perspective (see e.g., Widiger et al., 2023) point to the fact that "personality" is broader than self and social functioning, as is the full range of psychopathology currently captured in DSM's Section II 10 personality disorder diagnoses, and therefore focusing exclusively on interpersonal dysfunction is insufficient. They also argue that there is nothing particularly "interpersonal" about the current personality disorders; rather, interpersonal dysfunction is widespread in psychopathology. Finally, they argue that the data suggest that Criteria A and B of DSM-5 AMPD are problematically overlapping conceptually and as typically operationalized (i.e., via global retrospective self-report questionnaires) they are so highly correlated as to be problematically redundant, although the Criterion B traits typically cover more breadth and therefore typically explain more unique variance in external criteria. Therefore, parsimony would argue in favor of removing the Criterion A self and social impairments and recasting personality disorder entirely as a set of maladaptive traits. Each of these concerns are important to consider, and we address them in subsequent sections.

If Psychopathology Is Dimensional, What Are Personality Disorders?

At this stage in our understanding of psychopathology, DSM-5 and ICD-11 (World Health Organization, 2022) are primarily organized around major domains of mental and behavioral functioning. For instance, there are sections devoted to affective dysfunction, encompassing unipolar or bipolar mood disorders, or anxiety disorders. There are sections on conditions defined by grossly aberrant thinking (e.g., schizophrenia spectrum and other psychotic disorders), and others cover disorders of behavioral control (e.g., disruptive, impulse-control, and conduct disorders). There are even whole sections devoted to seemingly basic biological functions, not specific to humans, such as feeding and elimination. However, conspicuously absent from this organization are sections devoted to what are arguably the most human domains of functioning (Sharp & Wall, 2021), our sense of self and capacity for complex social relating (i.e., interpersonal dysfunction; Wright & Nielsen, 2025; Wright et al., 2022)—unless, of course, one recognizes that what most personality disorder diagnoses share and what most distinguishes them from other disorders is the preponderance of self and social impairments. These impairments include socially costly patterns of behavior that leave afflicted individuals in conflict with or withdrawn from others as well as a self-architecture or identity that lacks coherence and consistency in organization of experience and goals across time and circumstances. Consistent with this, most theoretical models of personality disorders emphasize the centrality of self and social functioning to the phenomena (Bender et al., 2011; Hopwood et al., 2013; Kernberg, 1984; Livesley, 1998; Parker et al., 2004; Wright et al., 2022). Thus, theorists from varying perspectives have highlighted the centrality of interpersonal dysfunction (both self and social) in personality disorder, and logically it would seem that this should be a major section of DSM-5 given the centrality of interpersonal functioning for the human species (e.g., Fiske, 1992).

Empirical quantitative structural research now confirms this longstanding theoretical perspective. Results of research on the structure of mental disorders show that at the higher-order level, it converges with the structure of maladaptive personality traits (e.g., Wright & Simms, 2015), which themselves correspond to the domains of basic personality (e.g., Wright & Simms, 2014). For convenience, we'll use the labels negative affectivity, antagonism, detachment, disinhibition, and psychoticism to referred to the spectra from the shared structure. However, when estimating the higher-order structure of mental disorder diagnoses, you only get the domains of antagonism and detachment when you include personality disorder diagnoses (Wright et al., 2022; Wright & Simms, 2015). Ringwald and colleagues' (2023) recent meta-analysis illustrates this phenomenon most clearly such that of the nine personality disorder diagnoses included in their model,[7] six (obsessive–compulsive, narcissistic, histrionic, avoidant, borderline, and paranoid) had their highest loading on either the detachment or antagonism domains and all but schizotypal had marked cross-loadings on one or both domains. Thus, the preponderance of the variance shared among these diagnoses is interpersonal. It is also the case that some diagnoses, like schizotypal, loaded only on thought disorder and antisocial loaded much more strongly on disinhibition than it did on antagonism, and others still, like schizoid, paranoid, borderline, and avoidant each had significant cross-loadings on the thought-disorder or negative-affectivity domains, as it may be.

The question is what to do with these findings? It is obvious that the 10 Section II personality disorder diagnoses contain content beyond self and social dysfunction. But it would seem most logical to us to say, as many have been for years, that many of these diagnoses are heterogenous constructs, poorly alloyed, that should be reorganized more logically based on the domains of impairments. There's no reason we should feel obliged to march along the narrow hegemony of the existing structure. That's been the whole point of the quantitative empirical approach to organizing psychopathology. To do so defeats the purpose of structural research. Instead, these diagnoses can and perhaps should be pulled apart, or at the very least reorganized. In fact, the ICD and DSM have already done so by either moving or cross-listing diagnoses like schizotypal and antisocial into or in other sections of the manuals (e.g., schizophrenia spectrum and other psychotic disorders or disruptive, impulse-control, and conduct disorders, respectively). But this could also be done with parts of traditional diagnoses that lack coherence, such as separating out problems with disinhibition from the self- and interpersonal dysfunction in the borderline diagnosis and coding these impairments in different sections of the manual. If one is committed to

[7]Dependent personality disorder was excluded for computational reasons likely due to low representation in studies.

reorganizing psychopathology using an empirically derived dimensional system, then one must imagine moving beyond the existing categorical diagnoses. The diagnoses can be reorganized, retaining most of it in an "interpersonal" or "self and social impairment" section and moving the remainder somewhere else.

If Personality and Psychopathology Share a Common Individual-Differences Structure, What Is Specific about Personality Disorders?

The second argument against recasting most of what is currently in the personality disorders diagnoses in a focal "self and social impairment" section is that interpersonal impairments are not specific to them. This is trivially true in the sense that it is rare for any clinically significant form of psychopathology to affect only a single domain of functioning. For instance, individuals with frank psychosis typically experience significant amounts of emotional distress, anguish even, because of their thought disorders but we typically do not refer to these as mood disorders. By the same token, individuals with major depression experience significant biases in their thinking and interpretation of events, but we do not classify these as thought disorders. In each of these examples, the focal pathologies often result in impairments in self and social impairments as well. Humans are systems of interacting domains, individuals are not composed of orthogonal factors, and in people these domains work together to function. Accordingly, as severity of impairment increases in any domain, the likelihood increases that additional domains are affected and exhibit their own dysfunction. Nonetheless, we can still differentiate forms of pathology based on the conceptual grounds of what type of or which domain of dysfunction is most central or definitional.

However, this is an almost impossible task when looking at covariance-based models in cross-sectional data using measures saturated with valence or general distress and dysfunction (e.g., Oltmanns et al., 2018). That is typically the type of evidence that is used to question the specificity of interpersonal impairments in personality disorder. Furthermore, most of the research used to support the contention that measures of the Criterion B traits outperform measures of Criterion A dysfunction in the prediction of outcomes is based on cross-sectional self-report data in convenience samples (see Sleep & Lynam, 2022, for a brief review). Setting aside the very limited explanatory value of this sort of study design and data, one should expect these findings. It would seem obvious that measures that are intended to tap 25 diverse constructs (e.g., the Personality Inventory for DSM-5) should predict more variance in outcomes than those that are intended to measure one (e.g., the Level of Personality Functioning Scale), especially when the outcomes are Section II personality disorder scales. The Criterion A content was intended to capture the source of the impairments but not necessarily recapitulate every feature of existing diagnoses, whereas that was the explicit goal of the trait scales. Therefore, this work is little more than a psychometric validation exercise, but it doesn't tell us much about the nature of personality disorder. Initial studies showing the overlap between the two systems were necessary (e.g., Hopwood et al., 2012), of course, but this sort of question would not seem to require repeated adjudication. One can also ask why it is so problematic that Criteria A and B are so overlapping in the AMPD, as good internal consistency is typically a virtue of diagnoses. It would be illogical for Criteria A and B to be uncorrelated and separately predict equal or large amounts of variance in the Section II diagnoses or other outcomes.

Other sources provide much more compelling arguments for the centrality of interpersonal dysfunction in personality disorder and its clinical importance. When you consider other classes of diagnosis, even those with significant interpersonal outcomes, they do not carry with them the same implications for clinical care. Clinicians generally expect patients with most diagnoses to establish an alliance and engage in treatment. Not so for patients with personality disorder diagnoses, who will typically struggle developing an alliance, which is a fundamentally interpersonal process (Bender, 2005). As a result, clinicians perceive these patients as challenging (Kernberg, 2007; Moukaddam et al., 2017; Nakamura & Koo, 2017; Stone, 2007). To combat this, treatments developed specifically for personality disorders incorporate features that provide structure and establish boundaries, deal with ruptures and impasses, support clinicians, and set expectations for extended treatments with elevated probabilities of dropout or reversals (Bateman et al., 2015). Clinically, the main point of diagnosis is to guide treatment. The interpersonal functioning associated with personality disorders is so central that it has implications for how treatment is delivered in a way that is not true of other diagnoses.

An alternative feature that was putatively specific to personality disorder, or at least distinguished them from other psychopathology, was the persistence, pervasiveness, and precociousness of the impairments. In the 1990s through early 2000s, several large prospective studies were undertaken to investigate just how stable the personality disorders were (see Skodol, 2008, for a summary). Although the results are somewhat nuanced, the surprising finding was that they were much less stable than was assumed. Not only are the DSM-5-defined personality disorders less stable than once thought, but it has also become clear that other forms of psychopathology are much more long-lasting. For instance, DSM-5 now offers persistent depressive disorder as a diagnosis to reflect long-term depressivity and it notes that the course of obsessive–compulsive disorder is "usually chronic" if left untreated and that the course of schizophrenia, at least as defined by periods of remission following first onset psychosis, is similar to that of personality disorder. Morey and Hopwood (2013) further review the stability of personality disorder as related to other constructs and determine that firm conclusions are difficult given methodological differences (e.g., clinical interviews vs. self-report scales). Pervasiveness is difficult to ascertain, and we are unaware of compelling data that address that point either way. Finally, precociousness is not definitional of personality disorder and many forms of psychopathology have their first manifestations in childhood or adolescence (see Casey et al., 2014). Thus, unfortunately the data just do not support persistence, pervasiveness, or precociousness as distinguishing features of personality disorder, although it would be a convenient solution were it the case.

Is There a Role for Personality Disorder in an Integrative Model of Personality and Psychopathology?

An integrative model of personality and psychopathology can be organized structurally around similar domains of content (e.g., the Big Five). From this perspective, the personality disorders might best be recast as interpersonal disorders, highlighting that self and social dysfunction is their core, and non-interpersonal content shifted to other domains. At least this is how we would suggest one should do it based on domains of dysfunction, which is how current diagnostic manuals do it now and how structural models of personality are organized. That said, this is a descriptive psychopathology approach, prioritizing the empirical structure of how dysfunction manifests. However, defining and explaining personality, psychopathology, and what distinguishes them goes far beyond their structural similarities (Hopwood et al., 2022; Wright & Hopwood, 2022). Space precludes fully delineating these distinctions, although this is what DSM-5's AMPD level of personality functioning (LPF) was designed to do (Bender et al., 2011). Conceptually we see a great deal of value in the LPF, but as we acknowledge below it has been very challenging to operationalize using existing assessment technologies.

If So, How Can the Distinct Features of Personality Disorders Be Conceptualized and Measured?

Isolating the core self and social dysfunction of personality disorders is easier said than done, and it has proven empirically difficult. Self and social impairments are not equivalent to one's standing on dimensional traits (Wright et al., 2022), even as they often manifest in elevated levels of antagonistic and detached behavior. Simply coding dimensional levels of antagonism and detachment would be straightforward and ready for implementation. In applied contexts, this would provide a much-needed shorthand for interpersonal dysfunction, which is often not assessed or coded. The expediency of this approach may be justified in many clinical settings, but this strategy comes with limitations, especially when considering mechanistic research. Most critically, it sidesteps the more challenging task of directly assessing the aspects of self and social dysfunction that are often the focus of clinical theories and interventions in personality disorders and as the LPF or Criterion A in the AMPD was designed to do. However, the defining impairments in personality disorder are notoriously challenging to assess validly. For instance, global retrospective self-report has proven unequal to the task and accumulating research suggests their theoretically diverse aspects typically collapse into an undifferentiated mass (Nielsen & Wright, 2025; Sleep et al., 2024). That cross-sectional global self-report is so limited for understanding processes and mechanisms may not be theoretically damning, but it is a practical challenge. Interviews, like the one developed for DSM-5's AMPD, are very lengthy and require specialized training, which limits their practical utility in clinical settings and may be why there has been very little uptake in systematic empirical studies. Because impairments in self and social functioning are defined mostly in terms of processes that occur in interpersonal situations, we believe this should be the focus of assessments—ideally over time and across contexts. This might best be achieved with intensive longitudinal data, either in patients' own naturalistic settings or in the context of the psychotherapeutic relationship. Nevertheless, these approaches also require more development before they are amenable for implementation in applied settings.

PART I REFERENCES

American Psychiatric Association. (2013). *Diagnostic and statistical manual of mental disorders* (5th ed.). Author.

Beckwith, H., Moran, P. F., & Reilly, J. (2014). Personality disorder prevalence in psychiatric outpatients: A systematic literature review. *Personality and Mental Health, 8*(2), 91–101.

Bode, K., Vogel, R., Walker, J., & Kröger, C. (2017). Health care costs of borderline personality disorder and matched controls with major depressive disorder: A comparative study based on anonymized claims data. *The European Journal of Health Economics, 18*, 1125–1135.

Chanen, A. M., & Thompson, K. N. (2019). The age of onset of personality disorders. In G. de Girolamo, P. McGorry, & N. Sartorius (Eds.), *Age of onset of mental disorders* (pp. 183–201) Springer International.

Clark, L. A. (2005). Stability and change in personality pathology: Revelations of three longitudinal studies. *Journal of Personality Disorders, 19*, 524–532.

Costa, P. T., Jr., & Widiger, T. A. (Eds.). (1994). *Personality disorders and the five-factor model of personality*. American Psychological Association.

D'Huart, D., Seker, S., Bürgin, D., Birkhölzer, M., Boonmann, C., Schmid, M., & Schmeck, K. (2023). The stability of personality disorders and personality disorder criteria: A systematic review and meta-analysis. *Clinical Psychology Review, 102*, 102284.

Eng, W., Heimberg, R. G., Hart, T. A., Schneier, F. R., & Liebowitz, M. R. (2001). Attachment in individuals with social anxiety disorder: The relationship among adult attachment styles, social anxiety, and depression. *Emotion, 1*(4), 365–380.

Few, L. R., Miller, J. D., Rothbaum, A., Meller, S., Maples, J., Terry, D., . . . MacKillop, J. (2013). Examination of the Section III DSM-5 diagnostic system for personality disorders in an outpatient clinical sample. *Journal of Abnormal Psychology, 22*, 1057–1069.

Gatner, D. T., Douglas, K. S., Almond, M. F., Hart, S. D., & Kropp, P. R. (2023). How much does that cost? Examining the economic costs of crime in North America attributable to people with psychopathic personality disorder. *Personality Disorders: Theory, Research, and Treatment, 14*(4), 391–400.

Green, M. F., Horan, W. P., & Lee, J. (2015). Social cognition in schizophrenia. *Nature Reviews Neuroscience, 16*(10), 620–631.

Gidhagen, Y., Holmqvist, R., & Philips, B. (2018). Attachment style among outpatients with substance use disorders in psychological treatment. *Psychology and Psychotherapy: Theory, Research and Practice, 91*(4), 490–508.

Jewell, T., Apostolidou, E., Sadikovic, K., Tahta-Wraith, K., Liston, S., Simic, M., . . . Yorke, I. (2023). Attachment in individuals with eating disorders compared to community controls: A systematic review and meta-analysis. *International Journal of Eating Disorders, 56*(5), 888–908.

Kerber, A., Ehrenthal, J. C., Zimmermann, J., Remmers, C., Nolte, T., Wendt, L. P., . . . Knaevelsrud, C. (2024). Examining the role of personality functioning in a hierarchical taxonomy of psychopathology using two years of ambulatory assessed data. *Translational Psychiatry, 14*, 340.

Kotov, R., Krueger, R. F., Watson, D., Achenbach, T. M., Althoff, R. R., Bagby, R. M., . . . Zimmerman, M. (2017). The hierarchical taxonomy of psychopathology (HiTOP): A dimensional alternative to traditional nosologies. *Journal of Abnormal Psychology, 126*(4), 454–477.

Lilienfeld, S. O., & Marino, L. (1995). Mental disorder as a Roschian concept:

A critique of Wakefield's "harmful dysfunction" analysis. *Journal of Abnormal Psychology, 104*(3), 411–420.

Lynam, D. R., & Widiger, T. A. (2001). Using the five-factor model to represent the DSM-IV personality disorders: An expert consensus approach. *Journal of Abnormal Psychology, 110*(3), 401–412.

Lynam, D. R., & Widiger, T. A. (2007). Using a general model of personality to understand sex differences in the personality disorders. *Journal of Personality Disorders, 21*(6), 583–602.

Miller, J. D., Reynolds, S. K., & Pilkonis, P. A. (2004). The validity of the five-factor model prototypes for personality disorders in two clinical samples. *Psychological Assessment, 16*(3), 310–322.

Mullins-Sweatt, S. N., & Widiger, T. A. (2010). Personality-related problems in living: An empirical approach. *Personality Disorders: Theory, Research, and Treatment, 1,* 230–238.

Muris, P., Meesters, C., Van Melick, M., & Zwambag, L. (2001). Self-reported attachment style, attachment quality, and symptoms of anxiety and depression in young adolescents. *Personality and Individual Differences, 30*(5), 809–818.

Nettle, D. (2006). The evolution of personality variation in humans and other animals. *American Psychologist, 61*(6), 622–631.

Oldehinkel, A. J., & Ormel, J. (2023). Annual research review: Stability of psychopathology: lessons learned from longitudinal population surveys. *Journal of Child Psychology and Psychiatry, 64*(4), 489–502.

Oltmanns, J. R., & Oltmanns, T. F. (2020). Self–other agreement on ratings of personality disorder symptoms and traits: Three meta-analyses. In T. D. Letzring & J. S. Spain (Eds.), *The Oxford handbook of accurate personality judgment* (pp. 276–293). Oxford University Press.

Pompili, M., Girardi, P., Ruberto, A., & Tatarelli, R. (2005). Suicide in borderline personality disorder: A meta-analysis. *Nordic Journal of Psychiatry, 59*(5), 319–324.

Powers, A., & Casey, B. J. (2015). The adolescent brain and the emergence and peak of psychopathology. *Journal of Infant, Child, and Adolescent Psychotherapy, 14*(1), 3–15.

Rose, L., Carter, N. T., Lynam, D. R., Miller, J. D., & Oltmanns, T. F. (2024). Validity, stability, and change in psychopathic traits in older adults: A registered report. *Clinical Psychological Science, 13*(3), 664–679.

Samuel, D. B., & Widiger, T. A. (2008). A meta-analytic review of the relationships between the five-factor model and DSM-IV-TR personality disorders: A facet level analysis. *Clinical Psychology Review, 28*(8), 1326–1342.

Sleep, C. E., Lamkin, J., Lynam, D. R., Campbell, W. K., & Miller, J. D. (2019). Personality disorder traits: Testing insight regarding presence of traits, impairment, and desire for change. *Personality Disorders: Theory, Research, and Treatment, 10,* 123–131.

Sleep, C. E., Lynam, D. R., & Miller, J. D. (2022). Understanding individuals' perceptions of desire for change, impairment, benefits, and barriers of change for pathological personality traits. *Personality Disorders: Theory, Research, and Treatment, 13,* 245–253.

Sleep, C. E., Lynam, D. R., Widiger, T. A., Crowe, M., & Miller, J. D. (2019). An evaluation of DSM-5 Section III Personality Disorder Criterion A (Impairment) in accounting for psychopathology. *Psychological Assessment, 31,* 1181–1191.

Stanton, K., Levin-Aspenson, H. F., Emery, N. N., Willis, L., Myntti, W., & McDonnell, C. G. (2025). Understanding participant perspectives on the scientific accuracy and stigma of personality trait labels. *Personality Disorders: Theory, Research, and Treatment, 16*(1), 91–102.

Trull, T. J., Widiger, T. A., Lynam, D. R., & Costa, P. T., Jr. (2003). Borderline personality disorder from the perspective of general personality functioning. *Journal of Abnormal Psychology, 112*(2), 193–202.

Whisman, M. A., Tolejko, N., & Chatav, Y. (2007). Social consequences of personality disorders: Probability and timing of marriage and probability of marital disruption. *Journal of Personality Disorders, 21*(6), 690–695.

Widiger, T. A. (2022). Personality traits are dynamic. *Personality Disorders: Theory, Research, and Treatment, 13,* 440–441.

Widiger, T. A., & Hines, A. (2022). The DSM-5 alternative model of personality disorder. *Personality Disorders: Theory, Research, and Treatment, 13,* 347–355.

Widiger, T. A., Miller, J. D., Lynam, D. R., & Samuel. D. B. (2023). Interpersonal and personality disorders: Comment on Wright, Ringwald, Hopwood, and Pincus (2023). *American Psychologist, 78,* 714–715.

Winsper, C., Bilgin, A., Thompson, A., Marwaha, S., Chanen, A. M., Singh, S. P., . . . Furtado, V. (2020). The prevalence of personality disorders in the community: A global systematic review and meta-analysis. *The British Journal of Psychiatry, 216*(2), 69–78.

Wright, A. G., Ringwald, W. R., Hopwood, C. J., & Pincus, A. L. (2022). It's time to replace the personality disorders with the interpersonal disorders. *American Psychologist, 77,* 1085–1099.

PART II REFERENCES

American Psychiatric Association. (2013). *Diagnostic and statistical manual of mental disorders* (5th ed.). Author.

Bateman, A. W., Gunderson, J., & Mulder, R. (2015). Treatment of personality disorder. *Lancet, 385*(9969), 735–743.

Bender, D. S. (2005). The therapeutic alliance in the treatment of personality disorders. *Journal of Psychiatric Practice, 11*(2), 73–87.

Bender, D. S., Morey, L. C., & Skodol, A. E. (2011). Toward a model for assessing level of personality functioning in DSM-5, part I: A review of theory and methods. *Journal of Personality Assessment, 93*(4), 332–346.

Casey, B. J., Oliveri, M. E., & Insel, T. (2014). A neurodevelopmental perspective on the Research Domain Criteria (RDoC) framework. *Biological Psychiatry, 76,* 350–353.

Fiske, A. P. (1992). The four elementary forms of sociality: Framework for a unified theory of social relations. *Psychological Review, 99*(4), 689–723.

Hopwood, C. J., Thomas, K. M., Markon, K. E., Wright, A. G. C., & Krueger, R. F. (2012). DSM-5 personality traits and DSM-IV personality disorders. *Journal of Abnormal Psychology, 121*(2), 424–432.

Hopwood, C. J., Wright, A. G. C., Ansell, E. B., & Pincus, A. L. (2013). The interpersonal core of personality pathology. *Journal of Personality Disorders, 27*(3), 271–295.

Hopwood, C. J., Wright, A. G. C., & Bleidorn, W. (2022). Person-environment transactions differentiate personality and psychopathology. *Nature Reviews Psychology,* 1(1), 55–63.

Kernberg, O. F. (1984). *Severe personality disorders: Psychotherapeutic strategies.* Yale University Press.

Kernberg, O. F. (2007). The almost untreatable narcissistic patient. *Journal of the American Psychoanalytic Association, 55*(2), 503–539.

Livesley, W. J. (1998). Suggestions for a framework for an empirically based classification of personality disorder. *Canadian Journal of Psychiatry, 43,* 137–147.

Moukaddam, N., Flores, A., Matorin, A., Hayden, N., & Tucci, V. T. (2017). Difficult patients in the Emergency Department: Personality disorders and beyond. *The Psychiatric Clinics of North America, 40*(3), 379–395.

Morey, L. C., & Hopwood, C. J. (2013). Stability and change in personality disorders. *Annual Review of Clinical Psychology, 9,* 499–528.

Nakamura, M., & Koo, J. (2017). Personality disorders and the difficult dermatology patient: Maximizing patient satisfaction. *Clinics in Dermatology, 35*(3), 312–318.

Nielsen, S. R., & Wright, A. G. C. (2025). The structure of identity dysfunction in self-report measures. *Journal of Personality Assessment, 107*(1), 12–27.

Oltmanns, J. R., Smith, G. T., Oltmanns, T. F., & Widiger, T. A. (2018). General factors of psychopathology, personality, and PD: Across domain comparisons. *Clinical Psychological Science, 6*(4), 581–589.

Parker, G., Hadzi-Pavlovic, D., Both, L., Kumar, S., Wilhelm, K., & Olley, A. (2004). Measuring disordered personality functioning: To love and work reprised. *Acta Psychiatrica Scandinavica, 110,* 230–239.

Ringwald, W. R., Forbes, M. K., & Wright, A. G. C. (2023). Meta-analysis of structural evidence for the hierarchical taxonomy of psychopathology (HiTOP) model. *Psychological Medicine, 53*(2), 533–546.

Sharp, C., & Wall, K. (2021). DSM-5 level of personality functioning: Refocusing PD on what it means to be human. *Annual Review of Clinical Psychology, 17,* 313–337.

Skodol, A. E. (2008). Longitudinal course and outcome of personality disorders. *Psychiatric Clinics of North America, 31*(3), 495–503.

Sleep, C. E., & Lynam, D. R. (2022). The problems with Criterion A: A comment on Morey et al.(2022). *Personality Disorders, 13*(4), 325–327.

Sleep, C. E., Phillips, N. L., Du, T. V., Vize, C., Lynam, D. R., & Miller, J. D. (2024). Examining the structure of personality dysfunction. *Personality Disorders, 15*(2), 110–121.

Stone, M. H. (2007). *Personality-disordered patients: Treatable and untreatable.* American Psychiatric Publishing.

Widiger, T. A., Miller, J. D., Lynam, D. R., & Samuel, D. B. (2023). Interpersonal and personality disorders: Commentary on Wright et al.(2022). *American Psychologist, 78*(5), 714–715.

World Health Organization. (2022). *International classification of diseases* (11th rev.). Author.

Wright, A. G. C., & Hopwood, C. J. (2022). Integrating and distinguishing personality and psychopathology. *Journal of Personality, 90*(1), 5–19.

Wright, A. G. C., & Nielsen, S. (2025). A contemporary integrative interpersonal theory of self and social pathology. In K. Banicki & P. Zachar (Eds.), *Conceptualizing personality disorder: Perspectives from philosophy, psychological science, and psychiatry* (pp. 108–129). Cambridge University Press.

Wright, A. G. C., Ringwald, W. R., Hopwood, C. J., & Pincus, A. L. (2022). It's time to replace the personality disorders with the interpersonal disorders. *American Psychologist, 77*(9), 1085–1099.

Wright, A. G. C., & Simms, L. J. (2014). On the structure of personality disorder traits: Conjoint analyses of the CAT-PD, PID-5, and NEO-PI-3 trait models. *Personality Disorders: Theory, Research, and Treatment, 5*(1), 43–54.

Wright, A. G. C., & Simms, L. J. (2015). A metastructural model of mental disorders and pathological personality traits. *Psychological Medicine, 45*(11), 2309–2319.

CHAPTER 15

What can we learn about psychopathology from personality change interventions in nonclinical populations?

Personality was once considered to be basically stable in adulthood. However, research over the past few decades has shown that personality can and does change, and some evidence suggests that with effort, people can change their personalities in intended directions. Given that personality traits are also closely linked to psychopathological constructs, these findings raise interesting questions about the clinical relevance of personality change interventions in nonclinical populations. We asked two sets of experts the following three questions:

What is the overall state of knowledge on the use of psychological interventions in nonclinical populations?

Does evidence suggest that interventions in nonclinical populations are quantitatively or qualitatively different from those in clinical populations?

How can evidence about personality change interventions inform clinical practice?

Both Thielmann and Casali and Jayawickreme et al. express optimism about the value of personality interventions and offer insights about how aspects of personality interventions could be imported to clinical practice. For instance, Thielmann and Casali emphasize the potential value of focusing on higher-order traits rather than narrower disorder or symptom categories and make a specific pitch for integrating discrepancy awareness in interventions. Jayawickreme and colleagues contextualize findings within dynamic approaches to personality like Whole-Trait Theory and stress the potential of micro-interventions that are narrow in scope, goal driven, and brief that can often be delivered via apps, particularly for younger populations who tend to have the highest rates of mental health problems. However, both authors also note that more work needs to be done to test the durability and applicability of personality-based interventions.

PART I

Personality psychology meets clinical practice

Insights from personality change interventions

ISABEL THIELMANN and NICOLE CASALI

Personality traits are commonly defined as "individuals' characteristic patterns of thought, emotion, and behavior" (Funder, 2001, p. 198). Traditionally, personality has been considered as largely stable once established in early adulthood—that is, at around age 30 (McCrae & Costa, 1999). This view has also been adopted for personality pathology: according to the latest version of the *Diagnostic and Statistical Manual of Mental Disorders* (DSM), a personality disorder denotes an "enduring pattern of inner experience and behavior that . . . is *pervasive* and *inflexible* . . . [and] *stable over time*" (American Psychiatric Association, 2022, p. 733, emphasis added). In contrast to this notion, meta-analyses consistently show that personality—including personality pathology—does change, even until very old age (e.g., Bleidorn et al., 2022; Ferguson, 2010). This has led to a paradigm shift in personality psychology advocating that personality is both stable and malleable.

In turn, if normal-range personality traits can change "just like that," the question of whether they can also be changed through tailored interventions is obvious. Indeed, within psychotherapy, personality change is a goal in and of itself (Allemand & Flückiger, 2017; Chapman et al., 2014). By definition, psychotherapy aims at "assisting people to modify their behaviors, cognitions, emotions, and/or other personal characteristics in directions that the participants deem desirable" (Norcross, 1990, p. 218). This goal to change personality traits through therapy is also in line with the relatively recent shift from a categorical to a dimensional conceptualization of personality disorders, according to which personality pathology can be understood as maladaptive variations of personality traits (e.g., Trull & Durrett, 2005).

Notably, the idea that personality may be amenable to volitional changes through tailored interventions is also gaining traction within contemporary personality psychology. In recent years, several personality change interventions have been proposed and tested (see Haehner et al., 2024, for a review). Here, we attempt to integrate these recent developments in personality psychology with evidence from clinical psychology on psychotherapy. Specifically, we (1) summarize the overall state of knowledge on the effectiveness of personality interventions in nonclinical populations; (2) elaborate on whether and, if so, how these findings may apply to clinical populations; and (3) discuss how clinical practice may profit from current developments in personality psychology and vice versa.

Personality Interventions in Nonclinical Populations

Scholars in personality psychology have recently started to develop tailored personality interventions to allow for a "focal treatment of one or more specific dispositions identified by a person who wants to change" (Chapman et al., 2014, p. 1429). Research on volitional personality change is, however, still in its infancy. Table 15.1 provides an overview of some interventions that have been proposed and initially tested in prior research (for a more comprehensive overview, see Haehner et al., 2024). Although the interventions differ in multiple respects, they also have much in common. For example, all interventions adopt a bottom-up approach, assuming that repeated enactment of trait-relevant behaviors will ultimately result in trait-level changes. Also, all interventions stress a motivation to change. Many people have goals to change certain aspects of their personality (Baranski et al., 2017)—for example, desires to increase in extraversion (e.g., become more sociable and outgoing) and decrease in neuroticism (e.g., become less anxious and worry less)—which often originate from a desire to increase one's well-being (Sun & Goodwin, 2020). In turn, changing one's personality is difficult and requires hard work and persistence, whereas changes are usually only small to moderate in size (Haehner et al., 2024). Thus, without sufficient motivation, individuals will likely not follow through, thereby hampering intervention effectiveness (Hudson et al., 2019). Motivation to change is also critical from an ethical point of view: Personality interventions do not intend to "fix" individuals; they seek to help them change in line with their desires. Then again, motivation to change alone is often insufficient for intentional personality change to occur (Haehner et al., 2024), highlighting the need for tailored interventions leveraging individuals' motivation.

TABLE 15.1. Overview of Personality Change Interventions

Intervention	Targeted traits	Intervention components	Application	Duration/ frequency
Intentional personality change coaching (Martin et al., 2014)	Big Five (domains and facets)	(1) trait and value assessment, (2) self-reflection and personality feedback, (3) exploration of gaps between current and ideal self, (4) selection of change goals, (5) assessment of attitudes toward change (and potential revision of change goals), (6) design and implementation of coaching strategies, (7) progress feedback, (8) continuation of coaching sessions, (9) progress feedback and maintenance plan, (10) 3-month follow-up (progress feedback, refinement of maintenance plan)	One-on-one coaching sessions	10 weeks, weekly sessions
Behavioral activation intervention (Magidson et al., 2014; Roberts et al., 2017)	Conscientiousness	(1) monitoring of daily behavior and trait-level assessment, (2) identification of values, (3) consideration of daily activities consistent with values, (4) establishing motivation to change, (5) structured plan for engaging in valued activities, (6) creating or leveraging broader environments that support changes, (7) behavioral activation (i.e., change conscientiousness-related states), (8) monitoring of progress	Individual sessions with therapist, coach, or teacher	Multiple weeks until changes have become automatic; concrete duration will differ across individuals
PErsonality coACH (PEACH; Stieger et al., 2018)	Big Five	(1) trait assessment, (2) personality feedback (identify gaps between current and ideal self), (3) selection of change goals, (4) individualized implementation intentions, (5) psychoeducation, (6) behavioral activation tasks, (7) self-reflection, (8) resource activation, (9) progress feedback	Smartphone application using a conversational agent; weekly core theme	10 weeks, two daily dialogues with conversational agent
Challenges (Hudson et al., 2019)[a]	Big Five	(1) selection of targeted traits (change goals); (2) selection of weekly challenges—that is, specific, concrete actions to think, feel, and behave (1–4 challenges each week); (3) weekly progress feedback on challenge completion	Web-based study	15–16 weeks, weekly surveys

Overall, initial evidence on the effectiveness of personality change interventions is promising. Besides yielding small to moderate trait changes, individuals who perceived having changed during an intervention also reported greater life satisfaction and satisfaction with oneself as a person (Olaru et al., 2023) as well as increases in self-esteem (Allemand et al., 2024). This supports that attaining desired personality changes may have positive effects on well-being. Critically, trait changes are usually documented in terms of self-reported trait levels, which may be prone to demand effects: Those who desire to change and complete a personality intervention may be motivated to report that they have changed. Indeed, recent evidence suggests that a meaningful portion of personality-change-intervention effects on self-reported changes of trait levels and well-being are attributable to demand effects (Krämer et al., 2025). Then again, the results from a study measuring observer reports of targeted traits suggest that some trait changes are also visible to others (Stieger et al., 2021). Another limitation of prior studies is the predominant reliance on relatively short follow-up periods of just a few weeks or months; only one study showed that certain trait changes may persist or even intensify after 1 year (Stieger et al., 2024). Thus, more research using observer reports or actual behavior to assess trait changes and studying the long-term effects of personality interventions is needed.

Personality Interventions in Clinical Populations

The personality change interventions summarized in Table 15.1 have, as of yet, only been tested in nonclinical populations. However, there are several reasons why these interventions can be expected to also be effective in clinical populations. First, personality interventions usually contain elements from psychotherapy, such as self-reflection and behavioral activation (see Table 15.1). Thus, personality interventions incorporate means that have proven effective in clinical populations. Second, trait changes are often reported in clinical populations as a result of clinical interventions: A meta-analysis including 207 studies found clinical interventions (including psychotherapy but also pharmacotherapy) to be associated with noteworthy increases in emotional stability and extraversion (Roberts, Luo, et al., 2017). Third, there are no systematic differences in the magnitude of naturally occurring personality change between clinical and nonclinical populations (Ferguson, 2010). Collectively, personality change interventions are thus likely effective in nonclinical and clinical samples alike.

Cross-Fertilization between Personality Change Interventions and Clinical Practice

Overall, we see great potential in the integration of clinical and nonclinical approaches to changing personality traits and related individual-differences variables. Thus, we concur with the notion that "there is a pressing need for collaborations between interventionists and personality researchers" (Chapman et al., 2014, p. 1435). This last section is therefore devoted to two questions: (1) How can evidence about personality change interventions inform clinical practice? and (2) How can clinical practice inform personality change interventions?

Regarding the first question—the transfer from personality to clinical interventions—we suggest that specific components from personality interventions—particularly those derived from trait theories rather than adopted from clinical practice—be added to clinical interventions to boost treatment effects. For example, components from an intervention to increase conscientiousness, such as if–then plans to increase one's self-discipline in daily life (Stieger et al., 2018), may have positive effects on abstinence from substances (Bucher et al., 2019). Likewise, intervention components that help to increase agreeableness, such as practicing friendly and cooperative behaviors (Hudson et al., 2019), may lead to an improvement in the therapeutic alliance (Bucher et al., 2019)—a primary factor underlying treatment effectiveness (Flückiger et al., 2018). That said, research is mute concerning which components of personality interventions are most effective in driving (what kind of) trait change and could, therefore, most usefully be integrated within psychotherapy. Therefore, future research is needed to test how clinical interventions can be most usefully complemented by personality interventions.

Moreover, certain clinical interventions could profit from shifting the focus away from disorders toward higher-order traits. To illustrate, neuroticism is an indicator of various forms of psychopathology and thus considered a transdiagnostic marker of psychopathology (Lynch et al., 2021). It follows that "higher-order temperamental factors . . . may be a more appropriate target for assessment and intervention than may symptom-level manifestations of these traits" (Barlow et al., 2013, p. 344). In line with this notion, the Unified Protocol for Transdiagnostic Treatment of Emotional Disorders—a cognitive-behavioral therapy of anxiety and mood disorders that specifically tackles maladaptive levels of related traits (including neuroticism)—has been found to yield desirable trait changes and, in turn, improvements in symptoms, functioning, and quality of life (Sauer-Zavala et al., 2021). A direct implication of this is that therapists may explain to their patients early on that personality change is a target of the therapy and why this is so and formulate concrete personality change goals. This is important, as most people consider personality as immutable and may be reluctant to change aspects of their personality (Dweck, 2008).

Regarding the second question—that is, the transfer from clinical to personality interventions—we have already summarized above that many personality interventions draw on concepts and principles from psychotherapy. For example, the behavioral activation intervention (Roberts, Hill, et al., 2017) to change conscientiousness synthesizes personality trait theory with a behavior activation approach to therapy. Similarly, Allemand and Flückiger (2017) draw on general change mechanisms of psychotherapy to propose four main change factors for personality change interventions that form the basis of the PEACH intervention (Stieger et al., 2018): discrepancy awareness, strength orientation, insight, and practice.

One of these change factors that we want to specifically elaborate on further is discrepancy awareness as derived from problem activation in psychotherapy. The tenet of problem activation is that "a patient must come into direct contact with painful emotions to overcome his or her problems" (Gassmann & Grawe, 2006, p. 1). Applied to personality interventions, discrepancy awareness means to see a mismatch between one's actual and desired trait levels. Interestingly, discrepancy awareness differs between traits: for morality-related traits (e.g., honesty, humility, fairness) in particular, individuals tend to overestimate their own trait levels (e.g., Tappin & McKay, 2017), thus often overlooking discrepancies from their desired trait levels. Consequently, individuals rarely report goals to change in desirable ways on morality-related traits, whereas they regularly do report such goals for other traits, for example, extraversion (Thielmann & De Vries, 2021).

An effective means to raise discrepancy awareness and thereby instill goals to change in desirable ways is personality feedback (e.g., Casali et al., 2025). Research shows that providing individuals with feedback about their actual trait levels (in terms of their relative standing on certain traits compared to others) can increase corresponding change goals, particularly for morality-related traits (Thielmann & De Vries, 2021). Feedback is also an integral part of therapy. According to Goldfried (1980), providing patients with feedback "whereby patients/clients are helped to become more aware of what they are doing and not doing, thinking and not thinking, and feeling and not feeling in various situations" (p. 5) is a strategy that is common to all psychotherapeutic approaches. Feedback is, however, only included in some personality interventions (see Table 15.1). Although self-reflection is more commonly implemented, it can also be based on introspection alone. We therefore advocate for the systematic consideration of personality feedback in personality interventions to help individuals see the discrepancies between their actual and desired trait levels and, thereby, promote change goals. That being said, it is important to emphasize again that a mere goal to change does not suffice to bring about change—similarly to problem activation being insufficient to achieve therapeutic success (Gassmann & Grawe, 2006).

Conclusion

The title of this chapter asks, "What can we learn about psychopathology from personality change interventions in nonclinical populations?" We hope to have shown that there is a lot to learn about psychopathology—especially how to treat it—from personality change interventions. Conversely, personality change interventions can profit considerably from clinical interventions. However, many open questions remain. Most critical in our view is that we know little about the processes involved in intentional personality change and about which components of personality interventions are most effective under which circumstances. This is problematic because "interventions will be most effective when they target the appropriate psychological process given the disposition of the participant" (Rebele et al., 2021, p. 623). Arguably, we have just started to scratch the surface, and more research is needed to fully exploit the potential of personality interventions in both nonclinical and clinical samples.

ACKNOWLEDGMENTS

This work was supported by a grant from the European Union (European Research Council) awarded to Isabel Thielmann (KNOW-THYSELF; Project No. 101039433). Views and opinions expressed are those of the authors only and do not necessarily reflect those of the European Union or the European Research Council Executive Agency. Neither the European Union nor the granting authority can be held responsible for them.

PART II

Insights from personality dynamics highlight opportunities and challenges of volitional personality change interventions to promote mental health

ERANDA JAYAWICKREME, STEPHEN M. SCHUELLER, ROWAN KEMMERLY, and JULIETTE L. RATCHFORD

Recent work highlighting the success of volitional personality change interventions is welcome given both that personality traits have been shown to be robustly linked to a variety of important life outcomes and measures of well-being (Ozer & Benet-Martínez, 2006) and that people desire to change their personality. Multiple studies have found that when prompted, between 67.5% (Baranski et al., 2017) and 95% (Robinson et al., 2015) of participants describe a desire to change at least one personality trait. Moreover, evidence suggests that individuals can change their levels of extraversion, conscientiousness, emotional stability, and openness to experience when participating in a structured personality change program (e.g., Hudson et al., 2019). In this chapter, we discuss how recent advances in personality dynamics are consistent with these findings as well as novel ways in which such programs could be deployed as "micro-interventions" using technology platforms. We also caution against thinking of these interventions as a panacea that can lead to sustained change.

Personality Dynamics Suggest That Volitional Change Is Possible

The success of volitional personality change interventions falls squarely in line with recent advances in conceptualizing and fostering personality change as a dynamic personality process (e.g., Mendonça et al., 2023;

Jayawickreme et al., 2021; Fleeson & Jayawickreme, 2021; Wright et al., 2021). For example, Whole-Trait Theory (WTT; Fleeson & Jayawickreme, 2021) notes that although an individual's behavior varies rapidly and frequently across different occasions, their behavior is both stable and distinct from that of other individuals when averaged across a larger period such as a few days or a week. Extending from this account, personality traits are stable in the sense that there is reliable between-person variation and flexible in the sense that substantial within-person variation occurs in an individual's behavior depending on momentary goals and situational cues.

WTT proposes that an individual's personality can be *described* in terms of a distribution of *personality states* (Fleeson & Jayawickreme, 2021), measuring the extent to which an individual manifests a given trait at a specific point. According to the model possessing a specific trait—such as the moral trait of compassion (Mendonça et al., 2023)—is simply akin to behaving in a compassionate manner (e.g., kind, empathetic, and warm) more often. For this reason, the model conceptualizes the descriptive side of traits in terms of "personality states," which are similar to traits in affective, cognitive, and behavioral content; however, states are manifested for a few minutes or hours rather than for months or years (Fleeson, 2001). Past research has used experience-sampling methodology (ESM) in which participants are asked to report to the extent to which they have manifested behavior consistent with a given personality state at regular time intervals across the duration of several days or weeks (note that such an approach lends itself to micro-interventions outside online spaces; Balaskas et al., 2021). These reports are then aggregated into a distribution to convey the frequency with which an individual enacted each level of a given state. By examining the full distribution of an individual's behaviors, the model has revealed that there are reliable between-person differences in individuals' aggregated behaviors and that individuals also respond flexibly in different situational contexts. Moreover, this within-person (or situational) variability has important and real affective consequences for the individual in that specific moment (Fleeson & Wilt, 2010).

In addition, WTT proposes that these distributions of states can be *explained* by social-cognitive mechanisms that lead to the person enacting the trait at different state levels. One core insight of WTT is therefore the functional nature of traits; that is, individuals enact trait manifestations to fulfill specific goals and thereby achieve specific outcomes (McCabe & Fleeson, 2012) and in response to specific opportunities afforded by the situation (Zachry et al., 2018). In other words, people modulate their manifestations of character traits to achieve specific goals and manage distinct environments. Given this framing of character in terms of a distribution of intentional states, WTT provides distinctive insight for personality interventions, as repeated exactments of specific states may support enduring personality change. More specifically, according to WTT momentary change can be achieved through self-regulated changes in one's manifestations of behavior and long-term more enduring change can be achieved through influencing the processes underlying the distribution.

Similar to behavioral activation interventions used to treat challenges to well-being (Blackie et al., 2014), the successful and repeated manifestation of specific personality states in different contexts can lead to successful personality formation through reinforcement. Specifically, such repeated manifestations can become habitual through the targeting of specific mechanisms such as skill building, behavioral goals activation, and goal implementation intentions (Duckworth et al., 2013). In other words, if people have clear goals to manifest these states, reflect and plan for specific obstacles to achieving those goals, and are able to reflect on the success of their behaviors on a regular basis, then personality development can be supported over time.

Use of Volitional Personality Change in Clinical Populations

Although the concept of volitional personality change in many ways stems from clinical and applied psychology (e.g., the view that people play an active role in their own personality development; Baranski et al., 2017), few studies have applied this work to clinical populations. The extant literature on volitional personality change predominately targets subclinical populations. However, a related field of research, that of implementation intentions, provides insights into how findings may play out in clinical populations. Implementation intentions (i.e., if–then plans) are a strategy often engaged in volitional personality change programs (e.g., Mendonça et al., 2023), as they can be applied to change goals. Participants identify a potential obstacle to their change goal (i.e., the "if" aspect of the plan) and then describe a plan of action should that obstacle arise (i.e., the "then" aspect of the plan). In a meta-analysis of clinical and analogue (i.e., participants scoring above the relevant cutoff on clinical measures) samples, creating implementation intentions was effective in achieving goals related to action intention, self-regulation, and cognitive skills and that these intentions were effective across different mental health concerns, goals, and methodological approaches (Toli et al., 2016). It is important to note that developing too many implementation intentions can decrease their efficacy and potency (Dalton & Spiller, 2012), suggesting that perhaps focusing on one goal and set of implementation intentions may be the best practice to facilitate long-term personality trait change.

Extending Dynamic Personality Change Principles to Technology-Delivered "Micro-Interventions"

One possible new frontier for personality interventions involves leveraging novel technologies to deliver interventions in the context of people's daily lives. People, especially youth, are increasingly interacting with technologies including smartphones, social technologies, and wearable devices. Similar to ESM that asks people to report on their behaviors across periods in their daily lives, "ecological momentary interventions" (EMIs) provide interventions in people's daily lives and in real-world contexts (Heron & Smyth, 2010). A recent review of EMIs found that most of these studies used smartphone apps to deliver such interventions, with many making use of sensor-collected data to trigger the deployment of the interventions (Balaskas et al., 2021). Smartphone ownership in the United States is nearly ubiquitous, with 90% of U.S. adults and 95% of U.S. teens having access to a smartphone (Pew Research Center, 2024). This growth of technology adoption has ushered in an exciting opportunity for effective and scalable personality interventions, especially if they can blend principles for psychological and behavior change theories with technological affordances for delivery.

The design of such interventions, however, must be appropriate for the delivery platform and interaction style of the target individual. An exciting avenue for future research on personality interventions following from theories of dynamic change are "micro-interventions" delivered through technology platforms.

Distinctive Features of Micro-Interventions

Micro-interventions are defined as brief highly focused interventions using in-the-moment elements to achieve specific emotional, cognitive, or behavioral change (Baumel et al., 2020). Micro-interventions differ from brief or standard interventions in their breadth, goals, and time frame.

- *Breadth.* Compared to standard interventions, which might have broad goals, micro-interventions are narrow in scope, with highly focused objectives.
- *Goals.* Each micro-intervention has a specific goal, such as education, feedback, skill acquisition, social/emotional support, emotional change, or behavioral change.
- *Time frame.* Micro-interventions are intended to elicit in-the-moment change and require seconds to minutes rather than hours to weeks.

Micro-interventions have been trialed on various technology platforms and targeting different behaviors such as activity suggestions delivered via smartphones to increase physical activity (Klasnja et al., 2018) or behavioral intervention strategies delivered via text messages to promote cognitive and emotional well-being (Kravitz et al., 2020). Approaching personality change from WTT is well suited to micro-interventions because they align in terms of time frame (seconds to minutes rather than hours to weeks) and breadth (a focused scope on specific behaviors or tendencies). Although micro-interventions have broad potential across various technologies and populations, we describe a specific use case—supporting youth mental health in online spaces.

Youth tend to be early adopters of new technologies, and they are increasingly using online platforms for connecting with other people, entertainment, and learning. As noted earlier, youth access to smartphones is even higher than adults (95% of teens vs. 90% of adults), and most teens report they use the internet daily, with 46% reporting they use it almost constantly and 48% reporting they use it multiple times per day. Most of the public dialogue on youth use of technology and its relation to mental health has focused on the negative consequences including reduced attention, higher levels of loneliness and depression, and lower overall well-being (Twenge & Campbell, 2018). However, if technology has the potential for such detrimental consequences, it likely also has the potential for meaningful positive change. Recent robust systematic reviews of evidence in the health sciences show an uncertain and complex relation between youth mental health and social media use (Heffer et al., 2019), highlighting small associations between digital media use and youth well-being in both negative and positive directions. On one hand, online spaces offer the potential to build connections and community, access information, and practice self-expression. On the other hand, they pose opportunities for exposure to harmful content, overuse of technologies, and exacerbation of issues such as depression, distorted body images, and disordered eating. In the context of personality, they offer the opportunity to reinforce or shape the personality traits people desire or take advantage of the personality shapes one would like to change.

Regardless of the well-being costs or personality influences, technologies play an increasingly important role in the lives of youth. Micro-interventions are especially well suited to use in online spaces because content in online spaces is often designed for brief engagement and distilled information, instruction, or calls to action. They also represent a cutting-edge tool in promoting the development of specific traits by taking advantage of specific online contexts and motivating specific in-the-moment goals (Jayawickreme & Fleeson, 2017). An important and exciting future direction for research would involve incorporating such micro-interventions into programs focused on personality formation (and by extension, mental health promotion).

Understanding how best to support youth in online spaces requires the consideration of what common risks youth face in these spaces as well as the technology design features that exacerbate or mitigate these risks. One team (Salen Tekinbaş et al., 2023) recently conducted a review of what is known about the risks and benefits of youth engagement with online social technologies. The review focused on ages 13–24 and synthesized available scholarly and gray literature from fields such as psychology, child development, learning sciences, game studies, and human–computer interaction (HCI). Of note, few of the observed risks were about the technologies themselves, with perhaps the exception of tendency to overuse technology or privacy concerns that result from technologies. Instead, they stem from how youth use technologies; thus, approaches that focus on supporting youth (i.e., potentially through personality change) could mitigate some of the specific harms that result from using technology. Other researchers have raised concerns about dark patterns in technology or technology features that are designed to manipulate users into behaviors that go against their best interests (Kollmer & Eckhardt, 2023). These two lines of inquiry suggest two potential areas of research. One is investigating volitional personality interventions that are directed at youth that could play an important role in improving their ability to navigate these spaces by supporting *desired* behaviors and personality change in the direction of their desired selves. The second is identifying design features that could align with users' desired personality change and support behaviors that are consistent with those interests. One study explored design features of YouTube that could help support user agency including increasing relevance, supporting microplanning, and enhancing user control (Lukoff et al., 2021).

Can Such Interventions Deliver Lasting Change?

Our enthusiasm aside, there remains uncertainty over the long-term effects of such interventions. We close by raising two concerns over the possibility that volitional interventions can promote durable change. One is that relatively nonintensive interventions will likely have only short-term effects on personality and well-being, despite their clear utility (e.g., ease of access and deployment). To provide one example, with the goal of fostering positive change in the wake of bereavement, Roepke and colleagues (2018) developed a group-format, day-long psychosocial intervention, which was named SecondStory. In a randomized controlled trial (RCT), adults (N = 112) who experienced bereavement within the past 5 years were randomly assigned to partake in SecondStory or in an active control, expressive writing. In the original RCT analyses, SecondStory participants did not experience significant increases in domains of posttraumatic growth (PTG). Although they did experience decreases in depressive symptoms postintervention, this decrease mostly dissipated by the first follow-up.

In supplementary analyses focused on personality characteristics, we found a moderate effect of the intervention on emotional stability (Kemmerly et al., 2024). The observed changes in emotional stability were consistent with effect sizes for personality change following therapeutic interventions (Roberts et al., 2017), suggesting that SecondStory could be a promising short-term intervention to address depression and emotional stability/neuroticism. However, we also found no effect on two "characteristic adaptations" associated with PTG (Weststrate et al., 2022): prosociality and communion. These results suggest that although SecondStory had a short-term effect on depression and emotional stability, it was less effective at promoting change in personality domains theoretically linked to PTG.

One possible reason for this finding is that when selecting traits to modify, people prioritize emotional stability, extraversion, and conscientiousness (Sun & Goodwin, 2020; Sun & Berman, 2023). Although these findings are consistent with research suggesting that people prefer agency-oriented traits to communion-focused traits (Abele & Wojciszke, 2007), prosocial character traits such as compassion (Dutton et al., 2014), intellectual humility (Porter et al., 2022), and honesty (Fleeson et al., 2022) are also desirable traits associated with positive life outcomes. However, people typically view nonmoral traits such as emotional stability, extraversion, and conscientiousness as having greater positive effects on their well-being than moral traits do (Sun & Berman, 2023). Whether people are able to improve such traits has implications for both societal progress and individual well-being, as there is now increasing evidence that enacting moral behaviors and possessing high levels of character virtues and prosocial traits (including the Big Five/HEXACO traits of Agreeableness and Honesty/Humility) is associated with greater happiness and meaning in life (Sun et al., 2025). Although recent work suggests that people can be induced to volitionally change moral character traits (Mendonça et al., 2023), more research is needed.

A second concern has to do with the transition from short-term (elastic) to long-term or enduring (pliable) change (Roberts & Bonner, 2024). WTT and other theoretical perspectives in personality dynamics have highlighted the "multipotency" of personality traits—specifically, that trait manifestations can change as needed to accomplish momentary goals (Fleeson & Jayawickreme, 2021). The effectiveness of many volitional personality change interventions confirms this multipotency, as people can successfully modulate their personality trait manifestations in the short-term with the goal of changing one's personality traits.

However, people can simultaneously vary meaningfully in their behavior in the short term while maintaining high levels of stability over time (Fleeson, 2001). WTT posits that intentional short-term change can lead to long-term change to the extent to which changes in one's state manifestations have positive consequences (Fleeson & Jayawickreme, 2021). For example, when people change their momentary states with the goal of changing their personality traits and this goal pursuit is successful, they will experience the positive benefits of possessing the new level of the trait. This in turn can lead to a shift in individuals' density distributions, given that the change in states led to positive outcomes (Fleeson & Jayawickreme, 2021). However, we caution that such "pliable" change will necessarily involve lasting shifts in multiple sociocognitive mechanisms, meaning that achieving long-lasting personality change will be more challenging that the current set of positive findings suggests.

At the moment, there are few studies using longitudinal designs that examine whether volitional personality change programs create lasting change (but see Stieger et al., 2024, for one exception). However, in a study investigating the desire to change personality traits related to the Big Five and its facets longitudinally, Baranski et al. (2020) found that, for the most part, personality change desires did not predict actual change in the follow-up either 6 months (college sample) or 1 year later (internet sample). Additionally, change desires did predict change such that desired increases in the traits of Extraversion, Agreeableness, and Conscientiousness related to decreases in those traits (Baranski et al., 2020). These findings are in line with those of other research among young adults that found that change goals to change conscientiousness and emotional stability predicted change in the direction opposite to that in the stated goal (Robinson et al., 2015). Conversely, several prospective studies of volitional personality change suggest that desire to change a trait predicts subsequent growth in that trait (Hudson et al., 2019). These mixed findings may relate to evidence that suggests that a desire to change is not sufficient to evoke actual change; rather, successful personality change comes from actively implementing trait-related behaviors to change oneself (Hudson et al., 2019). This finding suggests that successful long-term change may best occur within an intervention that scaffolds the desires to the implementation of trait-related behaviors.

Such long-term change will occur when the change in states results in changes to different social-cognitive processes (specifically to the links between inputs, intermediates, and/or outputs; Fleeson & Jayawickreme,

2021). Although this change is more likely when people desire to change their long-term manifestations and think such change is feasible and the changes exacted become habitual (Hennecke et al., 2014), it is likely that such long-term change will be harder to achieve than short-term shifts are. Although we are enthusiastic about new directions in volitional personality change, we also urge humility and caution about their long-term value.[1]

ACKNOWLEDGMENTS

This research was made possible through the support of Grant No. 63161 from the John Templeton Foundation. The opinions expressed in this presentation are those of the authors and do not necessarily reflect the views of the John Templeton Foundation.

PART I REFERENCES

Allemand, M., & Flückiger, C. (2017). Changing personality traits: Some considerations from psychotherapy process-outcome research for intervention efforts on intentional personality change. *Journal of Psychotherapy Integration, 27*(4), 476–494.

Allemand, M., Oalaru, G., Stieger, M., & Flückiger, C. (2024). Intervention-related correlated change between personality traits and self-esteem. *Consulting Psychology Journal, 76*(4), 367–386.

American Psychiatric Association. (2022). *Diagnostic and statistical manual of mental disorders* (5th ed., text rev.). American Psychiatric Publishing.

Baranski, E. N., Morse, P. J., & Dunlop, W. L. (2017). Lay conceptions of volitional personality change: From strategies pursued to stories told. *Journal of Personality, 85*(3), 285–299.

Barlow, D. H., Sauer-Zavala, S., Carl, J. R., Bullis, J. R., & Ellard, K. K. (2013). The nature, diagnosis, and treatment of neuroticism: Back to the future. *Clinical Psychological Science, 2*(3), 344–365.

Bleidorn, W., Schwaba, T., Zheng, A., Hopwood, C. J., Sosa, S. S., Roberts, B. W., & Briley, D. A. (2022). Personality stability and change: A meta-analysis of longitudinal studies. *Psychological Bulletin, 148*(7–8), 588–619.

Bucher, M. A., Suzuki, T., & Samuel, D. B. (2019). A meta-analytic review of personality traits and their associations with mental health treatment outcomes. *Clinical Psychology Review, 70*, 51–63.

Casali, N., Metselaar, C., & Thielmann, I. (2025). Personality feedback as an intervention to encourage positive changes on moral traits. *Identity, 25*(3), 428–438.

---

[1] See also the work of Krämer and colleagues (2024) suggesting that current effects of volitional personality change may be inflated.

Chapman, B. P., Hampson, S., & Clarkin, J. (2014). Personality-informed interventions for healthy aging: Conclusions from a National Institute on Aging work group. *Developmental Psychology, 50*(5), 1426–1441.

Dweck, C. S. (2008). Can personality be changed? The role of beliefs in personality and change. *Current Directions in Psychological Science, 17*(6), 391–394.

Ferguson, C. J. (2010). A meta-analysis of normal and disordered personality across the life span. *Journal of Personality and Social Psychology, 98*(4), 659–667.

Flückiger, C., Del Re, A. C., Wampold, B. E., & Horvath, A. O. (2018). The alliance in adult psychotherapy: A meta-analytic synthesis. *Psychotherapy, 55*(4), 316–340.

Funder, D. C. (2001). Personality. *Annual Review of Psychology, 52,* 197–221.

Gassmann, D., & Grawe, K. (2006). General change mechanisms: The relation between problem activation and resource activation in successful and unsuccessful therapeutic interactions. *Clinical Psychology & Psychotherapy, 13*(1), 1–11.

Goldfried, M. R. (1980). Toward the delineation of therapeutic change principles. *American Psychologist, 35*(11), 991–999.

Haehner, P., Wright, A. J., & Bleidorn, W. (2024, June 21). *A systematic review of volitional personality change research. https://doi.org/10.31234/osf.io/h5db2*

Hudson, N. W., Briley, D. A., Chopik, W. J., & Derringer, J. (2019). You have to follow through: Attaining behavioral change goals predicts volitional personality change. *Journal of Personality and Social Psychology, 117*(4), 839–857.

Krämer, M. D., Hopwood, C. J., Miller, T. J., & Bleidorn, W. (2025). What explains personality change intervention effects? *Journal of Personality and Social Psychology, 129*(5), 972–1005.

Lynch, S. J., Sunderland, M., Newton, N. C., & Chapman, C. (2021). A systematic review of transdiagnostic risk and protective factors for general and specific psychopathology in young people. *Clinical Psychology Review, 87,* 102036.

McCrae, R. R., & Costa, P. T. (1999). A five-factor theory of personality. In L. A. Pervin & O. P. John (Eds.), *Handbook of personality: Theory and research* (2nd ed., pp. 139–153). Guilford Press.

Norcross, J. C. (1990). An eclectic definition of psychotherapy. In J. K. Zeig & W. M. Munion (Eds.), *What is psychotherapy? Contemporary perspectives* (pp. 218–220). JosseyBass.

Olaru, G., van Scheppingen, M. A., Stieger, M., Kowatsch, T., Flückiger, C., & Allemand, M. (2023). The effects of a personality intervention on satisfaction in 10 domains of life: Evidence for increases and correlated change with personality traits. *Journal of Personality and Social Psychology, 125*(4), 902–924.

Rebele, R. W., Koval, P., & Smillie, L. D. (2021). Personality-informed intervention design: Examining how trait regulation can inform efforts to change behavior. *European Journal of Personality, 35*(4), 623–645.

Roberts, B. W., Hill, P. L., & Davis, J. P. (2017). How to change conscientiousness: The sociogenomic trait intervention model. *Personality Disorders: Theory, Research, and Treatment, 8*(3), 199–205.

Roberts, B. W., Luo, J., Briley, D. A., Chow, P. I., Su, R., & Hill, P. L. (2017). A systematic review of personality trait change through intervention. *Psychological Bulletin, 143*(2), 117–141.

Sauer-Zavala, S., Fournier, J. C., Jarvi Steele, S., Woods, B. K., Wang, M., Farchione, T. J., & Barlow, D. H. (2021). Does the unified protocol really change neuroticism? Results from a randomized trial. *Psychological Medicine, 51*(14), 2378–2387.

Stieger, M., Flückiger, C., & Allemand, M. (2024). One year later: Longer-term maintenance effects of a digital intervention to change personality traits. *Journal of Personality, 92*(5), 1424–1437.

Stieger, M., Flückiger, C., Rüegger, D., Kowatsch, T., Roberts, B. W., & Allemand, M. (2021). Changing personality traits with the help of a digital personality change intervention. *Proceedings of the National Academy of Sciences, 118*(8), e2017548118.

Stieger, M., Nißen, M., Rüegger, D., Kowatsch, T., Flückiger, C., & Allemand, M. (2018). PEACH, a smartphone- and conversational agent-based coaching intervention for intentional personality change: Study protocol of a randomized, wait-list controlled trial. *BMC Psychology, 6*(1), 43.

Sun, J., & Goodwin, G. P. (2020). Do people want to be more moral? *Psychological Science, 31*(3), 243–257.

Tappin, B. M., & McKay, R. T. (2017). The illusion of moral superiority. *Social Psychological and Personality Science, 8*(6), 623–631.

Thielmann, I., & De Vries, R. E. (2021). Who wants to change and how? On the trait-specificity of personality change goals. *Journal of Personality and Social Psychology, 121*(5), 1112–1139.

Trull, T. J., & Durrett, C. A. (2005). Categorical and dimensional models of personality disorder. *Annual Review of Clinical Psychology, 1*, 355–380.

PART II REFERENCES

Abele, A. E., & Wojciszke, B. (2007). Agency and communion from the perspective of self versus others. *Journal of Personality and Social Psychology, 93*(5), 751–763.

Balaskas, A., Schueller, S. M., Cox, A. L., & Doherty, G. (2021). Ecological momentary interventions for mental health: A scoping review. *PLOS One, 16*(3), e0248152.

Baranski, E., Gray, J., Morse, P., & Dunlop, W. (2020). From desire to development? A multi-sample, idiographic examination of volitional personality change. *Journal of Research in Personality, 85*, 103910.

Baranski, E. N., Morse, P. J., & Dunlop, W. L. (2017). Lay conceptions of volitional personality change: From strategies pursued to stories told. *Journal of Personality, 85*(3), 285–299.

Baumel, A., Fleming, T., & Schueller, S. M. (2020). Digital micro interventions for behavioral and mental health gains: Core components and conceptualization of digital micro intervention care. *Journal of Medical Internet Research, 22*(10), e20631.

Blackie, L. E. R., Roepke, A. M., Forgeard, M. J. C., Jayawickreme, E. & Fleeson, W. (2014). Act well to be well: The promise of changing personality states to promote well-being. In A. C. Parks & S. M. Schueller (Eds.), *Handbook of positive psychological interventions* (pp. 462–474). Wiley-Blackwell.

Dalton, A. N., & Spiller, S. A. (2012). Too much of a good thing: The benefits of implementation intentions depend on the number of goals. *Journal of Consumer Research, 39*(3), 600–614.

Duckworth, A. L., Kirby, T. A., Gollwitzer, A., & Oettingen, G. (2013). From fantasy to action: Mental contrasting with implementation intentions (MCII) improves academic performance in children. *Social Psychological and Personality Science, 4*(6), 745–753.

Dutton, J. E., Workman, K. M., & Hardin, A. E. (2014). Compassion at work. *Annual Review of Organizational Psychology and Organizational Behavior, 1,* 277–304.

Fleeson, W. (2001). Toward a structure- and process-integrated view of personality: Traits as density distributions of states. *Journal of Personality and Social Psychology, 80*(6), 1011–1027.

Fleeson, W., & Jayawickreme, E. (2021). Whole traits: Revealing the social-cognitive mechanisms constituting personality's central variable. *Advances in Experimental Social Psychology, 63,* 69–128.

Fleeson, W., Furr, R. M., Jayawickreme, E., & Hardin, B. (2022). Honesty as a trait. *Current Opinion in Psychology, 47,* 101418.

Fleeson, W., & Wilt, J. (2010). The relevance of Big Five trait content in behavior to subjective authenticity: Do high levels of within-person behavioral variability undermine or enable authenticity achievement? *Journal of Personality, 78*(4), 1353–1382.

Heffer, T., Good, M., Daly, O., MacDonell, E., & Willoughby, T. (2019). The longitudinal association between social-media use and depressive symptoms among adolescents and young adults: An empirical reply to Twenge et al. (2018). *Clinical Psychological Science, 7*(3), 462–470.

Hennecke, M., Bleidorn, W., Denissen, J. J., & Wood, D. (2014). A three–part framework for self–regulated personality development across adulthood. *European Journal of Personality, 28*(3), 289–299.

Heron, K. E., & Smyth, J. M. (2010). Ecological momentary interventions: Incorporating mobile technology into psychosocial and health behaviour treatments. *British Journal of Health Psychology, 15*(1), 1–39.

Hudson, N. W., Briley, D. A., Chopik, W. J., & Derringer, J. (2019). You have to follow through: Attaining behavioral change goals predicts volitional personality change. *Journal of Personality and Social Psychology, 117*(4), 839–857.

Jayawickreme, E., Fleeson, W., Beck, E. D., Baumert, A., & Adler, J. M. (2021). Personality dynamics. *Personality Science, 2,* 1–18.

Kemmerly, R., Collins, C., Roepke, A. M., & Jayawickreme, E. (2024, February 8–10). *Examining the impact of an intervention targeting posttraumatic growth on the personality characteristics of bereaved adults.* Poster presented at the Society for Personality and Social Psychology 2024 Annual Convention, San Diego, CA.

Klasnja, P., Smith, S., Seewald, N. J., Lee, A., Hall, K., Luers, B., . . . Murphy, S. A. (2019). Efficacy of contextually tailored suggestions for physical activity: A micro-randomized optimization trial of HeartSteps. *Annals of Behavioral Medicine, 53*(6), 573–582.

Kollmer, T., & Eckhardt, A. (2023). Dark patterns: Conceptualization and future research directions. *Business & Information Systems Engineering, 65*(2), 201–208.

Krämer, M. D., Hopwood, C. J., Miller, T. J., & Bleidorn, W. (2024, September 5). Personality change through self-improvement or self-acceptance: A multi-study approach accounting for expectancy and demand effects. *https://doi.org/10.31234/osf.io/eb6p7*

Kravitz, R. L., Aguilera, A., Chen, E. J., Choi, Y. K., Hekler, E., Karr, C., . . . Schmid, C. H. (2020). Feasibility, acceptability, and influence of mHealth-supported *N*-of-1 trials for enhanced cognitive and emotional well-being in US volunteers. *Frontiers in Public Health, 8,* 260.

Lukoff, K., Lyngs, U., Zade, H., Liao, J. V., Choi, J., Fan, K., . . . Hiniker, A. (2021, May). How the design of YouTube influences user sense of agency. In Yoshifumi Kitamura & Aaron Quigley (Gen. Chairs), *Proceedings of the 2021 CHI Conference on Human Factors in Computing Systems* (pp. 1–17). Association for Computing Machinery.

McCabe, K. O., & Fleeson, W. (2012). What is extraversion for? Integrating trait and motivational perspectives and identifying the purpose of extraversion. *Psychological Science, 23*(12), 1498–1505.

Mendonça, S. E., Murray Dykhuis, E., & Jayawickreme, E. (2023). Examining the possibilities for volitional character change in compassion and intellectual humility through a three-month online intervention. *Journal of Research in Personality, 104,* 104373.

Ozer, D. J., & Benet-Martínez, V. (2006). Personality and the prediction of consequential outcomes. *Annual Review of Psychology, 57,* 401–421.

Pew Research Center. (2024). Mobile fact sheet. *www.pewresearch.org/internet/fact-sheet/mobile*

Porter, T., Baldwin, C. R., Warren, M. T., Murray, E. D., Cotton Bronk, K., Forgeard, M. J., . . . Jayawickreme, E. (2022). Clarifying the content of intellectual humility: A systematic review and integrative framework. *Journal of Personality Assessment, 104*(5), 573–585.

Roberts, B. W., & Bonner, C. (2024). Life events may not change your personality, but life experiences probably will. *European Journal of Personality, 38*(3), 584–585.

Roberts, B. W., Luo, J., Briley, D. A., Chow, P. I., Su, R., & Hill, P. L. (2017). A systematic review of personality trait change through intervention. *Psychological Bulletin, 143*(2), 117–141.

Robinson, O. C., Noftle, E. E., Guo, J., Asadi, S., & Zhang, X. (2015). Goals and plans for Big Five personality trait change in young adults. *Journal of Research in Personality, 59,* 31–43.

Roepke, A. M., Tsukayama, E., Forgeard, M., Blackie, L., & Jayawickreme, E. (2018). Randomized controlled trial of SecondStory, an intervention targeting posttraumatic growth, with bereaved adults. *Journal of Consulting and Clinical Psychology, 86*(6), 518–532.

Salen Tekinbaş, Adame, A., Schueller, S. M., & Khan, F. R. (2023). *Youth, mental health, and the metaverse: Reviewing the literature.* Connected Learning Alliance.

Stieger, M., Flückiger, C., & Allemand, M. (2024). One year later: Longer-term maintenance effects of a digital intervention to change personality traits. *Journal of Personality, 92*(5),1424–1437.

Sun, J., & Berman, J. (2023). People prioritize personal fulfillment over morality in the context of self-improvement. Available at *https://osf.io/preprints/psyarxiv/gd5pw_v5*

Sun, J., & Goodwin, G. P. (2020). Do people want to be more moral? *Psychological Science, 31*(3), 243–257.

Sun, J., Wu, W., & Goodwin, G. P. (2025). Are moral people happier? Answers from reputation-based measures of moral character. *Journal of Personality and Social Psychology, 128*(5), 1160–1180.

Toli, A., Webb, T. L., & Hardy, G. E. (2016). Does forming implementation intentions help people with mental health problems to achieve goals? A meta-analysis of experimental studies with clinical and analogue samples. *British Journal of Clinical Psychology, 55*(1), 69–90.

Twenge, J. M., & Campbell, W. K. (2018). Associations between screen time and lower psychological well-being among children and adolescents: Evidence from a population-based study. *Preventive Medicine Reports, 12,* 271–283.

Weststrate, N. M., Jayawickreme, E., & Wrzus, C. (2022). Advancing a three-tier personality framework for posttraumatic growth. *European Journal of Personality, 36*(4), 704–725.

Zachry, C. E., Phan, L. V., Blackie, L. E. R., & Jayawickreme, E. (2018). Situation-based contingencies underlying wisdom-content manifestations: Examining intellectual humility in daily life. *The Journals of Gerontology. Series B, Psychological Sciences and Social Sciences, 73*(8), 1404–1415.

CHAPTER 16

Where do cognitive and neurodevelopmental disorders fit in dimensional models of psychopathology?

Most of the research on dimensional models of psychopathology has used questionnaire- or interview-based assessments, sampled young to middle-aged adults, and been conducted by people interested primarily in emotional and interpersonal problems. For these reasons, cognitive and neurodevelopmental disorders are often not fully represented in these models. In this section, we asked experts three questions about where cognitive and neurodevelopmental disorders fit into dimensional models of psychopathology:

Can and should dimensional models of personality and psychopathology include cognitive and neurodevelopmental disorders?

Do we need to think of different kinds of hierarchical models to account for such problems?

How can individual differences in personality and cognition be integrated to generate an efficient and effective diagnostic scheme?

In both chapters, the authors agree that dimensional diagnosis applies equally well to cognitive and neurodevelopmental disorders and integrate these disorders into a common system with personality and psychopathology. However, they use recent evidence about the covariance structure of mental health problems to propose somewhat different modifications to the HiTOP model. There are two main ingredients to Wilson and Michelini's proposal. First is that cognitive difficulties represent a separate higher-order factor distinct from psychopathology. Second is the incorporation of developmental considerations that have often been neglected in the advancement of hierarchical dimensional models. Forbes offers a different approach to fitting cognitive and neurodevelopmental disorders within general models of psychopathology, leading to an equally comprehensive but somewhat less drastic revision of HiTOP that includes such problems as an additional spectrum of psychopathology, rather than a separate higher-order factor.

PART I

Incorporating neurodevelopmental and neurocognitive conditions in transdiagnostic dimensional models of psychopathology

SYLIA WILSON and GIORGIA MICHELINI

Transdiagnostic dimensional models of psychopathology include constructs that span multiple psychiatric conditions and account for their high co-occurrence and heterogeneity. Specific clinical features of many psychiatric conditions are well situated within transdiagnostic frameworks—as internalizing, externalizing, and psychosis dimensions/spectra.[1] However, to date, few studies that inform current transdiagnostic frameworks have considered features of neurodevelopmental and neurocognitive conditions or studies have been narrowly limited (e.g., mainly to attention-deficit/hyperactivity disorder [ADHD]). This literature has also predominantly focused on early to middle-aged adult samples, with less attention to developmental processes earlier or later in life. As a result, our transdiagnostic dimensional models of psychopathology are limited in comprehensive coverage of the neurodevelopmental, neurocognitive, and psychiatric conditions that occur across the entire lifespan. The explicit inclusion of neurodevelopmental and neurocognitive conditions in transdiagnostic frameworks is crucial to promoting a new and expanded understanding of their etiology, developmental course,

[1] Other transdiagnostic spectra/dimensions are included in transdiagnostic dimensional models (somatoform, detachment) but are as-yet less well established, and we do not specifically consider them here.

co-occurrence/comorbidity, and the structure of psychopathology,[2] with important implications for transdiagnostic dimensional models, research, and clinical practice.

"Neurodevelopmental disorders"[3] are characterized by difficulties with attention, executive functions, learning, motor abilities, and social communication that emerge *early* in life and have a persistent developmental course. "Neurocognitive disorders"[4] are characterized by learning and memory problems as well as difficulties in attention, executive functions, language, perceptual motor problems, and social cognition that typically first emerge in *later* adulthood and reflect a decline from a previously attained level of cognitive function. The primary differentiation for the clinical features of neurodevelopmental and neurocognitive conditions is whether they are first evident in childhood or later in life and whether they reflect a decline from earlier functioning.

There has been growing recognition that individuals with neurodevelopmental conditions often experience psychiatric conditions, such as internalizing and externalizing problems, either concurrently or at later stages of development. To account for this comorbidity, we recently proposed a neurodevelopmental spectrum, situated within a broader transdiagnostic framework, and provided extensive evidence of its dimensional structure, validity, reliability, and clinical utility (Michelini et al., 2024). Conversely, to date the neurocognitive conditions remain noticeably absent from transdiagnostic frameworks despite also showing evidence of high co-occurrence and comorbidity with psychiatric conditions (e.g., Balanzá-Martínez et al., 2010; Kwak et al., 2017; Meyers, 1998).

The clinical features that characterize the neurodevelopmental conditions are typically present into and throughout adulthood, with

---

[2]We are mindful that incorporating neurodevelopmental and neurocognitive conditions into structural models of *psychopathology* implies that features of autism, ADHD, and other cognitive differences are pathological rather than reflecting neurodiversity. We suggest that future efforts move toward a focus on understanding the range of and differences in human experience that are captured in clinical features of neurodevelopmental, neurocognitive, and psychiatric conditions, with an emphasis on distress and functioning rather than pathology.

[3]Classified together in a chapter in the *Diagnostic and Statistical Manual of Mental Disorders—Fifth Edition* (DSM-5; American Psychiatric Association, 2013) that includes autism spectrum disorder (ASD), ADHD, intellectual and developmental disability, learning disorders, motor disorders (e.g., Tourette syndrome), and disorders of speech, language, and communication (e.g., social pragmatic communication disorder).

[4]Classified together in a chapter in the DSM-5 that includes dementia and major and mild neurocognitive disorders due to various medical conditions (e.g., Alzheimer's disease, frontotemporal degeneration) or exposures (e.g., traumatic brain injury, substance use).

potential implications for later aging and neurodegenerative processes (see Magnin, 2021). At the same time, differences in cognitive function are often evident well before the onset of a diagnosable neurocognitive condition (Geschwind et al., 2001; Seifan et al., 2015; Whalley et al., 2006). Notably, neurodevelopmental conditions, including autism, ADHD, and learning disabilities, have been found to be associated with later emerging neurocognitive conditions, particularly dementia (Golimstok et al., 2011; Klein et al., 2023) and case studies suggest that some neurocognitive conditions diagnosed in adulthood actually reflect previously undiagnosed neurodevelopmental conditions (Gossink et al., 2016). Other conditions, including schizophrenia and bipolar disorders, also show presymptomatic differences in cognitive function and post-onset cognitive decline (Jonas et al., 2022; Sheffield et al., 2018) and are associated with increased risk for later neurocognitive conditions (Cai & Huang, 2018). Similarly, internalizing and externalizing conditions including depression, anxiety, conduct problems, antisocial behavior, and substance use are also associated with premorbid and concurrent differences in cognitive function (Iacono et al., 2008; Snyder, 2013). Thus, differences in cognitive function appear to be a defining clinical feature of neurodevelopmental and neurocognitive conditions as well as psychiatric conditions.

To account for these widespread cognitive correlates, we propose that the differences in cognitive function that characterize the neurodevelopmental and neurocognitive conditions as well as psychiatric conditions are situated as spectra within transdiagnostic frameworks of psychopathology and captured by a "cognitive function" factor. Figure 16.1 provides a graphic representation that incorporates the neurodevelopmental and neurocognitive conditions and their clinical features alongside psychiatric conditions as well as the proposed cognitive function factor and neurodevelopmental and neurocognitive spectra. We suggest that the cognitive function factor is broad, general, nonspecific, and transdiagnostic, with loadings on the established internalizing, externalizing, psychosis, and proposed neurodevelopmental and neurocognitive spectra (see Michelini et al., 2024; Abramovitch et al., 2021). Although we see this cognitive function factor as conceptually similar to the general factor of intelligence, which has been found to be associated with general psychopathology (von Stumm et al., 2024), we consider it a broader factor that includes the full range of cognitive and executive functions that may influence and be influenced by psychiatric conditions.

Transdiagnostic models of psychopathology readily incorporate personality, and we suggest that it is necessary to also incorporate cognition. The proposed cognitive function factor is unique relative to already well-established spectra/dimensions in that age of onset, course, severity,

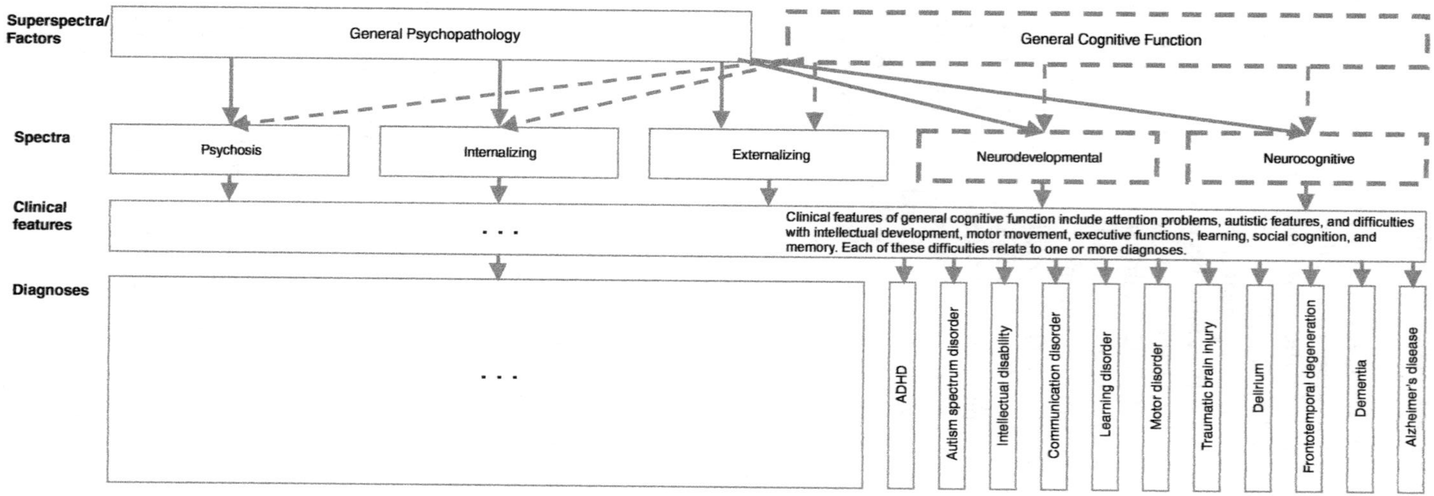

FIGURE 16.1. Proposed transdiagnostic model. Dashed lines indicate that the cognitive factor and neurodevelopmental and neurocognitive spectra are propositional. Ellipses indicate additional clinical features and diagnoses that are not illustrated here. ADHD = attention-deficit/hyperactivity disorder.

and the specific cognitive domains affected differentiate neurodevelopmental, neurocognitive, and psychiatric conditions (see Figure 16.2). Differences in cognitive function are a defining clinical feature of neurodevelopmental and neurocognitive disorders, but only when they emerge in early development or (typically) later in life and reflect a decline from previous functioning, respectively, whereas there is gradual and more general deterioration across adolescence and early adulthood in schizophrenia and more specific differences in cognitive and executive function processes for internalizing and externalizing disorders.

Evaluations of this proposed transdiagnostic dimensional model that incorporates cognitive function are necessary. Structural models must be conducted at different developmental stages to track the onset and course of clinical features of neurodevelopmental, neurocognitive, and psychiatric conditions. Although requiring considerable resources and time, lifespan longitudinal investigations that span from early childhood into later adulthood are needed to evaluate between- and within-person developmental processes, including changes in cognitive function over time. This work will require careful definition and measurement of "cognitive function" given the range of cognitive processes that may be affected and that some cognitive processes may be more or less specific to or be more or less severely affected in different neurodevelopmental, neurocognitive, and psychiatric conditions. However, despite the work that is needed to evaluate this more comprehensive proposed transdiagnostic dimensional model and the challenges in doing that work, considering and incorporating individual differences in both personality and cognitive function offers a better way of conceptualizing and diagnosing the full range of neurodevelopmental, neurocognitive, and psychiatric conditions and associated functioning. This in turn improves clinical practices by improving the efficiency and effectiveness of diagnosis and providing a fuller view of an individual's needs and strengths throughout the lifespan.

In conclusion, we suggest that transdiagnostic frameworks that include features of neurodevelopmental and neurocognitive conditions as well as the broader cognitive function factor we propose here have great potential to promote a new understanding of etiology, interplay, and developmental course, thereby directly influencing future research and clinical practices.

ACKNOWLEDGMENT

Giorgia Michelini was supported by a Klingenstein Third Generation Foundation fellowship (20212999).

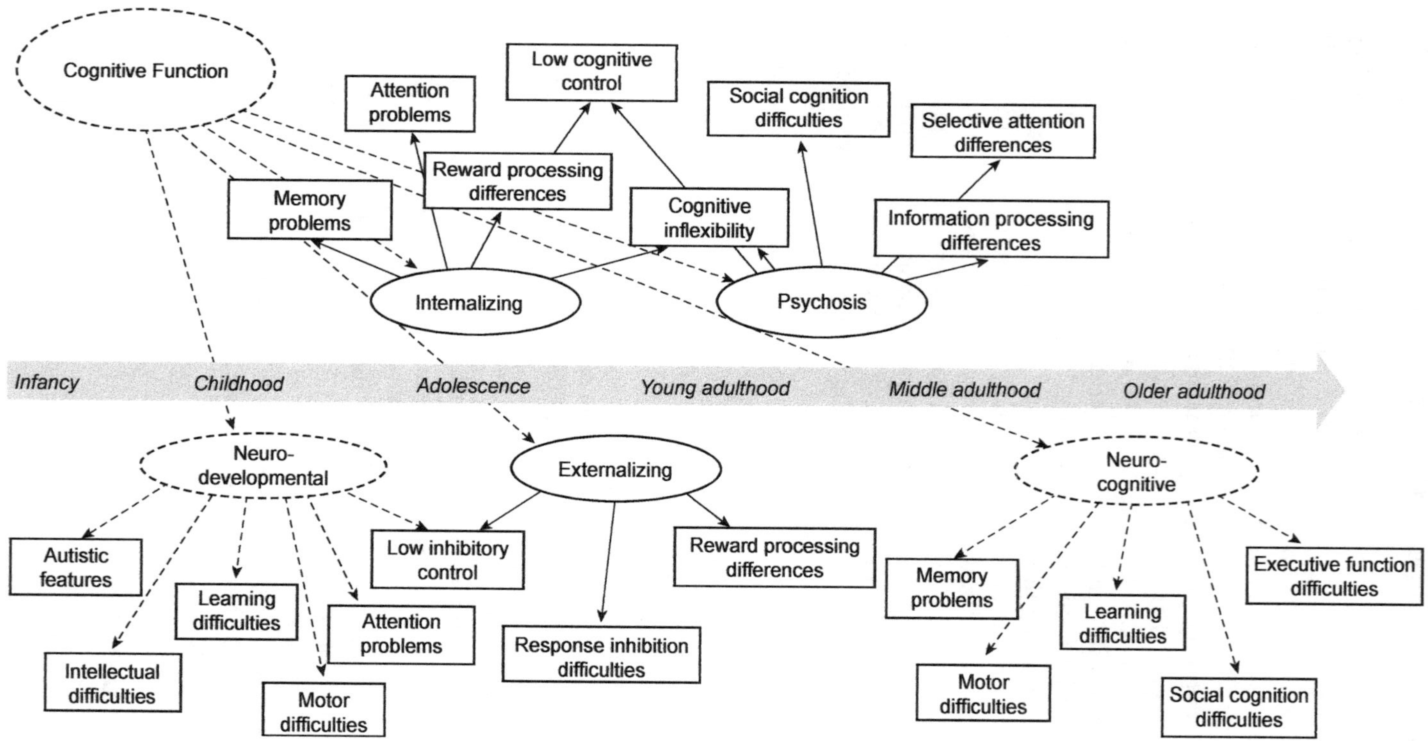

FIGURE 16.2. An illustration of common differences in cognitive function in neurodevelopmental, neurocognitive, and psychiatric conditions across the lifespan. The cognitive function factor has loadings on neurodevelopmental, internalizing, externalizing, psychosis, and neurocognitive spectra, and cognitive function differences are subsumed within each spectrum. Dashed lines indicate that the cognitive factor and neurodevelopmental and neurocognitive spectra are propositional.

PART II

Cognitive and neurodevelopmental disorders in dimensional models of psychopathology

MIRIAM K. FORBES

In contrast to the broad literature base informing the partner chapter in this section, my approach is quite self-indulgent, focusing on my own views and work on dimensional models of psychopathology. I hope it can be a useful complement to the rich information in Wilson and Michelini's companion chapter—and in Michelini et al. (2024)—by offering a perspective based on one of the types of data needed to fill the current gap in the literature (i.e., comprehensive and broad assessment of psychopathology that includes assessment of cognitive domains and neurodevelopmental disorder symptoms).

Models That Integrate Personality and Psychopathology Mostly Leave Out Cognitive and Neurodevelopmental Disorders: Does That Mean Dimensional Diagnosis Does Not Apply to Them?

I believe the reason these models leave out cognitive and neurodevelopmental disorders is because those disorders are usually not assessed in the studies that underpin the models, so they are largely missing in the literature synthesized in the Hierarchical Taxonomy of Psychopathology (HiTOP; Kotov et al., 2017), for example. However, the questions of (1) whether dimensional diagnosis can apply to cognitive and neurocognitive disorders and, relatedly, (2) whether these cognitive and neurodevelopmental disorders *should* be included in models of "psychopathology" are important to consider.

The first question is easy: Dimensional diagnosis can, and already does, apply to these disorders. Even the traditionally categorical DSM-5-TR (1) notes that neurodevelopmental disorders "demonstrate a range of severity, often without a very clear boundary with typical development" (American Psychiatric Association, 2022, p. 35); (2) includes dimensional assessment of the hallmark neurodevelopmental disorder, autism spectrum disorder; and (3) considers dimensional severity of cognitive and functional impairment in each of the six defined domains that compose the neurocognitive disorders (e.g., clinical thresholds are applied to determine the level of the diagnosis as "mild" versus "major" neurocognitive disorder; American Psychiatric Association, 2022). As for other classes of psychopathology, there does not seem to be any strong evidence for categorical distinctions along these continua (e.g., Harvey, 2019; Haslam et al., 2020; Thapar et al., 2017).

The second question is harder because including individual differences in neurodevelopmental and cognitive functioning domains in a model of "psychopathology" can be seen as pathologizing normative variation in the human experience. This is also the case for many, if not all, of the constructs in the current HiTOP model, which can be adaptive responses to the environment or a reflection of dysfunction in the environment rather than the individual. Thus, even very high levels of symptoms on a particular dimension do not necessarily indicate "pathology" at the level of the individual, which can be implied by a system developed to diagnose individuals—particularly one with the label "psychopathology" in its name. However, one benefit of dimensional classification is that dimensions can reduce stigma by removing the clean boundaries between "normal" and "abnormal" and describing all individuals' variations on the same set of dimensions (e.g., Lahey, 2021). We can then focus on distress or functional impairment to determine when intervention might be indicated (e.g., Üstün & Kennedy, 2009) and use dimensional symptom profiles for case formulation and treatment planning. In fact, this is similar to the approach already taken in the DSM-5-TR for both neurodevelopmental and neurocognitive disorders, as discussed further below.

Regardless, it is not my thoughts that matter here. There is a clear need for greater engagement with the end users of diagnostic systems to understand the implications and consequences of making these kinds of changes. What do people with neurodevelopmental or cognitive disorders think? How could their experiences be captured in a classification system that can facilitate access to neurodiversity-affirming care without stigmatizing or pathologizing the ways they experience and interact with the world?

Do We Need to Think of Different Kinds of Hierarchical Models to Account for Such Problems?

If we do consider how to incorporate neurodevelopmental and cognitive disorders into an existing hierarchical model like HiTOP, some points of disconnection are immediately clear. For example, neurodevelopmental disorders in DSM-5-TR are defined by their onset early in development (American Psychiatric Association, 2022). Not only is age of onset not included as a feature for diagnosis in the HiTOP framework, the framework itself is currently tested for only adults. This is an area of ongoing work in the literature and for the HiTOP Developmental Workgroup but a noteworthy obstacle. Similarly, the defining feature of neurocognitive disorders in DSM-5-TR is acquired deficits in cognitive functioning, as assessed by both (1) self-, informant-, or clinician-reported concern and (2) formal neuropsychological testing indicating a decline from previous functioning (American Psychiatric Association, 2022). HiTOP can incorporate data from standardized testing in theory but does not yet do so in practice, and although symptom change over time is a feature that can be tracked in a measurement-based care framework, HiTOP does not currently include course of illness (e.g., a change from usual functioning) as part of the diagnostic framework. Furthermore, the underlying pathophysiology of many neurocognitive disorders defined in DSM-5-TR is already known in many cases and HiTOP does not include such etiological factors, which in this case results in a loss of valuable diagnostic information. Finally, the absence of functional impairment in the HiTOP framework is another disconnect from the requirements for making neurodevelopmental or neurocognitive disorder diagnoses in DSM-5-TR (American Psychiatric Association, 2022).

In summary, to include these new domains in the HiTOP framework in the way they are currently conceptualized in the DSM, HiTOP would need to be expanded to incorporate age of onset, more types of evidence (e.g., standardized testing), course of illness, known etiology, and functional impairment—as well as being adapted to apply across the lifespan. Some of these are active projects underway in the HiTOP Consortium, but the foundation of the current model is cross-sectional symptom severity, so this lengthy list of disconnects suggest we might need a more complex hierarchical model to properly assess, classify, and diagnose cognitive and neurodevelopmental domains.

How Can Individual Differences in Personality and Cognition Be Integrated to Generate an Efficient and Effective Diagnostic Scheme?

If we proceed with integrating cognitive and neurodevelopmental domains into a model like HiTOP despite these points of disconnection, we might start by treating them the same way as the other classes of disorders in the DSM that are already in HiTOP—that is, in the first instance, relying on self-reported experiences of the symptoms that characterize the disorders. I recently led a study that offers some interesting results from this perspective: We analyzed the self-reported experiences of 14,762 individuals spanning every symptom described in DSM-5 to model the empirical structure of those symptoms based on the patterns of covariation among them (Forbes et al., 2025). Based on cross-method and cross-sample replication, we identified a set of transdiagnostic dimensions that closely resembled the current HiTOP models in many ways (see Figure 16.3).

Most relevant here, however, is the largest point of difference from the current HiTOP model: the novel "Neurodevelopmental and Cognitive Difficulties" spectrum (Figure 16.3). Figure 16.4 shows the lower levels of this branch in the model, splitting into narrower "Neurodevelopmental" and "Cognitive Difficulties" dimensions, which each included three nested subfactors—under "Neurodevelopmental": *social communication difficulties*, *altered sensation and attentional control*, and *ritualized behavior* and under "Cognitive Difficulties": *neurocognitive impairment*, *difficulties with organization*, and *forgetfulness*. In turn, these six subfactors were characterized by a variety of nested symptoms and syndromes that included many symptoms of prominent neurodevelopmental disorders like autism and ADHD and of the six cognitive domains that define neurocognitive disorders.

These results give us some ideas about how the DSM-defined symptom sets might fit into an empirical structure of psychopathology, and Figure 16.5 shows this perspective of translating DSM diagnoses into the empirical structure in more detail: Symptoms of autism primarily fell under "Neurodevelopmental," whereas ADHD symptoms split across the "Neurodevelopmental" and "Cognitive Difficulties" dimensions. Similarly, the cognitive domains of executive function, complex attention, and perceptual–motor functioning largely fell under the narrow *neurocognitive impairment* dimension, whereas the learning and memory, language, and social cognition domains were more heterogeneous with a subset of symptoms falling under the "Neurodevelopmental" dimensions of *social communication difficulties* and *altered sensation and attentional control*. We can also see in both panels of Figure 16.5

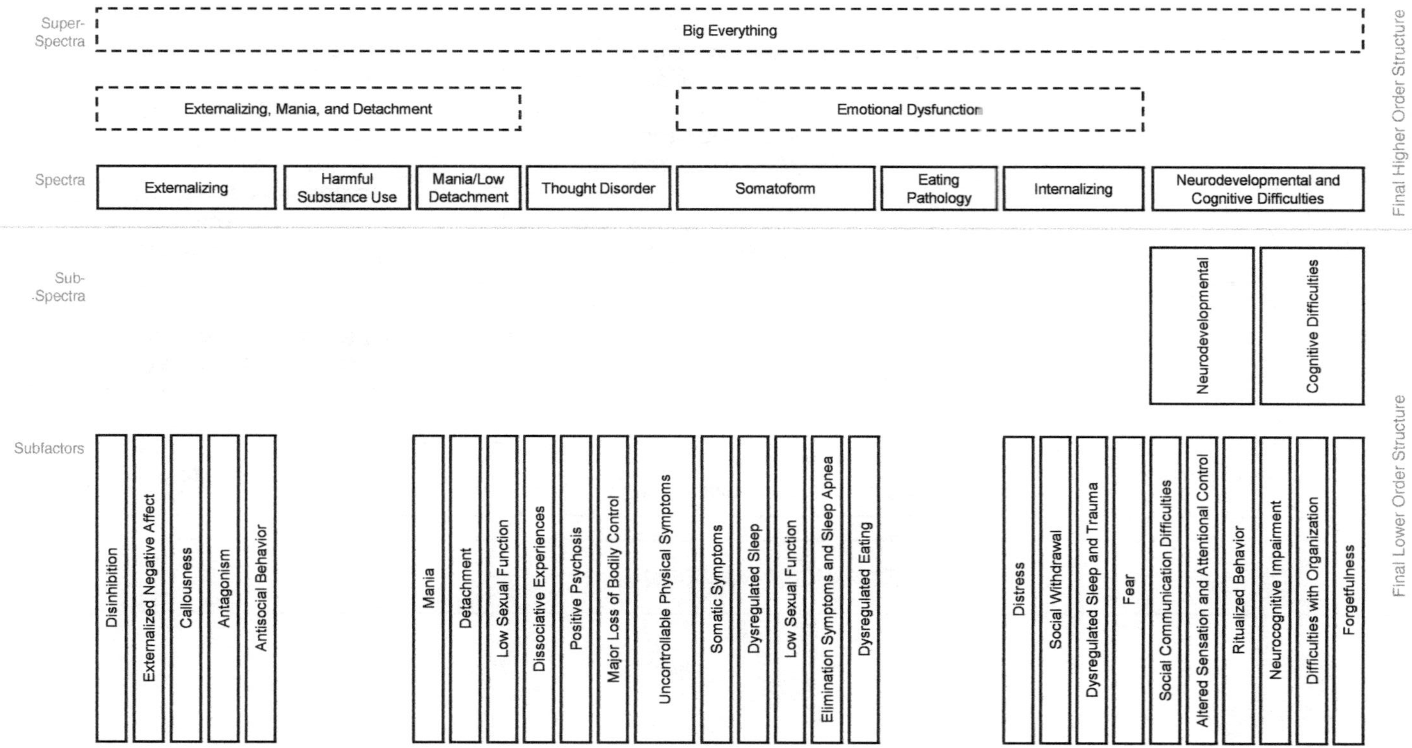

FIGURE 16.3. The upper levels of the results in Forbes et al. (2023). Adapted with permission. The lower levels of the model, including the individual symptoms that make up each construct are in the original article and supplementary materials. The next level down in the hierarchy for the "Neurodevelopmental and Cognitive Difficulties" branch of the model—the symptoms and syndromes—is shown in Figure 16.2.

Sub-Spectra	Neurodevelopmental		
Subfactors	Social Communication Difficulties	Altered Sensation and Attentional Control	Ritualized Behavior
Symptoms and Syndromes	**Low social engagement** **Disorganized speech** **Written communication difficulties** Selective mutism Difficulties with social communication Social non-responsiveness Language errors **Processing difficulties** Speech impediments Eccentricity* Name avoidance Nonspecific phrase use* **Behavioral perseveration**	Pressured speech Blurting Hyperactivity Fidgeting Unrestrained speech Speech perseveration Mimicry Fixations Specific food cravings* Nonspecific phrase use* Sensory sensitivity Eccentricity* **Excessive acquiring and saving**	Insistence on sameness Perfectionism Repetitive rituals and compulsions Ritualized greeting Specific food cravings*

Sub-Spectra	Cognitive Difficulties		
Subfactors	Neurocognitive Impairment	Difficulties with Organization	Forgetfulness
Symptoms and Syndromes	**Disorganized speech**	Excessive clutter	Cannot recall familiar names
	General cognitive difficulties	**Excessive acquiring and saving**	Reliance on reminders for memory*
	Processing difficulties	Lost track of finances*	Lost track of finances*
	Low social engagement	Lost track of possessions	Spatial navigation difficulty*
	Written communication difficulties	Difficulties with activities of daily living*	Reliance on lists for memory*
	Distractibility		Skill decline*
	Psychomotor impairment		(low) Difficulty awakening
	Behavioral perseveration		
	Difficulty awakening*		
	Sleepiness		
	Short-term memory impairment		
	Error proneness		
	Divided attention		
	Difficulties with activities of daily living*		
	Reliance on lists for memory*		
	Skill decline*		
	Spatial navigation difficulty*		
	Difficulties with arithmetic		
	Reliance on reminders for memory*		

* Denotes lower-order constructs that cross-load within the same panel. *Note.* **Bold** text denotes lower-order constructs that cross-load between the two panels.

FIGURE 16.4. The symptoms and syndromes that make up the six subfactors under the Neurodevelopmental (upper panel) and Cognitive Difficulties (lower panel) dimensions. Adapted from Forbes et al. (2025) with permission. The individual symptoms that make up each of these lower-order constructs are listed in Table S1 of Forbes et al. (2025).

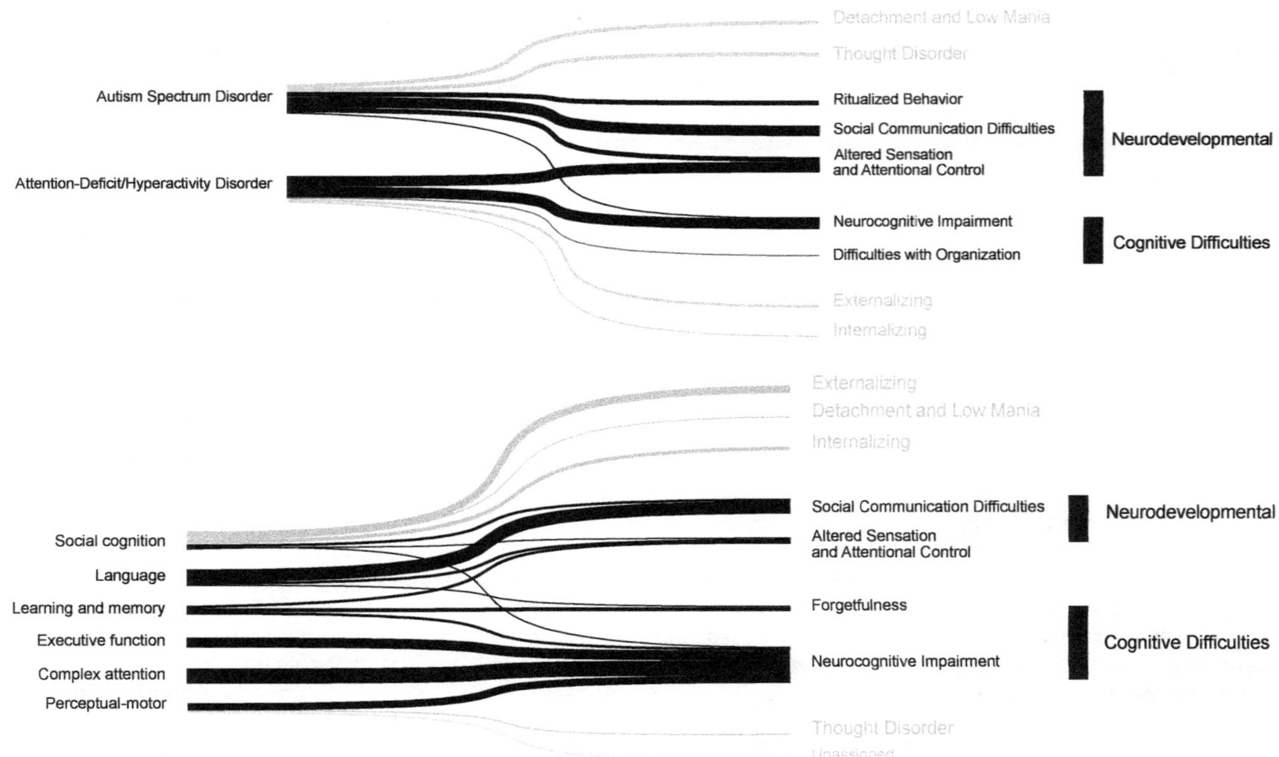

FIGURE 16.5. Sankey plots illustrating how symptoms that make up the diagnostic criteria of DSM-defined diagnoses split across the hierarchy of dimensions shown in Figure 16.1. Autism spectrum disorder and attention-deficit/hyperactivity disorder are shown in the upper panel as examples of neurodevelopmental disorders; the six cognitive domains that define the neurocognitive disorders are in the lower panel.

that there are symptoms that load elsewhere in the structure, suggesting a differentiation between "core" versus "nonspecific" symptoms in the DSM diagnostic criteria that may be more or less useful for differential diagnosis.

It is of course an important limitation that these data rely on self-report alone in a community sample and represent a single study. The sample had substantial representation of people in treatment for their mental health (63.7%) and prevalence of cognitive and neurodevelopmental symptoms (mean = 62.3% endorsement, ranging from 12.2% for "I started social interactions in an unusual way [e.g., touching the face of someone I don't know, or staring at them]" to 96.9% for "I felt frustrated"), but the observed patterns of symptom covariation would undoubtedly be different in people selected for cognitive or neurodevelopmental disorders or using other approaches to measurement—for example, a comprehensive neurocognitive battery. This makes it all the more important to interpret the results in the context of the broader literature, such as that reviewed in Michelini et al. (2024). There is also some recent brilliant work by early-career researchers in the field with (1) better measurement of neurodevelopmental disorders that aligns with the secondary associations seen in Figure 16.5 for autism with "Detachment" and ADHD with "Externalizing" (Dow, 2023) and (2) better measurement of cognitive domains showing patterns of correlations that align with the secondary associations found here for social cognition with "Externalizing" and "Detachment" (Lipsitz, 2023). However, other results in these theses diverged from those in Forbes et al. (2025), including the noteworthy absence of "Neurodevelopmental" and "cognitive difficulties" spectra, highlighting a clear need for replication and more work on how these domains might interleave with the empirical structure of psychopathology.

Beyond the implications for DSM-defined neurodevelopmental and neurocognitive disorders, the emergence of the "Neurodevelopmental" and "Cognitive Difficulties" dimensions in Forbes et al. (2025) had interesting implications for symptoms traditionally housed in other HiTOP dimensions and DSM diagnoses. For example, cognitive symptoms from the Somatoform spectrum; perseveration and restricted affect from the "Internalizing" spectrum; some symptoms of inexpressivity from the "Thought Disorder" spectrum, and distractibility from the Externalizing spectrum all shifted to these new spectra. Similarly, when considering DSM disorders from other chapters, symptoms from manic episodes (pressure to keep talking, flight of ideas, and psychomotor agitation all fell under *altered sensation and attentional control*; distractibility under *neurocognitive impairment*), schizophrenia (avolition under *neurocognitive impairment*), major depression (diminished ability to think or concentrate under *neurocognitive impairment*), and obsessive–compulsive disorder (repetitive rituals and compulsions under *ritualized behavior*) all loaded on these new dimensions in the broader framework. These findings will require replication and probing with richer and more varied methods but indicate that taking a more inclusive approach to the symptom domains included in modeling of individual differences could have broader implications for our understanding of quantitative nosology and models like HiTOP.

Further, future research should work to disentangle the "Neurodevelopmental" and "Cognitive Difficulties" subfactors of *social communication difficulties* versus *neurocognitive impairment*. These lower order dimensions had substantial overlap in their symptoms that was

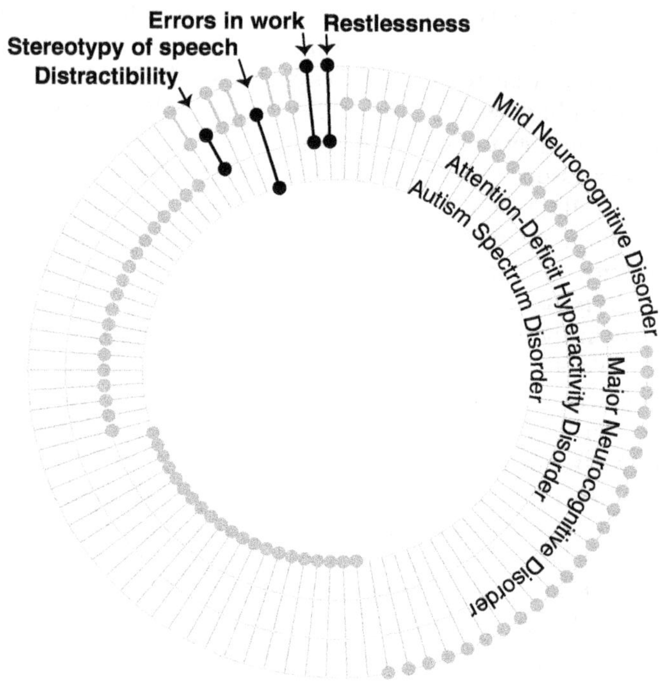

FIGURE 16.6. A map of the symptom overlap among core neurocognitive disorders (mild and major neurocognitive disorder) and neurodevelopmental disorders (autism spectrum disorder, attention-deficit/hyperactivity disorder). Each ring represents a diagnosis and the dots on the ring represent the symptoms of the diagnosis. Linked dots along the radii repeat between diagnoses, black linked dots repeat between the two chapters (i.e., spanning the neurocognitive and neurodevelopmental disorders chapters).

not related to overlap in the symptoms of diagnostic criteria of core neurodevelopmental and cognitive disorders (Forbes et al., 2024; e.g., mild and major neurocognitive disorder, ADHD, autism; see Figure 16.6). Instead, the overlap could indicate equifinality (i.e., capturing either social communication difficulties or cognitive impairment, depending on the underlying causes) or poor differentiation in the items we developed and a need for future research to determine whether different underlying causes can be differentiated at the phenotypic level for these constructs (Forbes et al., 2025).

Overall, I am optimistic that cognitive and neurodevelopmental domains could be included in a model like HiTOP with some further development and modifications. Embracing a hierarchical and dimensional approach to classification in these domains could offer the wide variety of advantages that this system offers—discussed elsewhere in this book—and overcome many of the same limitations posed by traditional diagnostic categories in other areas (e.g., frequent comorbidity, heterogeneity; APA, 2022). Although this work should be undertaken with careful co-design and consultation with individuals with lived experience of each domain, it has exciting implications for the future of quantitative psychopathology and dimensional diagnosis.

PART I REFERENCES

Abramovitch, A., Short, T., & Schweiger, A. (2021). The C Factor: Cognitive dysfunction as a transdiagnostic dimension in psychopathology. *Clinical Psychology Review, 86,* 102007.

American Psychiatric Association. (2013). *Diagnostic and statistical manual of mental disorders* (5th ed.). Author.

Astle, D. E., Holmes, J., Kievit, R., & Gathercole, S. E. (2022). Annual research review: The transdiagnostic revolution in neurodevelopmental disorders. *Journal of Child Psychology and Psychiatry, 63*(4), 397–417.

Balanzá-Martínez, V., Selva, G., Martínez-Arán, A., Prickaerts, J., Salazar, J., González-Pinto, A., . . . Tabarés-Seisdedos, R. (2010). Neurocognition in bipolar disorders—A closer look at comorbidities and medications. *European Journal of Pharmacology, 626*(1), 87–96.

Cai, L., & Huang, J. (2018). Schizophrenia and risk of dementia: A meta-analysis study. *Neuropsychiatric Disease and Treatment, 14,* 2047–2055.

Geschwind, D. H., Robidoux, J., Alarcón, M., Miller, B. L., Wilhelmsen, K. C., Cummings, J. L., & Nasreddine, Z. S. (2001). Dementia and neurodevelopmental predisposition: Cognitive dysfunction in presymptomatic subjects precedes dementia by decades in frontotemporal dementia. *Annals of Neurology, 50*(6), 741–746.

Golimstok, A., Rojas, J. I., Romano, M., Zurru, M. C., Doctorovich, D., & Cristiano, E. (2011). Previous adult attention-deficit and hyperactivity disorder symptoms and risk of dementia with Lewy bodies: A case–control study. *European Journal of Neurology, 18*(1), 78–84.

Gossink, F. T., Dols, A., Kerssens, C. J., Krudop, W. A., Kerklaan, B. J., Scheltens, P., . . . Pijnenburg, Y. A. L. (2016). Psychiatric diagnoses underlying the phenocopy syndrome of behavioural variant frontotemporal dementia. *Journal of Neurology, Neurosurgery & Psychiatry, 87*(1), 64–68.

Iacono, W. G., Malone, S. M., & McGue, M. (2008). Behavioral disinhibition and the development of early-onset addiction: Common and specific influences. *Annual Review of Clinical Psychology, 4*, 325–348.

Jonas, K., Lian, W., Callahan, J., Ruggero, C. J., Clouston, S., Reichenberg, A., . . . Kotov, R. (2022). The course of general cognitive ability in individuals with psychotic disorders. *JAMA Psychiatry, 79*(7), 659–666.

Klein, C. B., McQuaid, G. A., Charlton, R. A., Klinger, L. G., & Wallace, G. L. (2023). Self-reported cognitive decline among middle and older age autistic adults. *Autism Research, 16*(3), 605–616.

Kwak, Y. T., Yang, Y., & Koo, M.-S. (2017). Anxiety in dementia. *Dementia and Neurocognitive Disorders, 16*(2), 33.

Magnin, E. (2021). Neurodevelopmental and neurodegenerative similarities and interactions: A point of view about lifelong neurocognitive trajectories. *Journal of Alzheimer's Disease, 79*(4), 1397–1407.

Meyers, B. S. (1998). Depression and dementia: Comorbidities, identification, and treatment. *Journal of Geriatric Psychiatry and Neurology, 11*(4), 201–205.

Michelini, G., Carlisi, C. O., Eaton, N. R., Elison, J. T., Haltigan, J. D., . . . Wilson, S. (2024). Where do neurodevelopment conditions fit in trans diagnostic psychiatric frameworks: Incorporating a new neurodevelopmental spectrum. *World Psychiatry, 23*, 333–357.

Seifan, A., Schelke, M., Obeng-Aduasare, Y., & Isaacson, R. (2015). Early life epidemiology of Alzheimer's disease-a critical review. *Neuroepidemiology, 45*(4), 237–254.

Sheffield, J. M., Karcher, N. R., & Barch, D. M. (2018). Cognitive deficits in psychotic disorders: A lifespan perspective. *Neuropsychology Review, 28*, 509–533.

Snyder, H. R. (2013). Major depressive disorder is associated with broad impairments on neuropsychological measures of executive function: A meta-analysis and review. *Psychological Bulletin, 139*(1), 81–132.

von Stumm, S., Malanchini, M., & Fisher, H. L. (2024). The developmental interplay between the p-factor of psychopathology and the g-factor of intelligence from age 7 through 16 years. *Development and Psychopathology, 36*, 1479–1488.

Whalley, L. J., Dick, F. D., & McNeill, G. (2006). A life-course approach to the aetiology of late-onset dementias. *The Lancet Neurology, 5*(1), 87–96.

PART II REFERENCES

American Psychiatric Association. (2022). *Diagnostic and statistical manual of mental disorders* (5th ed., text rev.). Author.

Dow, K. S. (2023). *Using the hierarchical taxonomy of psychopathology (HiTOP) as a framework to dimensionally map neurodevelopmental disorders*. Doctoral dissertation, Curtin University.

Forbes, M. K., Baillie, A., Batterham, P. J., Calear, A., Kotov, R., Krueger, R. F., . . . Clark, L. A. (2025). Reconstructing psychopathology: A data-driven reorganization of the symptoms in the *Diagnostic and Statistical Manual of Mental Disorders. Clinical Psychological Science, 13*(3), 462–488.

Forbes, M. K., Neo, B., Nezami, O. M., Fried, E. I., Faure, K., Michelsen, B., . . . Dras, M. (2024). Elemental psychopathology: Distilling constituent symptoms and patterns of repetition in the diagnostic criteria of the DSM-5. *Psychological Medicine, 54*(5), 886–894.

Harvey, P. D. (2019). Domains of cognition and their assessment. *Dialogues in Clinical Neuroscience, 21*(3), 227–237.

Haslam, N., McGrath, M. J., Viechtbauer, W., & Kuppens, P. (2020). Dimensions over categories: A meta-analysis of taxometric research. *Psychological Medicine, 50*(9), 1418–1432.

Kotov, R., Krueger, R. F., Watson, D., Achenbach, T. M., Althoff, R. R., Bagby, R. M., . . . Zimmerman, M. (2017). The hierarchical taxonomy of psychopathology (HiTOP): A dimensional alternative to traditional nosologies. *Journal of Abnormal Psychology, 126*(4), 454.

Lahey, B. B. (2021). *Dimensions of psychological problems: Replacing diagnostic categories with a more science-based and less stigmatizing alternative.* Oxford University Press.

Lipsitz, O. (2023). *Uncovering general and specific relationships between psychopathology and neurocognition: A hierarchical, dimensional approach using latent variable models.* Doctoral dissertation, University of Toronto.

Michelini, G., Carlisi, C. O., Eaton, N. R., Elison, J. T., Haltigan, J. D., . . . Wilson, S. (2024). Where do neurodevelopment conditions fit in trans diagnostic psychiatric frameworks: Incorporating a new neurodevelopmental spectrum. *World Psychiatry, 23*, 333–357.

Thapar, A., Cooper, M., & Rutter, M. (2017). Neurodevelopmental disorders. *The Lancet Psychiatry, 4*(4), 339–346.

Üstün, B., & Kennedy, C. (2009). What is "functional impairment"Disentangling disability from clinical significance. *World Psychiatry, 8*(2), 82.

Author Index

C

D

E

F

G

H

I

J

K

L

M

N

O

P

R

S

T

U

V

W

Y

Z

Subject Index

Note. *f*, *t*, or *n* following a page number indicates a figure, a table, or a note.

B

C

D

E

H

I

L

O

P

T

U

V

W